D1294191

Epidemiology and Quantitation of Environmental Risk in Humans from Radiation and Other Agents

NATO ASI Series

Advanced Science Institutes Series

A series presenting the results of activities sponsored by the NATO Science Committee, which aims at the dissemination of advanced scientific and technological knowledge, with a view to strengthening links between scientific communities.

The series is published by an international board of publishers in conjunction with the NATO Scientific Affairs Division

A	Life Sciences	Plenum Publishing Corporation
B	Physics	New York and London
C	Mathematical and Physical Sciences	D Reidel Publishing Company Dordrecht, Boston, and Lancaster
D	Behavioral and Social Sciences	Martinus Nijhoff Publishers
E	Engineering and Materials Sciences	The Hague, Boston, and Lancaster
F	Computer and Systems Sciences	Springer-Verlag
G	Ecological Sciences	Berlin, Heidelberg, New York, and Tokyo

Recent Volumes in this Series

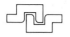

Series A: Life Sciences

Epidemiology and Quantitation of Environmental Risk in Humans from Radiation and Other Agents

Edited by

A. Castellani

ENEA, Energy Research Center, Casaccia
Rome, Italy

Plenum Press
New York and London
Published in cooperation with NATO Scientific Affairs Division

MIDDLEBURY COLLEGE LIBRARY

AA2-5827

5/1987
Biol

Proceedings of a NATO Advanced Study Institute on
Epidemiology and Quantitation of Environmental Risk in Humans
from Radiation and Other Agents,
held September 2–11, 1984,
in San Miniato, Italy

Sci.Ctr.
RA
1231
R2
N363
1984

Library of Congress Cataloging in Publication Data

NATO Advanced Study Institute on Epidemiology and Quantitation of Environ-
   Risk in Humans from Radiation and Other Agents (1984: San Miniato, Italy)
   Epidemiology and quantitation of environmental risk in humans from radiation
and other agents.

   (NATO ASI series. Series A, Life sciences; v. 96)
   "Proceedings of a NATO Advanced Study Insitute on Epidemiology and Quan-
titation of Environmental Risk in Humans from Radiation and other Agents, held
September 2–11, 1984, in San Miniato, Italy"
   Bibliography: p.
   Includes index.
   1. Radiation—Toxicology—Congresses. 2. Toxicology—Congresses. 3. Health
risk assessment—Congresses. I. Castellani, Amleto. II. Title. III. Series.
RA1231.R2N363   1984   616.9′89707   85-19117
ISBN 0-306-42093-7

©1985 Plenum Press, New York
A Division of Plenum Publishing Corporation
233 Spring Street, New York, N.Y. 10013

All rights reserved

No part of this book may be reproduced, stored in a retrieval system, or transmitted,
in any form or by any means, electronic, mechanical, photocopying, microfilming,
recording, or otherwise, without written permission from the Publisher

Printed in the United States of America

PREFACE

The identification and quantitation of environmental risk in humans is one of the main problems to be solved in order to improve the protection of individuals and of human populations against physical and chemical pollutants. Epidemiology plays a central role in the evaluation of health risk directly in human populations.

In this volume are collected 33 lectures presented at the ASI course on "Epidemiology and quantitation of environmental risk in humans from radiation and other agents: potential and limitations", sponsored by NATO and Italian Association of Radiobiology and organized by ENEA.

The course has been devoted to a number of aspects of environmental risk analysis and evaluation based on epidemiological investigation.

Basic epidemiological concepts and methods have been reviewed. Fundamentals of dosimetry and microdosimetry were presented in relation to the contribution of epidemiology in defining the dose-effect relationships for radiation carcinogenesis and its relation with age, sex and ethnicity. The mechanisms of carcinogenesis as a multi-stage process were illustrated.

One of the main topics was 'cancer epidemiology' and its correlation with: - occupational and non-occupational exposure to radiation - diagnostic and therapeutic irradiation - cancer proneness - hereditary and familiar diseases - abnormal response to carcinogens - environmental pollution in air and water - exposure to radon in mines and in building material - atomic bomb explosion - chemotherapy - dioxin and related compounds.

The combination of molecular and cellular biologists and epidemiologists was successfully achieved in the presentation of what we called 'biochemical epidemiology' mostly in the field of characterization of individual factors suspected to be associated with increased radiosensitivity and increased incidence of cancer (risk of cancer in humans).

v

In the same line were presented the analysis of proto-oncogene and the biochemical detection of molecular markers of carcinogenesis. The potential cancer inducers in human populations and the unsuspected hazards due to industrial agents were also presented and correlated with occupational and non-occupational exposure.

Large part was dedicated to the results from the atomic bomb survivors in Hiroshima and Nagasaki, with consequences at the level of the intelligence of children exposed in utero.

The ASI course has provided an up-to-date overview of existing knowledge and/or controversial issues, potential and limitation of the epidemiological approach to quantitation of health risk from environmental agents, the main focus being on radiation hazards from ionizing and non-ionizing radiation (microwaves and U.V.), particularly from low-dose and low dose-rate exposure.

My appreciation to Pieranita and Alberto Castellani for the assistance during the meeting and to Giuseppe Biondi for his help in some of the editorial work.

Amleto Castellani

Department for Environmental
Protection and Health
ENEA, CRE, Casaccia
Rome, Italy

CONTENTS

RADIATION CARCINOGENESIS

Edward E. Pochin

National Radiological Protection Board
Chilton, Didcot
Oxfordshire OX11 ORQ England

ABSTRACT

Estimates have been obtained, by epidemiological investigations in man, of the frequency with which different forms of cancer
may be induced by radiation exposure of the body or of the
individual body organs. The risk estimates which have been obtained
for over 20 organs are particularly important, since some organs may
be selectively irradiated by the concentration of certain radionuclides in them. The estimates depend upon the comparison of
cancer incidence or mortality between groups of people or populations which have or have not been exposed to increased radiation,
and in which the frequency of cancer is recorded comprehensively
for long periods of time following the exposures. The source of
these estimates, and the need for exact comparisons between the
irradiated and unirradiated populations, are reviewed.

INTRODUCTION

It has been known, in a qualitative way, for 80 years that
high doses of ionizing radiation could cause cancer[1]. The
quantitative study of this carcinogenic effect of radiation, and
of the frequency with which cancer is caused at different dose
levels and in different body tissues, is, however, particularly
necessary for a number of reasons.

This is not primarily because of its overall importance. It
can be estimated that about 1 per cent of all cancers may be caused
by radiation, and mainly by the natural sources to which the race
has always been exposed[2]. The importance of assessing these
carcinogenic risks numerically is, I think, mainly because this is

1

the major - and perhaps the only - harmful effect on the individual exposed at low doses. Genetic effects are induced also, and are of concern to the exposed individual, at least when expressed in his or her children or grand-children. Some forms of developmental abnormality also are likely to be caused by low radiation exposures of the child at certain stages of its development in utero[3]. At least a main component of the harm or detriment resulting from an individual's radiation exposure, however, must be the risk that the exposure, even at the lowest doses, may cause cancer. And if so, a reliable assessment of this carcinogenic risk must be a major consideration in ensuring that an appropriately high degree of safety is being achieved in different conditions of occupational and public exposures.

In practice it would be desirable to attempt this kind of assessment of the levels of safety or risk that result from all potentially harmful chemical or physical agents in the environment. This is particularly important, however, when, as in the case of ionizing radiation, it is not justifiable to assume that there is an entirely safe threshold dose, below which no harmful effects are caused. We then no longer have only the purely technical problem of assessing the amounts and kinds of risk that are incurred in different circumstances. The question now requires an opinion also from the community and from its decision-makers, on how low a level of risk must be ensured under conditions in which complete safety can never be attainable.

The presence of some level of risk in all occupations, and indeed in all human activities, makes such a question realistic, provided that information is available on the size and the nature of the risks involved in conventional occupations and activities, as well as on the risks from environmental contaminants.

A later paper (p 551) reviews the comparisons that can be made between the level of risk that is estimated for occupations involving radiation exposure, and that observed in a range of other occupations. Meanwhile, it is necessary to examine the evidence on which radiation risk estimates are based. This evidence relies partly upon epidemiological studies of human populations exposed at moderate doses of up to a few sieverts to the body or to individual organs. It also depends upon inference from radiobiological evidence indicating the risks expected from dose rates of only a few millisieverts per year, since these are the rates to which most of the population is exposed from natural sources[4], and most groups of workers may be exposed from occupational sources (Table 1).

The earliest evidence of radiation carcinogenesis was obtained following exposures which caused microscopically obvious damage to the tissues exposed. No consistent measurements were possible, however, of the doses involved, or therefore of the damage or cancer

2

following any particular dose. Moreover, it was known that cancer might sometimes follow such gross tissue damage, however caused. It was reasonable to assume that cancer might only follow doses which were high enough to cause such effects on the tissues, and that there might be a threshold dose, below which cancer would never be caused.

The likelihood that there might be a safe threshold dose was reduced, however, when a survey of the causes of death of early radiologists showed an excess of cancer to have occurred after radiation exposures which were not reliably known, but which were certainly insufficient to cause structural damage in the tissues in which an excess of malignancies was observed. Moreover, no evidence of a threshold was found during certain investigations on animals in which some increase of cancer was observed down to doses of only moderate size. Also, in the genetic field, the frequency with which mutations were induced in the fruit fly continued to be about proportional to the dose delivered, as the dose levels examined were progressively reduced (Table 2).

The series of human epidemiological studies which give the present rather full evidence on risk estimates, however, began in the 1950's, with investigations in which adequate dose measurements or assessments were made, and in which large groups of exposed individuals were followed for long periods of time to determine any excess of cancers developing in the tissues that had been exposed to radiation[5].

The present evidence identifies 20 or more different body organs or tissues as being susceptible to cancer induction by radiation, and indicates the histological type or types of cancer induced in them. (The term cancer is here used to cover all forms of malignant growth, including sarcomas, leukaemias, and forms of disseminated malignancies such as multiple myeloma and lymphomas.) In most of these cases, the detection of an increased frequency of cancers of an organ, and an assessment of the dose which the organ received, allows some estimate of the risk of cancer induction in that organ[6]; for example, as the excess number of cancers (or fatal cancers) per thousand people exposed and per year following the exposure, at the level of dose at which they (or the organs concerned) were exposed. An expression of a risk as "per million person-year-sieverts" (per 10^6PYSv), however, requires qualification in terms of the doses or mean dose following which the frequency was observed, since the frequency may not, and in general will not, remain proportional to dose over a range of doses.

The precision of these estimates of risk to an organ, or for a particular type of cancer, varies considerably according to the size of the survey on which the estimate is based, and the frequency of "naturally occurring" cancers from which the induced cancers of the same type needed to be discriminated. The importance of even approximate risk estimates for such a large number of body organs, however, results from the fact that many of the radio-nuclides that may be taken into the body, by being inhaled or swallowed, become selectively concentrated only in certain body organs and may not deliver significant doses to the rest of the body. The radiation risk from various forms of environmental exposure may therefore depend upon sensitivities of individual organs rather than of the body as a whole.(The so-called "effective" dose equivalent recognises this[7], by giving a weighting factor to the actual dose to particular organs such that the effective dose indicates the dose to the whole body which would cause the same number of severe effects as do the actual doses to the individual organs that are irradiated.)

Much further, and more accurate, information is still needed on the sensitivity to cancer induction of many of these 20 organs or tissues. It is some indication of the scope of the present evidence, that a much shorter list can be suggested of the types of malignancy which appear not to be induced by radiation (or not in detectable numbers, or perhaps just not yet, in continuing surveys). Thus there is no clear evidence of the induction of one type of leukaemia (the chronic lymphatic type), of skin cancer (malignant melanoma), or of thyroid cancer (the medullary, and perhaps the anaplastic forms).

The epidemiological evidence, whether positive or negative, is based upon the study of human populations or groups of people who have been exposed to radiation for various reasons - and the quantification of these risk estimates depends necessarily upon the effects of human exposure, since the frequency of cancers induced in other species cannot be used in any quantitative way in infer the human sensitivity, even to the induction of identical types of cancer. Subsequent papers discuss information that has been obtained following different forms of exposure: in radiotherapy, and in certain diagnostic uses of x-rays; from occupational exposure in uranium miners and in uses of luminous paints; in populations of Hiroshima and Nagasaki who were exposed to atomic bombs; and studies have been made on populations exposed to unusually high levels of radiation from natural sources.

These various forms of exposure involve different advantages and disadvantages in their epidemiological study. All quantitative assessments of the carcinogenic effects of radiation face certain common problems. These arise from four main causes. Firstly, the cancers that are induced are identical in their clinical behaviour and microscopic appearance to the cancers of the same organ or tissue that occur naturally. The estimation of the excess must therefore be made on statistical rather than on clinical grounds. Secondly, most of the cancers induced by a given radiation exposure

4

only develop many years after the exposure[8]. Thirdly, and in consequence, the detection and measurement of any excess depends upon a comparison of cancer rates, over prolonged periods of time, with those over the same period of time in a population which has not been equally exposed to radiation, but which is otherwise comparable. And, fourthly, any estimate of risk depends upon reliable assessment of the dose received by the organ or organs exposed; or in some cases, by the types of cell within the organ which are responsible for the cancer development[9].

Some of these factors cause particular problems in certain types of survey, even in studies of the increased numbers of cancers developing after moderate radiation doses of a few sieverts to body organs. The difficulties, and possible sources of error, are much greater when studies are made to detect any increases occurring after low doses, of a tenth of these levels or less.

Evidence from radiotherapy

Much of the most important evidence on the risks of cancer induction in different organs has come from studies on patients in whom these organs have needed to be irradiated as treatment for existing disease[6]. Investigation of the risks of such irradiation is facilitated by the fact that these patients will ordinarily need to be under some degree of medical surveillance for long times after the treatment, so that abnormal effects of treatment are likely to be detected. Moreover, the size of the doses delivered to different organs will have been determined, and any increase of cancer incidence can therefore be related to dose, and the relevant risk estimated.

However, radiotherapy is most commonly used in the treatment of cancer, and there may therefore be uncertainty whether the subsequent development of a malignant growth represents a possible induced cancer or a recurrence of the original disease. Moreover, the doses normally used in such treatments are, of course, intended to be sufficiently large to kill most or all cells of the treated cancer; and there is evidence that such high doses reduce the frequency with which cancer is induced by radiation, presumably by killing also some of the cells which the radiation has transformed to have a cancer-forming potentiality. For both these reasons, such surveys may be reliable only on cancers occurring in organs which have been indirectly irradiated at lower dose by scattered radiation during the treatment.

A further difficulty in such cases arises from the fact that the majority of all cancers induced by radiation only develop or become detectable at more than 10 years after the radiation, and induced cancers of most types continue to appear after 20 or 30 years. Risk estimates based on the radiotherapy of cancer are

5

therefore likely to be useful mainly in conditions in which the treatment is ordinarily curative and is followed by survival for a normal lifetime, and for forms of cancer which occur and are treated at younger ages than in the case of most cancers.

For these reasons, risk estimates have usually been derived from the radiotherapy of non-malignant disease, when survival times are ordinarily long and the administered doses are lower. For the very reason, however, that such doses may be carcinogenic, the treatment of benign disease by radiation is now infrequent, and likely to be limited to conditions in which the benefits outweigh the small risks involved, and are not more safely obtainable otherwise. But, in general, the benign conditions that have been treated do not in themselves require the continuous medical surveillance after therapy that applies to the treated cancers. Records of cancers developing many years after the radiation exposure have thus needed to be derived by review, for example, of national death certificates rather than of available clinical records from hospital follow-up clinics. It is in this situation that any national treatment of death certificates as confidential documents can be a bar to epidemiological investigations. This difficulty can, however, be resolved if the national authority which maintains records of deaths and causes of death is itself equipped and empowered to release to the investigator the various causes of death in a group of named individuals, without identifying the cause in the case of any one of the individuals.

In basing risk estimates on the effects of any form of radiotherapy, it is important to review the possibility that the disease which has been treated may in itself be associated with a liability to subsequent cancer development, since even a small association of this sort could be misinterpreted as being due to a considerable cancer induction rate. Such an association might be due to a direct effect of the disease, or possibly to a genetically determined predisposition to both diseases. Moreover, any medicines also used in treatment might in some cases have a small carcinogenic effect.

In some instances it has been possible to study directly the cancer incidence in patients with the same disease which had been treated by other means than by radiation[10]. It still remains possible that in some circumstances the need to use radiotherapy was determined by the severity of the disease, and that a subsequent cancer frequency was influenced by the severity. At least, however, the likelihood of a genetic association is reduced by such control determinations.

Evidence from radiodiagnosis

The tissue doses of radiation that are needed in diagnosis

are typically of the order of 100 times smaller than those used for treatment of benign conditions, and perhaps 1000 times lower than in cancer therapy. Cancer induction has only been detected, and is only likely to be detectable, in circumstances in which very large numbers of diagnostic x rays are given to each individual, or when very large numbers of individuals are studied. Moreover, the doses delivered, although their average value can commonly be estimated, are usually not known with the confidence that applies to those used in therapy.

Risk estimates for cancer induction in the breast have been derived from studies of female patients with pulmonary tuberculosis who required repeated injections of air into the chest to cause collapse and healing of the affected lung segments[6]. The monitoring of the degree of collapse and healing often required up to several hundred x-ray examinations. Such examinations are best made by fluoroscopy rather than by x-ray films so that the contour of the collapsed lung can be examined, although the dose per screening is greater than with film.

In these cases the average doses delivered to breast tissues could be estimated retrospectively by testing the rate at which radiation was emitted by the kinds of x-ray equipment that had been used, and by records, or memories, of whether patients ordinarily faced the x-ray tube or the doctor during the screening. A greater uncertainty was involved in estimating the duration of the x-ray exposure per examination, using memories and reconstructions of the kind of examinations made. The uncertainties of dose estimation, however, may not have added appreciably to the statistical uncertainty of discriminating a small excess of induced breast cancers from a much larger number that would have occurred naturally in the absence of the fluoroscopies.

Risk estimates for irradiation of the liver and the bone marrow have also been obtained from the diagnostic use of a thorium preparation[11]. Thorotrast was at one time used to give x rays which could define the presence and position of arterial disease, after injection of the preparation into cranial or other arteries. The radioactivity of the thorium, however, and the long retention of its insoluble oxide in liver and bone marrow, delivered high doses to these tissues, and caused an increase of liver cancer and leukaemia subsequently. In this case, the estimate of tissue dose was complex, since much of the (alpha) radiation emitted from the thorium was absorbed in the thorium oxide particles, and more was delivered only to cells already killed by the radiation from these particles. It was necessary also to confirm that thorium did not have a chemical, as well as a radiation, effect in causing cancer; and this was done by tests in animals using an injection having the same concentration of thorium but a lower radioactivity (by using a different thorium radioisotope)[12].

By these means, consistent risk estimates have been obtained from clinics in a number of countries in which Thorotrast was formerly used.

Evidence from occupational exposures

Clear evidence has been obtained of cancer induction by radiation following two forms of occupational exposure, in addition to that in early radiologists, as mentioned above.

In uranium miners, an increased mortality from lung cancer has been recognised for many years, and has been related to the radiation dose to lung tissues. Rather consistent estimates have been obtained, in a number of countries, of the lung cancer risk per unit radiation dose, despite various difficulties in the estimation. For example:-

1. The dose to lung tissue comes essentially from the radioactive decay products of the radioactive gas radon that is inhaled, and from gamma radiation from the rock that is being mined. The concentration of the radon in the air and the gamma radiation levels have ordinarily been sampled at fixed positions in the mine galleries, and only recently by measuring devices carried by individual miners. Doses to individuals or to groups of miners have thus usually been inferred from the positions and mines in which they worked, and from the estimated durations of work in each.

2. Furthermore, the doses that are relevant to the induction of cancers developing now, are those delivered during mining 20 or more years ago.

3. The atmosphere, at least in underground mines, is likely to contain materials such as arsenic or diesel fumes which might have a significant carcinogenic effect, either by themselves, or acting in combination with radiation.

4. Cigarette smoking has such a powerful effect in causing lung cancer that the type and frequency of smoking by miners needs to be known and strictly compared with that in the population with which the lung cancer rates are contrasted.

5. The dose to lung tissues in fact depends, not on the concentration of radon itself in the air, but on the concentration of products of the continuous radioactive decay of the radon, and on the

proportion of these short-lived products which are adsorbed onto particles in the air.

6. Even so, it is the deposition and retention of these daughter products of radon on different regions of the lung, and the sensitivity for cancer induction of these tracheal, bronchial or alveolar regions of the lung, which will determine the number of cancers which may develop[13].

7. And finally, since the radiation delivered is essentially in the form of alpha particles, the risk estimates depend on the different effectiveness of alpha radiation and commoner forms of exposure, and so need to be corrected for this difference before they can be used for lung irradiation in general.

It is perhaps a measure of the careful analysis that these factors have received, that the radiation risks delivered from experience in different uranium and other mines have such a high degree of consistency and value[14].

The study of radium dial painters illustrates a further important aspect of radiation carcinogenesis: namely, that the detection and quantification of an effect is facilitated when a radionuclide is relatively highly concentrated in an organ in which cancer normally develops rarely. The similarity between radium and calcium in their chemical properties, and therefore in their metabolic behaviour in the body, has the consequence that radium becomes concentrated in bone, so that much higher doses are delivered to bone cells than to other body tissues. As a result, and because bone cancers are normally uncommon, the risk of bone cancer induction by radiation was determined earlier than that for many other forms of cancer[15]; and this was despite the fact that the induction rate per unit dose is low for cancer of bone.

Evidence from Hiroshima and Nagasaki

The opposite applies to the risk for induction of stomach cancer in the survey of Japanese atomic bomb survivors. Stomach cancer has a high natural incidence in Japan, and its induction by moderate doses of uniform whole body radiation from the bombs was not at first detected, despite this cancer having a substantial induction rate per unit dose. For leukaemia the position is reversed, this form of malignancy having a higher induction rate per unit dose relative to the natural incidence. An excess of leukaemia thus became detectable soon after the bombing - owing in part also to the shorter average latency between exposure and development of the disease for leukaemia than for most other forms of cancer.

The prolonged and careful studies that have been carried out in Hiroshima and Nagasaki illustrate also the complexities of estimating the radiation doses received by individuals, according to their exact positions within the town and within buildings, and the penetration through the atmosphere and through the buildings of the radiations caused in the explosions or emitted by the fission products immediately formed by them.

It has been necessary also to compare the cancer rates in those who survived exposure at different dose levels, without introducing bias due to any effects that these doses may have had otherwise upon the health or conditions of life of the individuals surviving, or by the "selection" of those individuals who were capable of surviving them.

The detailed, clinical and statistical study of large numbers of survivors of the atomic bombing of these cities has yielded essential evidence of the risks of cancer induction by radiation, and the risk estimates for many individual body organs[16]. Dr. Jablon's paper (p. 413) describes the progress of this important work and the epidemiological problems involved.

Evidence from areas of high natural radiation

Several studies have been made of the frequency of cancer or other conditions in areas in which the natural background levels of radiation are higher than normal. Such studies are of potential importance, since, if effective, they could give valuable direct evidence on the frequency of effects produced at low dose rates. Hirtherto, however, none has yielded unequivocal results, essentially for two reasons.

Firstly, when the natural exposure is increased in communities living at high altitude, with a raised dose rate from cosmic radiation, or in hill or mountain areas of volcanic origin, with increased terrestrial radioactivity, differences in dietary, cultural and economic conditions have made it difficult to establish valid comparisons, either with national statistics or with those of neighbouring communities in low lying areas.

Secondly, however, very large populations are likely to be needed to show significant increases of harmful effects at these relatively low dose rates. An example makes this clear.

The number of deaths from cancer per year, and per million population, varies considerably in different countries, largely because of differences in the average life expectancy of the populations. The average value for 39 countries for which these figures are available[17] is about 1400 per million person-years (median 1470, quartiles 550 and 2250). In a survey extending over N million person years, a typical expected number of cancer deaths in an area of normal background radiation would thus be 1400 N.

It is likely that approximately 1% of all cancers may be caused by normal background radiation levels. In an area where the total radiation from all natural sources was q times normal, therefore, (q - 1)% of 1400 N additional cancers would be induced. To be statistically detectable, this excess, of 14 (q - 1)N, would need to exceed about twice the standard error of the 1400 N that would be expected in the absence of increased radiation, or

$$14(q - 1)N > 2 \sqrt{1400N}$$

indicating that N should be greater than

$$\frac{4 \times 1400}{196 \ (q-1)^2} = \frac{28}{(q-1)^2} \text{ million person years}$$

One of the highest natural exposures occurs in Kerala[18], where a population of about 70,000 receives an average annual dose of about 4 mSv from the local monazite sands. This is about 12 times the dose normally received from terrestrial sources, and would raise the total from all natural sources to about 3 times its normal value. Cancer statistics are not currently available in Kerala. On the basis of the calculations given above, however, a study of total cancer mortality would need to involve some 7 million person years (assuming an average value of 1400 cancer deaths per million person years). With 70,000 people exposed, a 100 year survey of all cancer deaths would be required to show a significant increase, and about twice this duration to estimate the size of the increase. Even if the natural mortality rate were as high as 2000 per million person years, an increase would only be detectable after 70 years.

In other regions, in which surveys have been made, the terrestrial component of natural exposure has been 3 or 4 times the normal value[19], raising the total natural dose rate to about twice normal. This implies a likely need for a 25 to 30 million person-year survey, and no surveys have approached one-tenth of this figure.

The requirements might be less prohibitive in any regions of long life expectancy in which the annual cancer mortality was high and in which adequate medical records were available. The necessary size of survey might also be less if the study were focussed upon one particular type of cancer, for which the induction rate was high relative to the natural incidence, although then the reduction in numbers of cases would ordinarily offset the advantage gained by examining a greater relative risk. Or an increase might be detectable if mortality in a particular age group only was compared with the normal rate. Alternatively, a study of the numbers of cancers diagnosed, rather than only of those causing death, would yield considerably larger numbers of induced cases of some types of cancer, and particularly those of the thyroid and of the skin. Here, however, problems would result from the even greater difficulty of ensuring a comprehensive record of all diagnoses, rather than of all deaths, in a large population over many years, and particularly in areas in which clinical records or tumour registries were inadequate.

These factors, and their quantitative implications on the size of survey likely to be required, clearly need review when such surveys are undertaken. At least in regard to total cancer mortality, however, it seems unlikely that studies in any known high background areas can do more than indicate or exclude the possibility that rates of cancer induction at low dose are much higher than at present supposed; an objective which may be of substantial value in itself.

Difficulties in epidemiological assessment of low dose risks

The problems involved in studies of high background areas have indicated some of the needs and difficulties involved in any attempt to assess the risks of low doses epidemiologically. In most studies on which risk estimates for organs can be based, these estimates are derived from a population of one or more hundred people, in which an organ has been exposed to a dose of one or a few sieverts. To detect the effects of one or a few millisieverts, however, would require a population of one or more hundred <u>million</u> people, if the frequency of induced effects per unit dose remained the same, since the size of population required varies inversely as the square of the dose to which it was exposed. Even if the effect per unit dose were 10 times greater at very low doses, one or more millions would need to be studied[20].

Even at moderately low doses, of tenths of a sievert to the body or to particular organs, inefficiency in ascertainment of the population exposed, of the dose delivered, or of the nature of the medical effects produced, have caused unreliable results to be reported. The families of workers who have died of cancer may believe the worker to have been exposed occupationally to radiation when monitoring records show this not to have been the case; and a few such errors can suggest a high cancer incidence in supposedly exposed individuals. Failure to verify the cause of death from medical records may similarly introduce error, as may any method of collecting data which tends, however slightly, to increase the chance of deaths being reported more fully than deaths from other causes in the exposed population. And, quite generally, when small differences in cancer frequency are attributed to small radiation exposures, the confidence limits of the results need to be accurately assessed, stated, and examined. Otherwise the statistical variability of conclusions based upon small numbers will tend to result in random high variations being reported as positive effects, while the random low variations will remain unreported.

The normal variations of cancer incidence with age, with sex, with locality, with time and in some cases with race, require also that comparisons between exposed and comparison populations should be exact in these respects, as well as with regard to other known carcinogenic agents such as smoking and occupational exposure to chemicals; and that they should be analysed by modern statistical techniques which make correct allowances for the simultaneous action of many such sources of variation. Errors have arisen in the past by analysis of separate sources of carcinogenicity in isolation, by the use of different methods of ascertainment or classification of cancers in exposed and comparison groups, or by comparing populations of the same average age but in which the variations of age round this average were found to differ. It is inevitable that, at progressively lower doses, the results of epidemiological studies become increasingly subject to statistical uncertainty; and that the risk from very low doses can be more reliably inferred by appropriate interpolation, in the light of radiobiological evidence, between the risks observed at higher dose, and the safe presumption that there will be zero added risk at zero added dose.

Table 1
Average annual dose rates

(current UK values, effective dose equivalents)

Whole population   mSv per year

From

radon and thoron	0.8
all other natural sources	1.1
medical exposures	0.5
all other sources	0.03
From all sources	2.4 mSv y^{-1}

Local groups in the population

(maximum estimates for liquid discharges
from nuclear facilities)

From

Sellafields (from fish consumption)	3.4
Heysham (" " ")	0.95
Trawsfynydd (to fishermen)	0.55
Springfields (to houseboat dwellers)	0.35
Capenhurst (from fish consumption)	0.2
Chapelcross (to fishermen)	0.2
Others	less than 0.2

Occupational exposure rates

Nuclear fuel cycle	2.7
Ministry of defence	2.4
Research	1.5
Industrial uses	1.0
Medical and dental staff	0.7
Average, all occupations	1.5 mSv y^{-1}

Table 2

Frequency of mutations in drosophila

1930	Oliver	linear down to	3 Gy
1949	Uphoff & Stern	" " "	0.25 Gy
1961	Glass	" " "	0.05 Gy

References

1. A. Frieben, Demonstration eines Cancroids des rechten
    Handrücken, das sich nach langdauernder Einwirkung von
    Röntgenstrahlen entwickelt hat. Fortschr.Röntgenstr. 6:
    106 (1902).
2. E.E. Pochin, Radiation Protection, The Radiographer 30:89 (1983).
3. M. Otake and W.J. Schull, In utero exposure to A bomb radiation
    and mental retardation, Brit. J. Radiol. 57:409 (1984).
4. J.S. Hughes and G.C. Roberts, The radiation exposure of the UK
    population – a further review, National Radiological
    Protection Board, report in course of publication. NRPB,
    Chilton, Oxon. England.
5. E.E. Pochin, Sieverts and Safety, Health Physics 46:1173 (1984).
6. United Nations Scientific Committee on the Effects of Atomic
    Radiation, Sources and Effects of Ionizing Radiation – 1977
    report to the General Assembly, United Nations, New York
    (1977).
7. International Commission on Radiological Protection,
    Recommendations of the ICRP: ICRP Publications 26 and 28,
    Annals of the ICRP, Pergamon, Oxford, 1 (No. 3), (1977) and
    2 (No. 1):i (1978).
8. C.E. Land and M. Tokunaga, Induction Periods, in "Radiation
    Carcinogenesis: epidemiology and biological significance",
    J.D. Boice and J.F. Fraumeni, eds., Raven Press, New York
    (1984).
9. E.E. Pochin, Needs for further epidemiological studies of
    radiation effects, in "Radiation Carcinogenesis:
    epidemiology and biological significance", J.D. Boice and
    J.F. Fraumeni, eds., Raven Press, New York (1984).
10. P.G. Smith, R. Doll and E.P. Radford, Cancer mortality among
    patients with ankylosing spondylitis not given x-ray
    therapy, Brit. J. Radiol., 50:728 (1977).
11. G. van Kaick, H. Muth, A. Kaul, H. Immich, D. Liebermann,
    D. Lorenz, W.J. Lorenz, H. Lührs, K.E. Scheer, G. Wagner,
    K. Wegener and H. Wesch, Results of the German Thorotrast
    Study, in "Radiation Carcinogenesis: epidemiology and
    biological significance", J.D. Boice and J.F. Fraumeni,
    eds.., Raven Press, New York (1984).

12. H. Wesch, W. Riedel, K. Wegener, A. Kaul, H. Immich,
    K. Hasenöhrl, H. Muth and G. van Kaick, Recent results of
    the German Thorotrast Study - statistical evaluation of
    animal experiments with regard to the non radiation
    effects in human Thorotrastosis, Health Physics 44 (Suppl.
    1):317 (1983).

13. International Commission on Radiological Protection, ICRP
    Publication 32 : limits for inhalation of radon daughters
    by workers, Annals of the ICRP 6 (No. 1), Pergamon,
    Oxford (1981).

14. W. Jacobi, Carcinogenic effects of radiation on the human
    respiratory tract, in "Radiation Carcinogenesis",
    A.C. Upton, ed., Elvesier North Holland Inc., New York,
    in press.

15. H.S. Martland, The occurrence of malignancy in radioactive
    persons, Amer. J. Cancer 15:2435 (1931).

16. H. Kato and W.J. Schull, Studies of the mortality of A-bomb
    survivors. 7, Mortality, 1950-1978: part 1. Cancer
    Mortality, Radiation Research 90:395 (1982).

17. World Health Organization, World Health Statistics 1983, WHO,
    Geneva (1983).

18. A.R. Gopal-Ayengar, K. Sundaram, K.B. Mistry and K.P. George,
    Current status of investigations on biological effects of
    high background radioactivity in the monazite bearing
    areas of Kerala coast in south-west India, in Proceedings
    of International Symposium on areas of high natural
    radioactivity, June 1975, T.L. Cullen and E. Penna Franca
    eds., Academica Brasileira de Ciências, Rio de Janeiro
    (1977).

19. High Background Radiation Research Group, China, Health Survey
    in high background radiation areas in China, Science
    209:877 (1980).

20. E.E. Pochin, The epidemiology of radiation carcinogenesis in
    man, in "Radiation - Risk - Protection", Compacts Vol. 1,
    Proceedings of the 6th International Congress of the
    International Radiation Protection Association, Berlin
    1984, A. Kaul, R. Neider, J. Pensko, F-E. Stieve and
    H. Brunner, eds., Verlag TÜV Rheinland, Köln (1984).

STRATEGY OF ASSESSMENT OF HEALTH RISKS IN ENVIRONMENTAL AND

OCCUPATIONAL HEALTH

Reinier L. Zielhuis

Chair of occupational and environmental health
University of Amsterdam
Academic Medical Center
Meibergdreef 15, 1105 AZ Amsterdam, The Netherlands

INTRODUCTION

In the last decade fear of adverse health risks from environmental pollution has considerably increased. Consequently, the public demands a health surveillance study in the case of more or less insidious "normal" emissions from static or mobile sources ǒr incidental/accidental release from e.g. chemical waste dumps. Moreover, this also applies to occupational health. Activities which have been accepted as an asset in our (post)industrial age, are increasingly regarded as a liability.

The most important question put to local authorities and industries is: "Does this exposure carry (specified) health risks?" Another question is: "Are specified diseases caused by exposure?" Moreover, both questions may also be asked by individuals: "Do *I* run a health risk, is *my* disease caused by pollution?"

For sake of simplicity, I will mainly discuss the establishment of health risk in exposure to chemicals for groups of human beings. We should realize from the start that assessment of health risks not only has to do with establishment of increased health risks, but also and even maybe more frequently, with establishment of non-risks.

GENERAL ASPECTS OF STRATEGIES

A sequence of steps

The term *strategy* may be defined as: the *logical sequence of steps to achieve a valid answer to a specified question*. Each step determines whether it is feasible to carry out the next step.

17

The total sequence is: at first a maybe vaguely specified question (1) → translated into a more specified question after literature search, discussion with experts (2) → qualitative assessment of exposure and groups at risk (3) → maybe further specification of the question (4) → quantitative assessment of actual intake or uptake (5) → assessment of relative health risks (6) → assessment of the state of health (7) → report and recommendation, (8) → implementation of preventive/corrective measures (9) → follow-up (10). The last two steps will not be discussed.

It is important to distinguish between assessment of the "health *risk*", i.e. the *probability* that adverse health effects *may* occur, and of the "*state* of health", i.e. whether health effects *do* occur. The subjects examined usually do not make this distinction. In daily health care physicians answer in a yes/no-manner: you have not this disease, you run a risk of lungcancer, you are healthy. Physicians do not burden their patients with probabilities, although it serves the interests of the patients, when the physicians themselves remain thinking in terms of probabilities.

Non specificity of health effects

Man responds to a multitude of exogeneous or endogeneous stimuli with a limited number of biologic responses. The signs and symptoms of health impairment usually do not point to the cause itself. Lung cancer may be due to smoking, exposure to asbestos, chromium, nickel or arsenic compounds, bischloromethylether, ionizing radiation, etc.

Because the same signs and symptoms observed also occur in non-exposed subjects, one *always* has to examine *non-exposed control groups*. One estimates the *Relative Risks* (RR).

This may appear to be beating upon an open door, but too often authorities tend to bend under political pressure, and carry out a sloppy assessment of environment exposure or even only of the state of health of those who claim to be affected, without assessment of the relative risks or the relative state of health. Knowledge of the principles of epidemiology is still poor, even in government health services.

Variability of exposure and response

Even when living and/or working under apparent similar conditions of exposure, the actual individual exposure is much more variable than that of animals exposed in an experimental setting. The same applies to susceptibility. A "standard" man/women and standard living or working conditions do not exist. Nevertheless, data on exposure and on graded health effects are still expressed as arithmetric averages, suggesting a normal distribution, although the standard deviation may even exceed the mean. Quantal effects, e.g. abortion, malformation, cancer, cannot be averaged. Environmental and occupational epidemiology usually cannot rely on average *exposure*-average *effects* relationships, but we have to estimate *exposure-response* relationships, i.e. the *percentage* of humans affected with a specified intensity of a specified graded effect or with a specified quantal response at specified exposure levels.

Assessment of exposure itself is beset with at least three types of error: in sampling and analysis, in selection of sampling place and time, and in fractional uptake. Particularly in long lasting exposure in occupational health, retrospective assessment of past exposure may lead to an overestimate of exposure and consequently to an underestimate of risk (Ulfvarson 1983).

Assessment of health effects has to take into account (1) accuracy and precision of measurements and interobserver variability; (2) intra-individual variability. In repeated measurement of 12 clinico-chemical parameters in 68 healthy subjects Williams et al (1970) observed that the individual prophiles differed widely; the intra-individual variability usually is much smaller than the interindividual variability (3). We still rely too much on the interindividual range, treating humans as homogeneous highly selected well-bred experimental animals: this leads to an underestimation of individual health risks.

Moreover, the time of measurement of health effects has to be geared to exposure: assessment of subjective responses in relation to measured exposure levels in the case of acute effects, such as dizziness, headache, drowsiness, highly increases the sensitivity and specificity of the study (Zielhuis et al, 1963). In assessment of exposure and of health effects one has to follow a strict design (WHO, 1984).

In addition, one too often relies on socalled "reference values", established in clinical settings in maybe highly biased groups of subjects and with methods which may differ in detection level, accuracy and precision from the methods used in the study.

Clinical versus epidemiological studies

Clinical medicine usually has to deal with pathology, i.e. with large deviations from "normal". Clinicians apply highly sophisticated techniques, which allow catching large fishes with a net of fine mazes. In epidemiological studies we often cannot apply such techniques, which may even carry health risks, e.g. liverpunction, sampling of intraspinal fluid. Although the deviations of biological parameters from normal may be much smaller than in patients, we may have to use a net with wide mazes to catch small fishes. This draw-back can be overcome by increasing the size of the groups examined. An increase of the percentage of subjects with a β_2M level >300 μg/l or of Retinol Binding Protein (RBP) > 300 μg/l urine may indicate an increased risk of impaired renal tubulus function within this group, although a clinician might discard various individual levels at most as borderline.

Size of the group

In practice, we encounter a new drawback. The groups exposed may be rather small. Selevan (1980) estimated the variation in popu-lation size required to plan a cohort study of varying reproductive outcomes, given otherwise identical assumptions ($\alpha(P)=0.05$; $\beta=0.10$; RR=2, sex ratio = 1.1). For fetal loss (15% of recognized pregnan-cies expected) the size of index and of control group is for each group 160 pregnancies, for major birth defects (2%) 1525 live births; for club foot (most frequent major defect, 0.6%) 5199 live births; minor defect (10%) 266 live births. With decreasing expected inci-dence in the control groups, the minimum size of the exposed and the control group increases. However, when we apply a more sophis-ticated longitudinal method (immunologic assay of the pregnancy hor-mone human chorionic gonadotropin), which also permits to measure the extent of early unrecognized pregnancy loss, the total "normal" incidence is 33% of conceptions;most conceptions occurring before the 20th week are not recognized as such by the mother (Wilcox, 1983).

Decreasing the detection level and increasing the accuracy of measurement together with a strategy fully geared to the specified question to be answered, increases the sensitivity of the study.

Individuals vary both in exposure and in susceptibility. How-ever, this variation may also be treated as a group phenomenon. Some groups may be more exposed and/or more susceptible. When we carried out a study on environmental exposure to inorganic lead around a secundary smelter, we did not observe any relation between lead levels in blood and distance from the smelter in adult women. However, we observed this in their 2-3 year old children. The children constitute the group actually at risk, both in regard to exposure and to susceptibility. Moreover, we also observed increa-sing blood lead levels with decreasing socio-economic status (Zielhuis et al, 1979): young children of low socio-economic class clearly constitute the *actual group at risk*. In the 1979 and 1981 lead studies carried out within the CEC, most countries carried out studies mainly in adults and/or in relatively old primary school children. The WHO-study (Vahter, 1982) in 10 countries to assess exposure to lead and to cadmium, sampled blood from adult teachers (about 200 per country), living in an urban area. Both international studies may have underestimated actual exposure to the groups most at risk.

The choice of groups at risk differs according to the type of exposure: in exposure to lead dust the young children; in exposure to carbon monoxide adults over 40 yrs of age (decreased cardiovascular capacity in 5-10%; in the case of respiratory irritants those with chronic non-specific lung impairment (10-20%); in exposure to persistent halogenated hydrocarbons (e.g. PCB's, PBB's) pregnant and lactating women; in the case of short chain organic mercury pregnant women and infants.

MENTAL HEALTH

Recently the Dutch Environmental Defense Association organized a symposium: "You may not become ill, but you certainly become crazy". Mental health problems tend to overrule signs and symptoms of somatic impairment. Kotala (1980) and Holden (1980) described the serious mental health problems in the Love Canal region. Panicky reactions occurred; EPA-officials were even taken as hostages. Various often contradictory official reports and, not to forget, press and television made Love Canal into a "neighbourhood of fear". Scientists gave their conclusions with all scientific reservations, which were not understood by the laymen, and even increased anxiety. In the case of natural disasters a well planned rescue organization usually is in charge; however, in the case of waste dumps incidences (e.g. Love Canal), industrial accidents (e.g. Harrisburg) data on actual exposure and on health risks become slowly available over a too long period of uncertainty. Local and central government responds to outbreaks of anxiety, to pression groups. Some studies were quickly critisized by other scientists, which diminished the confidence in government sponsored studies. In Love Canal the inhabitants themselves founded pression groups and rescue teams. Moreover, within the families the men employed locally did not want to migrate and to loose their job, whereas the women could not endure the uncertainty, particularly because they wanted to protect the health of their children. Particularly the lack of a consistent government policy created a lack of confidence. Similar observations have been made in the Netherlands. Our government also had no clear strategy; it started studies more to ease public tension instead of assessing exposure and health risk according to basic principles of environmental epidemiology.

HEALTH STUDIES

Pression groups from "the neighbourhood of fear" or from workers demand study of health risks and/or the actual state of health: "what risks do we actually run? Is an alleged excess of lung cancer, infertility, liver disease due to *this* environmental or occupational pollution?" In this paper the emphasis will be put upon the first question: assessment of *health risks*.

The population is acquainted with hospitals and general practitioners and in addition with screening programs for early detection of cancer, cardiovascular or respiratory diseases. Each subject receives the answer: yes or no, and not: you may run a risk; the probability is 1.10^{-3} per year. The patient in clinical medicine is not burdened with probabilities.

However, because most non-infectious diseases are multi-causal, they may also occur in non-exposed groups. One can only assess *relative* risks between exposed and controls; one cannot make a specific cause-related diagnosis in individuals. Therefore, an essentially different study program has to be carried out in the case of exposure to chemicals.

We may distinguish three types of study programs (Zielhuis et al, 1982):
A. *Individual-directed study*, i.e. a *screening* program as outlined above. No control group is examined; the cause is irrelevant.
B. *Cause-directed study*, i.e. a *research* study to expand knowledge of exposure-response-relationships. Study of a control group is essential. Potential causes and the state of health have to be examined.
C. *Situation-directed study* to assess health risks in a specified location. The probable cause (exposure to specified chemicals) is known; reasonably valid exposure-response-relationships are available. Again, study of a control group is essential. Quantitative assessment of exposure takes priority.

The population is only acquainted with program A, whereas programs B or C are necessary. In this paper attention is focussed on study-program C.

The decision to start a study B or C raises many problems: (1) It may consolidate and even increase anxiety: "when the government starts a study, there certainly will be something wrong". (2) The anxiety may affect participation (positive or negative bias) and also the frequency and intensity of symptoms (positive or negative bias). (3) Because one cannot conclude whether observed health impairment in individuals is caused by his/her exposure to pollutants, the subject will not be reassured. Even an increased prevalence of chromosomal abnormalities does not permit to conclude that *this* individual runs a higher risk of e.g. cancer, abortion. (4) The size of the group exposed is often limited. (5) It may be difficult to find a control group; moreover, the study has no advantage for the non-exposed themselves. (6) The interpretation of data may be hampered by the fact that an alleged or real observation of e.g.

abortion, cancer, within a locality/factory department formed the original signal for starting the study. This may lead to an over-estimated relative risk. A casual agglomeration of specific diseases tends to be regarded as a significant excess. (7) The study may easily lead to false-negative data in regard to diseases with a long latency period, particularly when the alleged period of exposure is relatively short. A cohort study may have to be carried out, both in exposed and in controls. (8) An expected low incidence of specific diseases among the non-exposed group requires very large groups of exposed and non-exposed subjects.

Assessment of health risks requires a *consistent* and *logical* strategy. When the relevant pollutants can be defined, and reasonably valid exposure-response relationships are known, a situation-directed study C appears to be the program of choice.

A LOGICAL STRATEGY—STUDY C

In 1983 Landrigan outlined the basic epidemiological tenets, which ought to guide the evaluation of persons exposed to chemical waste dumps: (1) documenting exposure; (2) defining the population exposed; (3) diagnosing disease and dysfunction as unequivocally as possible; (4) application of rigorous statistical methodology to establish the relations between exposure and disease. These overall tenets apply both to studies B and C.

We recently worked out a strategy for assessment of health *risks*, which presents a logical *sequence of steps* to be taken(Zielhuis et al, 1982). This strategy can be applied to accidental, incidental and also to "normal" everyday exposure to chemicals in the ambient and the working environment.

The proposal presents a series of ten subsequent steps, mentioned already in the introduction. *Each* step determines the *feasibility* of the next *step*.

Question to be answered: the five W's (steps 1, 2, 4)

Any strategy should start with a specified question. At least five W's have to be taken into account: "who, what, where, when, why" (referring to the English, German and Dutch languages).

Who: Define the exposed group (particularly those probably *most at risk*) and the non-exposed otherwise comparable *control group*.

Where: Define the location: e.g. factory departments, location of waste disposal, urban versus rural.

What: Define the relevant sources of exposure and the chemicals to be measured; moreover, define whether the study aims to assess "external exposure in general sense" (*concentrations* in air, food, drinking water, etc.), "exposure in a narrow sense" (the actual *intake* = amount) or "internal exposure" (*uptake*, by means of biological monitoring) (WHO, 1983).

When: Define the relevant points of time of sampling in relation to the potential health effects.

Why: Define the ultimate aim of the study: a cause-directed study or a situation-directed study? Is the occurrence of health effects already evident, and have we to study also the state of health?

A maybe vaguely specified question (step 1) may have to be translated into a more specified question (step 2). Literature research and discussion with other experts may lead to further specification. Step 4 should define the final question.

Qualitative assessment of exposure (step 3)

We may distinguish several types of exposure (Zielhuis, 1977): (1) *Occupational exposure*, (a) indoor, direct from the workers' own occupation, (b) indirect from work carried out by other workers, even in other departments, or by passive smoking (offices, restaurants); (c) as the result of poor hygiene. In a recent study by Hassler (1983) in 18 workers exposed to cadmium in air (about av.7 µg Cd/m^3) the Cd in blood level (4 to 60 µg Cd/1) proved to be highly related to the personal hygiene score, and did not depend on the Cd-level in air. Occupational exposure may also be due to background environmental pollution outdoors (d) e.g. custom officials, traffic wardens.
(2) *Paraoccupational exposure*, (a) due to hobby work or a second job; (b) exposure of wife and children from polluted shoes/clothes carried home, of infants from breast milk when the mother is occupationally exposed.
(3) *Environmental exposure* from "normal" ambient air, food, drinking water (a) may be the result of neighbourhood exposure from industrial emission (b) or waste dump emission (c). Particularly young children may have a relatively high oral intake from polluted soil and objects (d).
(4) *Indoor exposure at home*, which increasingly receives attention (e.g. WHO, 1977): passive smoking, cooking, making beds.
(5) Exposure through *personal life style*, e.g. active smoking, food habits, consumption of beverages, use of cosmetics.
(6) Intake of *drugs*, pharmaceutical or as dopes.

In assessing exposure, one may have to assess *all* types of exposure. Subjects may be exposed to the same chemical at work, in the outdoor environment, at home; moreover, they may be exposed to different combinations of maybe interacting chemicals, differing according to the source of exposure.

In the second place a *qualitative* assessment of groups of chemicals has to take place: one should know which exposure to which chemicals has to be measured and from which sources.

In the third place the exposed group probably most at risk and the control group have to be precisely defined. This third step should give enough information to define the final question (step 4).

It is particularly important to assess whether the allegedly exposed population is in *actual* contact with the chemicals. Too often living above/near a waste dump or a factory creates the fear that one is being exposed, whereas careful qualitative assessment may show that direct contact by e.g. air, food, drinking water not or hardly exists. In that case, the subsequent step 5 does not need to be carried out. The same applies when the qualitative assessment only discovers chemicals, which can hardly be regarded as toxic.

Quantitative assessment of exposure (step 5)

This includes in the first place *measurement* of the *concentration* of pollutants in all relevant sources of intake. It should be emphasized that the sampling strategy should lead to a *representative* assessment of the pollutant levels. In the second place measurement or at least estimation of the volumes/weights of air, food, water, soil in inhaled and/or ingested air should be made. Man does not respond to a concentration, but to an *amount (intake)*. In estimating risks of air pollution, one usually essumes a respiratory volume of 24 m^3/24 h, as also is done for the ICRP-standard man. However, in fact the respiratory volume may be considerably lower, and subjects are never exposed continuously to ambient air pollution. This is illustrated inter alia by Fugas (1976, 1977). It is not possible to measure/estimate the intake for each subject separately, but one should take the estimated amounts/volumes, covering e.g. 80-90% of subjects. The following volumes/weights may serve as guidelines for adults: women 15 m^3 air/24 h, workers (moderate activity) and not employed men 20 m^3/24 h, workers (high activity)(10 m^3/8 h) drinking water 2 1/24 h; polluted food stuffs 100-500 g/day.

In addition, one should also take the highest (or maybe the 80-90% upper limit of) concentration(s) actually measured. Particularly for dust (children) one should take about 50 mg per day (from swimming, polluted hands, etc.). Summarizing the products of concentration and volume/weight/day allows to estimate the *total* intake. By taking high cut-off points, one *maximizes* the actual intake/day.

For several pollutants one may rely on *biological monitoring*, which permits to estimate the actual *uptake*. The advantages and limitations of this approach are discussed in the second paper.

It should be emphasized that assessment of the actual intake should be carried out both for the exposed group most at risk and the control group.

When even the maximized intakes do not or only little differ between both groups, further study is not feasible.

Assessment of relative health risks (step 6)

We assume that for the relevant chemicals reasonably valid exposure (dose)-response relationships have been established. If not, then one has to follow the full sequence (study B). In study C the relative health risk on the basis of the established intakes/uptakes has to be estimated. We may make a short cut, by comparing the exposure with accepted regulatory quality limits for e.g. workroom air (TLV, MAC) or Acceptable Daily Intakes (ADI), applying the maximized estimated intake.

Two examples from the Netherlands may illustrate this. In the first case of pollution of a housing site built upon a chemical waste dump exposure occurred inter alia to toluene and xylene. The highest concentration of toluene measured was 0,42 mg/m^3 in indoor air and 0,1 mg/l in drinking water. Assuming for the general public a respiratory volume of 15 m^3/24 h, and a drinking water consumption of 2 l/day, the maximized total intake per week is about 45 mg: 7 d x 0,42 mg/m^3 x 15 m^3/24 h = 44 mg (inhaled) + 7 d x 0,1 mg/l x 2 l/24 h = 1,4 mg (ingested). The TLV (and the Dutch MAC) is 375 mg/m^3 (8 h/d, 40 h/wk). Assuming a respiratory volume at work of 10 m^3/8 h the total intake for a worker (inhaled and ingested) is about 20.000 mg/week. For adult workers this exposure is expected not to lead to health impairment, even when exposed for 30-40 yr. This intake is about 20.000:45 = 450 times the maximized intake for the general public. Even when we assume that the general public might be 10 times more susceptible than adult workers, then there still is no reason to expect any increased health risk.

In the 1960's chemical waste of a pesticide factory was dumped; this was discovered in 1980, leading to a "neighbourhood of fear". Chlorinated benzenes and phenols, hexachlorocyclohexane and even TCDD were measured in vegetables, meat (fishes, rabbits, grazing cattle, etc.) and sludge. Taking the highest concentrations measured and assuming a relatively high consumption, the *maximized* intake from surface water was 2% of the exposure weighted total ADI (for all chemicals combined), sludge 21%, soil 0,6%, milk 10%, vegetables 7%, ale 50%, adipose tissue of cattle 93%, when the population should have consumed the chemicals from each source daily for about 15 years. It should be realized that the highest levels did not occur in the same samples and that the subjects did not consume all samples each day. Moreover, only about 30 members of farmer families might have achieved this maximized intake.

Both examples, taken from two highly publicized "neighbourhoods of fear", illustrate that it is possible to derive a reasonably valid estimate of exposure, when one follows a consistent logical step-wise strategy. In both cases the alleged public health risks could largely be refuted. Urged by public pression groups the government laboratory carried out a health surveillance study in the first location. No deviation of various biochemical and haematological parameters from "official" reference values were observed. This negative finding could have been predicted. However, the study was deficient in design, because a non-exposed control group was not examined.

We published our proposal for a strategy in 1982. In recent years the Dutch government has become much more reticent in giving in to public pression to carry out studies, which might be classified as individual-directed screening programs (A), which never can lead to a conclusive answer on exposure-effect-relationshups in such a location.

Further steps (7-10)

Only when according to a logical strategy a clearly increased risk has been established, may there be reason to carry out *step 7*: examination of the *state* of health, and then only according to the criteria of the WHO (Wilson and Junguer, 1968) set for screening studies A.

Of course a report should always be made public (*step 8*), in terms to be understood by the layman. Moreover, even when no health risks appear to exist for the general public, there may be other reasons (e.g. risks of drinking water pollution in the future, risks to ecosystem) to take sometime even costly corrective and preventive measures (*step 9*). There may also be reasons for follow-up studies (*step 10*), but discussion of these steps is outside the scope of this paper.

INFORMATION CONTENT AND CONFIDENCE INTERVAL

The strategy should aim at "informative" answers: the study should permit to conclude that health risks very probably do not exist or do exist, and if so, to what extent, and in which groups of the general public or workers concerned.

The information-content depends upon (Verberk, 1984):
a) *subjects*
  - selection of exposed subjects (at risk groups)
  - selection of controls
  - dropout (healthy subjects/workers' effect)

b) *measurements*
- exposure (type, intensity, frequency, duration)
- signs and symptoms (type, intensity) (study A, B)
- confounders and disease promoting factors

c) *treatment of data*
- translation of measurements into indices of exposure and of effects
- taking account of confounders
- sensitivity of the statistics applied

d) *size of the study*: number of exposure data, person-years of exposure, incidence/prevalence of diseases.

The confidence interval of the relative risk is more decisive for the information-content than the level of significance (P). This can be illustrated as follows:

Examples of "non-significant" relative risks: "negative" studies

RR	90% confidence interval	
1.04	0.98 - 1.10	*informative*: probably no increased risk
1.04	0.25 - 4.3	*not informative*; there may be a decreased or an increased risk
4.0	0.96 - 17	rather *informative*: there may be an increased risk; probably significant when the study size had been larger

Examples of "significant" relative risks: "positive" studies

RR	90% confidence interval	
1.04	1.02 - 1.06	*informative*: a weak effect has been established
4.0	1.02 - 16	rather *informative*: there is an effect, but the actual increased risk cannot be established
4.0	3.9 - 4.1	*informative*: an increased risk has been defined.

Too much reliance on the P as such, not taking the confidence interval into account, may lead to conclusions, and consequently to actions not warranted by the data: either too much, or too little action is undertaken.

CONCLUSION

A logical and consistent strategy has been proposed which permits to derive an informative and conclusive answer. The general public or the workers exposed to chemicals, accidental, incidental or in their "normal" life/work situation expect answers from medical health authorities, which cannot be given. Studies often are carried out in an emotionaly disturbed situation; pression groups and the media often tend to exaggerate health risks, even may present misleading information. The strategy proposed should be accompanied by a thorough and trustworthy health education program. Authorities have to form a group of experts, which should have the confidence of the public and the workers. This at least requires training in assessment of exposure, and particularly for medical officers of health extensive training in matters of environmental/occupational epidemiology and toxicology.

SUMMARY

Groups of the general population loudly clamour for health examinations in the case of environmental pollution. The recent discoveries of large chemical waste dumps create much anxiety. Similar demands are raised by groups of workers.

One should distinguish three types of health studies:
A) *individual*-directed study, e.g. screening for carcinoma, cardiac disease. No controls are examined; the cause is not relevant.
B) *cause*-directed study, i.e. a research study to expand knowledge of exposure response-relationships. A control group is essential.
C) *situation*-directed study, i.e. the probable cause is known, exposure-response relationships are available. A control group is essential.

The population demands study A, whereas studies B or C are needed. This discrepancy in expectation raises difficulties and should fully be explained.

When the probable causative agent is known and exposure-response relationships are available (study C), the following *step by step strategy* is proposed: A maybe vaguely stated question (1) to be translated into a more specified question after literature search and consultation (2); this leads to a qualitative assessment of exposure and groups at risk (3), followed by further specification of the question (4). Subsequently exposure to the group at risk and the control group should be quantitatively assessed (intake, uptake) (5), which allows to estimate the relative risk (6). This may have to be followed by a health surveillance study (7). A report with recommendations should be published (8), followed by implementation of preventive/corrective measures (9) and a follow up (10). Each step determines the feasibility of the subsequent step. Carrying out such a study in a "neighbourhood of fear" seems to be the only logical and consistent approach to come to an informative study, which permits a conclusive answer. This strategy can be applied both in environmental and in occupational environments.

This logical strategy should be accompanied by a thorough and trustworthy health education program in order to create a base of confidence between experts, the exposed population and the authorities. Moreover, much attention should be paid to prevention of mental health disturbances which are often more serious than somatic health risks.

REFERENCES

Fugas, M., 1976, Assessment of total exposure to an air pollutant, in: Proc. Int. Conf. on Environm. Sensing and Assessment, Las Vegas 1975, Vol 2, 1-3, Inst. Electron. Eng., New York.

Fugas, M., 1977, Biological significance of some metals as air pollutants, Part I: Lead, US Environ. Protection Agency, Research Triangle Park NC.

Hassler, E., 1983, Exposure to cadmium and nickel in an alkaline battery factory - as evaluated from measurements in air and biological material, Karolinska Institute, Dept. Environ. Hygiene, Stockholm.

Holden, C., 1980, Love Canal residents under stress , Science, 208: 1242-1244.

Kotala, G.B., Love Canal: false alarm caused by botched study, Science, 208:1239-1242.

Landrigan, Ph.J., 1983, Epidemiologic approach to persons with exposures to waste chemicals, Environm. Health Perspect., 48: 93-97.

Selevan, S.G., 1980, Evaluation of data sources for occupational pregnancy outcome studies, University Microfilms Intern., Ann Arbor.

Ulfvarson, U., 1983, Limitations of the use of employee exposure data on air contaminants in epidemiologic studies. Int. Arch. Occup. Environ. Health, 52:285-300.

Vahter, M., 1982, Assessment of human exposure in lead and cadmium through biological monitoring, Nat. Swed. Inst. of Environ. Med., Karolinska Institute, Dept. of Environ. Hyg., Stockholm.

Verberk, M.M., 1984, Strategy of measurement, some epidemiological and statistical aspects (in Dutch), Symposium on strategies of measurement at work, Coronel Laboratory, Univ. of Amsterdam, Amsterdam.

Wilcox, A.J., 1983, Surveillance of pregnancy loss in human populations, Am. J. Ind. Med., 4:285-291.

Williams, G.Z., Young, D.S., Stein, M.R. and Cotlove, E., 1970, Biological and analytic components of variation in long-term studies of serum constituents in normal subjects: objectives, subject selection, laboratory procedures and estimation of analytic deviation, Clin. Chem., 12:1016-1021.

Wilson, J.M.G. and Jungner, G., 1968, Principles and practice of screening for diseases, WHO, Geneva, Public Health papers 34.

World Health Organization (WHO), 1977, Health aspects related to indoor air quality, Euro Reports and studies, 21, WHO, Regional Office for Europe, Copenhagen.

World Health Organization (WHO), 1983, Guidelines on studies in environmental epidemiology, Environ. Health Criteria 27, WHO, Geneva.

Zielhuis, R.L., Hartogensis, F., Jongh, J., Kalsbeek, J.H.W. and Rees, H. van, 1963, The health of workers processing reinforced polyesters, in: Proc. XIVth Int. Conf. Occup. Health, vol III, 1092-1097, Excerpta Medica, Amsterdam, International Congress Series 62, vol III.

Zielhuis, R.L. (ed), 1977, Public health risks of exposure to asbestos. Pergamon Press, Oxford.

Zielhuis, R.L., Castilho, P. del, Herber, R.F.M., Wibowo, A.A.E. and Sallé, H.J.A., 1979, Concentration of lead and other metals in blood of two and three-year old children living near a secondary smelter, Int. Arch. Occup. Environ. Health 42:231-239.

Zielhuis, R.L., Verberk, M.M. and Wijnen, J.H. van, 1982, Environmental pollution and health studies (in Dutch), Ned. Tijdschr. Geneesk., 126:1595-1597.

CHOICE OF COMPARISON GROUPS IN ENVIRONMENTAL STUDIES AND DEALING WITH BACKGROUND MORBIDITY IN VARIOUS SUBPOPULATIONS

Olav Axelson

Department of Occupational Medicine
University Hospital
S-581 85 Linköping, Sweden

INTRODUCTION

The influence of occupational, environmental, nutritional, behavioural and genetic factors on health create a complex situation for epidemiologic evaluations of causes of disease. Such determinants of disease may also interact so as to jointly increase or decrease the morbidity, or can operate independently of one another. Strong and moderately widespread determinants can be revealed even by rather crude and simple study designs, e.g. smoking with regard to lungcancer, but the evaluation of weaker effects from more rare as well as from extremely common exposures are more demanding on the epidemiologic technique, both in design and analysis. The intention is here to discuss some design issues with regard to environmental studies, particularly in reference to background morbidity in various subpopulations along with the implications for the choice of comparison groups.

MORBIDITY IN SUBPOPULATIONS AND ESTIMATIONS OF EFFECT

Various subpopulations are characterized by different morbidity due to the influence of both recognized and unknown determinants of disease. Some of these determinants are general and fundamental like gender and age, whereas others are more specific like those of occupational origin, e.g. exposure to asbestos or wood dust with regard to respiratory cancers. Still others are behavioural like smoking and drinking, and there are also nutritional ones, say, intake of retinoids, selenium, etc. Finally, genetically determined characteristics might be of importance, like enzymatic activities. Rather ill-defined aggregates of such various factors are often taken as social determinants of disease and given considerable emphasis and allowed for in epidemiologic research. Furthermore, also certain selectional phenomena contribute to the creation of subpopulations with a particular morbidity or mortality pattern. The so-called "healthy worker effect" (McMichael, 1976) might be recalled in this context as referring to an undermortality seen in occupational cohorts, when compared to the general population. This relative undermortality is mainly dependent on the fact that the general population includes many individuals, who are unable to work for such medical or social reasons, that also impose a high mortality. Although common in occupational health epidemiology that a particular worker group is followed over time, and the cause-specific deaths are compared with expected numbers as derived from the general population, this approach has also been seriously criticized (Wang and Miettinen, 1982) because of the lacking comparability between a particular worker group and the general population.

However, before a further discussion of the influence of various determinants in different subpopulations on the estimation of the effect of a particular exposure, it might be helpful to here introduce a rather recent concept in epidemiology, namely the study base (Miettinen, 1982). This concept refers to the health experience over time of a particular study population and can be illustrated as in figure 1.The cases are symbolized with the plus signs and the total area with its subdivisions might be taken

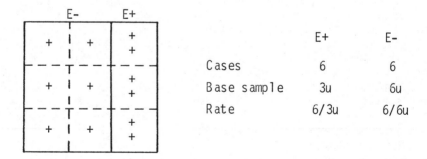

	E+	E-
Cases	6	6
Base sample	3u	6u
Rate	6/3u	6/6u

Fig. 1   Study base, either open or closed, with sectors of exposure and non-exposure. The plus-signs denote the cases and the squares symbolize units, u, of the study base, which might be represented either through a census or through a sample of the population, the latter characterizing the case-referent approach. The rate ratio is obtained as (6/3u)/(6/6u) = 2, irrespective of type of approach.

as representing the underlying population over time as delivering the cases. The study base might be either closed or open, i.e., either consisting of once defined individuals, e.g. an occupational cohort, or being a population with a turnover in membership like that of an administrative unit, a parish, etc.

The various measures of occurrence of disease relate to the particular type of study base. Thus, the incidence rate (or incidence density) is primarily applicable to an open study base, the cumulative incidence refers to a closed base, whereas the prevalence rate can be used in both situations. It should be noted also, that a sampling of the base is characteristic for the case-referent (case-control) type of study, i.e., the referents (controls) are supposed to reflect the base with regard to the distribution of the exposure under study as well as other determinants of interest. Usually a case-referent study has an open base, but this type of approach might also be taken to a closed study base, resulting in a so-called nested case-referent study (or a case-referent study within a cohort). Moreover, the traditional cohort study represents what might preferably be thought of as a census approach (i.e., "a complete sample") to a closed study base. Further aspects on study designs can be obtained elsewhere (Miettinen, 1982; Axelson, 1983), but the brief remarks given here might serve as a background for the various issues to be dealt with in this context.

The pictorial representation of the study base is quite useful also for the illustration of a study situation, where an attempt is made to study the effect of a rather weak determinant, or exposure, in the presence of another, more widespread and stronger one or an aggregate of various other such factors. As can be seen in figure 2, an increased background morbidity leads to a less impressive rate ratio for the exposure at issue, unless there is a more or less multiplicative interaction between the exposure and the determinant(s) of the background morbidity. The rate difference would be less affeced, however, but is not directly available if the study design is of the case-referent type.

In the example of fig. 2, the other determinant(s) formally cause(s) a modification of the effect under study in terms of the rate ratio, but without any biological implications. However, a true biological modification or interaction, stronger or weaker than just exactly causing a multiplicative situation, would also result in some effect-modification in terms of a variation in the rate ratio over categories of the(se) other determinant(s), whereas, interactions of any strength would result in an effect-modification in terms of the rate difference. Hence, an effect-modification might in the first place be looked upon as a phenomenon in the data as primarily dependent on the measure of effect that is involved, and may or may not represent also a biological phenomenon.

35

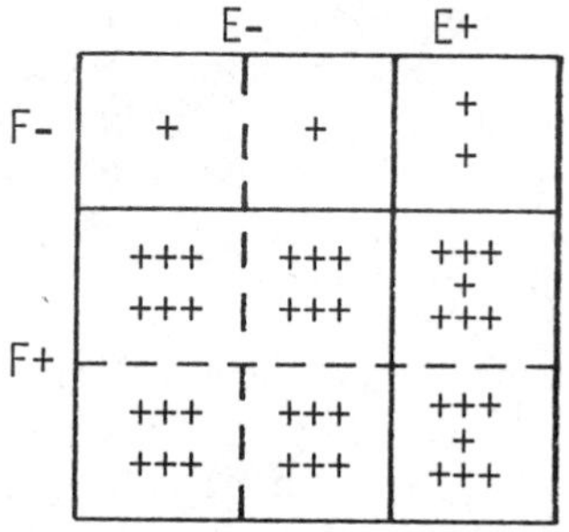

	E−	E+
F−	+ ¦ +	+ +
F+	+++ ¦ +++ +++ ¦ +++	+++ + +++
	+++ ¦ +++ +++ ¦ +++	+++ + +++

	E+	E−	RR
F−	$\dfrac{2}{u}$	$\dfrac{2}{2u}$	2
F+	$\dfrac{14}{2u}$	$\dfrac{24}{4u}$	1.$\underline{2}$
F±	$\dfrac{16}{3u}$	$\dfrac{26}{6u}$	1.2

Fig. 2   Study base with a strong and relatively widespread determinant (F) for the disease, which is
primarily studied with regard to the exposure (E),
however. Note how the increased background morbidity
from F tends to reduce and obscure the effect of E
in terms of the rate ratio, RR.

Multiple exposures and confounding effects

There are further aspects than the aforementioned effect-modification to consider, when determinants for the disease are associated to some degree with the exposure, or, alternatively, operate
more or less in the absence of the exposure. Such situations would
lead to so-called confounding, positive or negative, the first
spuriously increasing and the second reducing the effect of the
exposure under study. Usually the concerns about confounding in
epidemiologic studies relate merely to the positive (exaggerating)
effects, whereas negative confounding is given little attention
even when perhaps masking an existing effect, as illustrated in
figure 3. To the extent that other determinants than the potential
one under study, the exposure, operate exclusively in a subset
of the nonexposed, then there is rather incomparability than confounding in the study base. Such a situation would require, that
this subpopulation with the other determinants is left out, i.e.,
in principle a new study base would have to be created. Similarly,
when focusing etiological questions, a study base involving strong
confounders might preferably be further restricted so as to leave
out subjects with the confounding determinants, especially as there
usually would remain strong negative effect-modification even after
the control of the confounding qualities of the factors. Again,
such effect-modification would tend to make the effect of the exposure to appear less convincing. Restrictions are not always ad-
visable, however, as reducing the material that is available and

thereby the power of the study, although often less than feared because the power is already limited in such sectors of the base, where negative effect-modification is at hand.

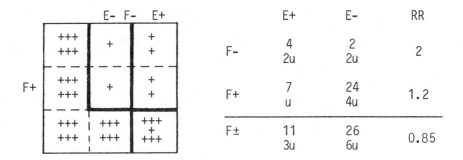

	E+	E-	RR
F-	4 2u	2 2u	2
F+	7 u	24 4u	1.2
F±	11 3u	26 6u	0.85

Fig. 3   Study base with exposed and non-exposed sector and with a strong, additional determinant for the disease exerting a strong negative confounding effect in addition to effect-modification as masking the role of the exposure (E). The SMR, taken as (observed)/(expected), is needed to distinguish an overall effect of the exposure, i.e.
SMR = 11/(2x2u/2u + 24xu/4u) = 11/(2+6) = 1.6.

The identification of various determinants, that are extraneous and disturbing with regard to the exposure under study, is a difficult task and no ideal and infallible method can be proposed. Evidently, existing epidemiologic and toxicologic knowledge is most important for the recoginition of such determinants, about which information has to be collected in the first phase of a study, preferably in a liberal way, because of the problems involved in the primary judgements about what factors of interest might operate in the study population. A further problem is then to decide which factors would be of sufficient importance to finally require consideration in the analysis of the data as likely to exaggerate or obscure the effect under study. One possibility here could be to calculate crude rate ratios for a number of these factors and to select for further control those which are associated with some risk or prevention, for practical purposes, say crude rate ratios of 1.2 and above or about 0.8 or below. In such a crude analysis, there is the risk, however, that some of these factors might be negatively confounded by another factor and even by the specific exposure under study, so that they appear rather weak and therefore get overlooked. Further aspects on the detection of confounders can be found elsewhere (Miettinen and Cook, 1981).

An approach similar to what has been described was taken in a study of various determinants for acute myeloid leukemia, there-among the possible effect of background radiation, c.f. table 1 (Flodin et al., 1981). After the identification of factors, for which the rate ratios were elevated, a second step was then to investigate if those factors also were associated with one another, i.e., if they really had the characteristics of confounders, especially with regard to the potential effect of background radiation.

Table 1. Status or exposure (especially identified or otherwise interesting determinants were selected for this table) among cases of myeloid leukemia and referents along with estimates of the crude rate ratio.

Status or exposure	Number of individuals exposed or with status		Crude rate ratio
	Cases (N=42)	Referents (N=244)	
Male gender	23	121	1.2
Pesticides	3	6	3.1
X-ray treatment	4	20	1.2
X-ray examination	12	68	1.0
Animal contacts	16	79	1.3
- cats	14	62	1.5
- poultry	8	36	1.4
- cattle	10	43	1.5
Solvent exposure	11	13	6.3
Smoker	19	117	0.9
Rural domicile	11	59	1.1

Table from Flodin et al., 1981.

One technique of checking the degree of association, as utilized in this particular study, can be to calculate the odds ratio between the various determinants occurring in the base population or in the base sample (i.e., among the referents in a case-referent study), as shown in table 2 (note that this odds ratio calculation has nothing to do with odds ratio equalling the incidence rate ratio in a case-referent study).

Table 2.   A suggested approach to studying a potential association between two determinants, A and B, by means of an odds ratio. The base population only should be involved (i.e. referents in case-referent studies).

Exposure to	A+	A-
B+	α	β
B-	γ	δ

If $\alpha\delta/\beta\gamma \neq 1$, some association is at hand, the magnitude of which and its significance have to be considered in the light of other information, especially with regard to the strength of the factors as determinants for the disease under study.

After an identification of potential or actual confounders, either before the study has started or in the data of the study, there is the further question whether to restrict the base population to such sub-domains, where the influence from various extraneous factors would be small, or to rather involve different sub-populations for the purpose of studying interaction phenomena and the relative importance of the particular exposure for the morbidity in a larger and more representative population. The first approach would be the most attractive for early studies of a particular topic, as more clearly elucidating if there are causal relations or not between an exposure and a disease. In later phases of epidemiologic research, the latter approach would be of increasing importance, however, especially for judgements about the relative effect of preventive measures in quantitative terms. Then, the etiologic fraction* tends to become the measure of greatest interest rather than the rate ratio or the rate difference as demonstrated in a recent study by Pastorino et al. (1984) about the (rather considerable) contribution of occupational exposures to the lung cancer morbidity in a population.

---

*The etiologic fraction, EF, is obtained through multiplying the fraction of exposed cases in the base, i.e. the case fraction, CF, by a quantity representing the relative effect of the exposure as derived by means of the rate ratio, RR, namely (RR-1)/RR. Hence, EF = CF x (RR-1)/RR (Miettinen, 1976a).

Comparability of the reference population

From the discussion above it is obvious that considerable problems are involved in the choice of comparison groups for obtaining an optimal study design in environmental studies, especially with regard to homogeneity in the background morbidity for both the exposed and non-exposed subpopulations. Even if particular industrial exposures may occur in rather well-defined occupational groups without too many other disturbing exposures, there might instead be problems to find an adequate reference population for comparison with regard to interfering determinants of, say, socio-economic and behavioural character but without involving other specific or different industrial exposures. This is to say, that a worker population from another factory without the particular exposure of interest might be thought of as attractive for comparison, but there could be some other exposure instead, that might influence or cause the morbidity under study.

There are actually very few studies with an ideal design in this particular respect, but a good and illustrative example of the requirements involved has been provided by Ott et al. (1983), when they were able to find two factories with the same type of production but one of them not using the agent of interest, namely methylene chloride. Both populations showed nothing but strong "healthy worker effects" in comparisons to the national cause-specific mortality, but the population with exposure had a higher cardio-vascular mortality compared to the other. Although the numbers were small and the two factories located in different states in the US, this comparison of two seemingly well comparable populations indicated the possibility, that the metabolism of methylene chloride through carbon monoxide could be a risk factor for cardiovascular disease.

With regard to studies of more generally operating environmental factors such as background radiation, drinking water pollutants or intake of trace metals of nutritional importance, etc, it might be even more difficult to deal with background morbidity and comparability requirements than in the context of industrial exposures. The reason is that environmental factors first of all tend to have a relatively weaker effect, especially when so widespread that there is not even any truly unexposed reference group. Therefore it is also obvious that comparisons with the general population would be inadequate, since the general population to a great extent would be exposed to the particular agent under study, i.e., there is no correspondance at all to the occupational cohort, which, properly or not, is compared to the general population.

A reasonable solution of the design problem in studying general, environmental factors could be to allocate a study of such exposures to a particular geographical area, where relatively few other health hazards are likely to operate in the population. An example of this principle can be found in some pilot studies of lung cancer and indoor radon daughter exposure, when the study populations were chosen to be as rural as possible to avoid the influence of various industrial risk factors, which might exert a modifying and even a potentially confounding effect (Axelson et al., 1978; Edling et al., 1984). Furthermore, in one of the studies (Edling et al., 1979), the study base could be restricted to encompass only those subjects, who had lived for a long time in the same houses. Then, estimates and measurements had to be done about the different levels of radon daughter concentrations due to building materials and emanation of radon from the ground into the houses from a particular and well localized geologic struc- ture of alum shale. In view of the allocation and design of this study, it is likely that the compared subpopulations with various degrees of exposure should be quite homogeneous and low in other risk factors for lung cancer, smoking included as less prevalent in a rural population.

Although necessary for the validity of a study, the selection of a particular subpopulation for comparison purposes tends to be expensive, therefore setting economic limitations to epidemio- logic research. The case-referent approach can compensate to some extent in this respect, however, as relatively cheap, because a large population is represented through a limited number of re- ferents. Therefore relatively more sophisticated comparisons and evaluations can be achieved than in the more demanding and expensive follow-up studies. The guideline for a case-referent study should then be to try and allocate the base of the study to a particular setting, where the exposure of interest not only is relatively frequent but also well assessable, whereas other, interfering deter- minants affecting the comparability in the base should be less prominent. If the researcher is successful in such attempts, the subsequent analysis is also simplified, but still, allowance is usually necessary for age, gender and perhaps also for some other remaining determinants, that might exert confounding effects or at least act as modifiers. The methods for such control would be stratification or multivariate analysis, but an attractive alter- native can be to stratify by a multivariate confounder score (Miettinen, 1976 b). Matching is useful in cohort studies as creat- ing good comparability in the study base between exposed and non- exposed subjects but is quite useless and sometimes dangerous in case-rereferent studies, as not influencing the base itself but distorting the representation of it through recruting the refer- ents from domains, where the matching factor has determined many of the cases to appear (cf. Miettinen and Cook, 1981; Axelson, 1983). Furthermore, matching might cause the case-referent study to become more or less ineffective, namely when matching is done on a factor which has a strong association with the exposure, especially if this factor is not even a determinant for the disease, i.e. overmatching has then been obtained.

DOSE-RESPONSE AND DETERMINANTS OF BACKGROUND MORBIDITY

The assessment of a dose-response relationship is strongly supportive of a causal connection between exposure and disease, and such relationships are necessary to study for the quantification of health hazards. Not only is the documentation of the presence of a dose-response relationship desirable, but also the shape of the dose-response curve needs to be known for the proper evaluation of a certain health hazard. As an example, the discussions about the shape of the dose-response curve for low-LET radiation might be recalled, i.e. whether a linear or a linear-quadratic relationship is at hand (BEIR III, 1980). Interestingly, however, rather limited discussions have been devoted to the epidemiologic issues involved in the establishment of dose-response curves for radiation, namely the need for a standardization with regards various interfering determinants, at least for age.

To somewhat illustrate and emphasize such needs, fig 4 was constructed. The various populations in the table of fig. 4 are differentially distributed with regard to a given determinant. Furthermore, the basic rate for each population is multiplied for the respective dose levels; the same principles might also be applied to rate differences. Then, by choosing the specific dose-level rates (or rate differences) from some of the populations, it is possible to obtain various shapes of the dose-response curve. This is now tantamount to the practice of utlizing data from various more or less incomparable subpopulations with greater or lesser exposure, as even obtained from different studies, and without taking the needs for standardization into consideration.

The solution here is to apply a so-called direct standardization, i.e. the rates of the particular exposure levels and subpopulations should be transferred to the same standard population, for which the rates then would be comparable (Miettinen, 1972). Suppose that the first population is taken as the standard population, and then the standardization procedure would be to multiply the dose-level specific rate with the denominator (persons or person-years) of this standard population, which would give the number of cases with a denominator equal to that of the standard population. A standardization of this type is obviously not possible unless the distribution of the population over the relevant determinants is available, e.g. over age, and, say, in the context of radon daughter exposure and lung cancer, also over smoking categories. Luckily, however, such strong effects as shown in this constructed example are less likely to occur in practice, but still there is often some lacking comparability between various subpopula-

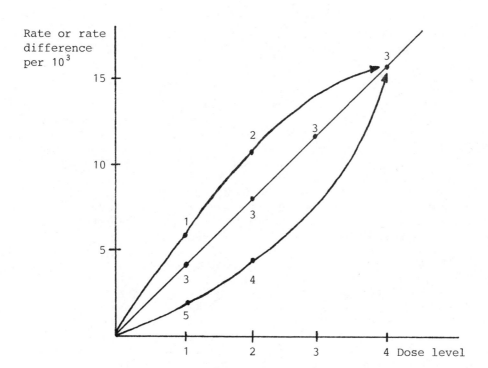

Rate or rate difference per 10^3

Stratum	Rates or rate differences for various populations				
of determ.	Popul 1	Popul 2	Popul 3	Popul 4	Popul 5
1	1:1000	1:1000	1:1000	6:6000	16:16000
2	8:4000	4:2000	2:1000	8:4000	16:8000
3	32:8000	16:4000	4:1000	8:2000	16:4000
4	128:16000	48:6000	8:1000	8:1000	8:1000
1-4	169:29000 $=5.8 \times 10^{-3}$	69:13000 $=5.3 \times 10^{-3}$	15:4000 $=3.8 \times 10^{-3}$	30:13000 $=2.3 \times 10^{-3}$	56:29000 $=1.9 \times 10^{-3}$

Dose		Popul 1	Popul 2	Popul 3	Popul 4	Popul 5
Dose	1	5.8	5.3	3.8	2.3	1.9
level	2	11.6	10.6	7.6	4.6	3.8
	3	17.4	15.9	11.4	6.9	5.7
	4	23.2	21.2	15.2	9.2	7.6

Underlined rates were chosen for the various dose levels to construct the curves, cf. pointer figures.

Fig. 4 The effect on the dose-response curve due to variation in distribution of the population over a determinant such as age or smoking. The example is exaggerated, but note that the rate or rate difference is the same across the populations within the same stratum.

tions from which information on radiation hazards (and other risks) is drawn, and therefore, the risk evaluations might sometimes be questioned on this ground.

EPILOGUE

The choice of adequate comparison groups is one of the key issues in epidemiologic research. The more subtle the effect under study, the more important is the need to achieve a good comparability between exposed and non-exposed sectors of the study base in order to avoid bias and even for obtaining any results at all. Furthermore, an effect tends to be fully outspoken in terms of the rate ratio only in relative absence of other determinants, i.e. in practice when there is minimum influence from other known and unknown determinants of the disease. Hence, etiological studies in the first phase of establishing an effect should be restricted to encompass only carefully selected subpopulations so as to achieve good comparability in the study base and as little effect-modification as possible. This view is particularly relevant for case-referent studies, where the measure of effect primarily is the rate ratio. Furthermore, the referents should first of all be representative of the base rather than be similar to the cases and in contrast to the situation in follow-up studies, a comparability between the exposed and non-exposed subpopulations involved in case-referent studies cannot be achieved through matching.

REFERENCES

Axelson, O., 1983, Elucidation of some epidemiologic principles Scand. J. Work Environ. Health, 9:231.

Axelson, O., Edling, C., and Kling, H., 1979, Lung cancer and residency - A case-referent study on the possible impact of exposure to radon and its daughters in dwellings. Scand. J. Work Environ. Health, 5:10.

BEIR III, i.e., Committee on the biological effects of ionizing radiation:, 1980, "The effects on populations of exposures to low levels of ionizing radiation," National Academy of Sciences, Washington DC.

Edling, C., Kling, H., and Axelson, O., 1984, Radon in homes - A possible cause of lung cancer. Scand. J. Work Environ. Health, 10:25.

Flodin, U., Andersson, L., Anjou, C. G., Palm, U. B., Vikrot, O., and Axelson, O., 1981, A case-referent study on acute myeloid leukemia, background radiation and exposure to solvents and other agents. Scand. J. Work Environ. Health, 7:169.

McMichael, A. J., 1976, Standardized mortality ratios and the "healthy worker effect": Scratching beneath the surface. J. Occup.Med. 18:165.

Miettinen, O. S., 1972, Standardization of risk ratios. Am. J. Epidemiol., 96:383.

Miettinen, O. S., 1976 a, Estimability and estimation in case-referent studies, Am. J. Epidemiol., 103:226.

Miettinen, O. S., 1976 b, Stratification by a multivariate confounder score, Am. J. Epidemiol. 104:609.

Miettinen, O. S., 1982, Design options in epidemiologic research - An update, Scand. J. Work Environ. Health, 8: suppl. 1:7.

Miettinen, O. S., and Cook, E. F., 1981, Confounding: Essence and detection, Am. J. Epidemiol., 114:593.

Ott, M. G., Skory, L. K., Holder, B. B., Bronson, J. M., and Williams, P. R., 1983, Health evaluation of employees occupationally exposed methylene chloride. Mortality, Scand. J. Work Environ. Health, 9: suppl. 1:8.

Pastorino, U., Berrino, F., Gervasio, A., Presenti, V., and Riboli E., 1984, Proportion of lung cancers due to occupational exposure, Int. J. Cancer, 33:231.

Wang, J. D., and Miettinen, O. S., 1982, Occupational mortality studies. Principles of validity. Scand. J. Work Environ. Health, 89:153.

THE PROBABILITY OF CAUSATION: AN APPROACH TO THE PROBLEM OF TOXIC TORTS, ESPECIALLY WITH RESPECT TO EXPOSURES TO IONIZING RADIATION

Seymour Jablon

National Research Council
2101 Constitution Avenue, N. W.
Washington, D. C. 20418

During the past several years an important issue has arisen
with respect to claims that exposure to ionizing radiation has,
in individual cases, caused subsequent cancer. Such allega-
tions are made in connection with suits for damages under what
the lawyers in the United States, and I believe in Britain
also, call "tort law". Typically in such a case leukemia or
other cancer has been diagnosed and a previous exposure to
ionizing radiation can be more or less well documented. Over a
thousand such suits have been filed against the government of
the United States by persons who allege cancer caused by
exposure to fallout from weapons tests at the Nevada test site
during the 1950's and who were then resident in the south-
western part of Utah or northern Arizona or southeastern
Nevada. Other cases involve employees of national laboratories
and of nuclear power plants. There is at least one case in
which it is claimed that the cause of the cancer was exposure
to releases from the nuclear electric generating plant at Three
Mile Island in Pennsylvania.

The characteristics of the cases vary widely: nuclear
power plant or national laboratory employees have well-
documented records of personal dosimeter readings and, while
there may be some difficulty in translating such numbers into
the dose to the organ which gave rise to the cancer, one does
know approximately where one stands. The other extreme is
represented by the residents of Utah; although rough estimates
can be made of possible doses, those estimates are marked by
considerable uncertainty. Such uncertainty is greatest when
the issue concerns dose to the thyroid gland of a child from
I-131, since the dose depends upon the amount of milk drunk,

the source of the milk, whether the cows were feeding on pasture or stored feed, how much fallout adhered to vegetation, and on and on. An uncertainty factor of ten would not be unusual in such a case.

Ignoring the problem of uncertain dosimetry, however, how is a claim for radiation injury in the form of cancer induction to be settled? It has been customary under the U. S. tort law to conduct a trial in which the plaintiff and the defendants each submits evidence and each brings his own "expert witnesses" to testify. Depressingly often, one set of experts testifies that, in their opinion, the cancer was in fact caused by the radiation which was received, or which is claimed to have been received. The other experts stoutly deny this, and assert that there was no connection between the cancer and the exposure. After this, a jury and, sometimes a judge, has to decide which experts to believe and render a decision on that basis.

Although the situation is no different, in principle, from that which might arise in relation to exposures to other toxic substances, radiation is unique in that, not only are estimates (more or less good) of dose available, but dose-response coefficients, also more or less good are available. Neither are normally available in other situations, such as exposure to benzene fumes or, to take a more extreme example, residence in an area which has been contaminated by waste chemicals such as at the Love Canal. In that case not even the specific substance that might have caused the injury can be specified. Ionizing radiation, then, is the potentially injurious agent which seems most appropriate as a candidate for a more rational way of deciding issues of damage and compensation than is provided by traditional tort law.

The great importance of the problem stems from the fact that cancer, generally, is not a rare disease: cancer is listed as the underlying cause of death in about 20 percent of all deaths in the developed countries and, taking account of non-fatal cancers, at least 30 percent of all persons have a cancer at some time during their lives. These cancers occur primarily at the advanced ages – when persons are between 50 and 80 years of age. Some hundreds of thousands of U. S. servicemen participated at atmospheric tests of nuclear weapons between 1946 and 1957. Those men are just now beginning to generate large numbers of cases of cancer and it is clear that the potential for claims is enormous.

The current interest in this subject follows from two, initially independent, but convergent efforts. The U. S. Department of Labor, some years ago, requested the National Council for Radiation Protection and Measurements (NCRP) for advice on how to respond to claims by radiation workers for compensation for alleged occupationally related cancers. At the same time Senator Orrin Hatch, from the state of Utah, was making efforts to achieve legislation which would be responsive to the claims for damages being made by his Utah constituents. Learning from Victor Bond, who was leading the NCRP effort about the possibilities of the PC approach, Senator Hatch was successful in obtaining legislation that required the Department of Health and Human Services to prepare official, governmental tables of the Probability of Causation. This is being done by a committee in the National Institutes of Health, which is chaired by Dr. Joseph Rall. Whether the tables, once completed, will have life breathed into them by legislation amending the Federal Tort Claims Act, is a question that only the future can decide.

With this as background, what is a Probability of Causation, or PC?

$$PC = \frac{\text{Excess radiation-induced risk}}{\text{Total Risk.}}$$

The essential idea is simple enough. The PC is a ratio; the numerator is the excess risk of the cancer which can be attributed to the radiation, while the denominator is the total risk, that is to say the baseline or background or "normal" risk plus the radiation risk. For example, if we were to assume that the radiation-induced leukemia risk at a certain age was 2 cases per million per annum per rad mean dose to the bone marrow, and if the baseline leukemia risk at a certain age is 30 cases per million per annum, then if someone had a history of a 0.5 marrow dose, and developed leukemia the PC would be

$$PC = \frac{2 \times 0.5}{2 \times 0.5 + 30} = .032,$$

or 3 percent.

So much for generalities. The PC approach is designed to apply to an instance when a cancer is diagnosed in a person previously exposed to ionizing radiation and the question is what is the chance that the radiation was, in fact, the "cause" of that cancer. The chance that the cancer was caused by the exposure in question depends on many factors, including estimates of the cancer induction rate per rad of organ dose,

the type of radiation and the organ dose received. The total
risk of the cancer includes (1) the above risk plus (2) the
risk for "natural" causes characterizing the exposed individual.

   Incidence, not mortality is used as the criterion for
cancer, for three reasons:

> o It is at the time that a cancer is first diagnosed
> in a person that the question will arise concerning
> the possible causal connection between that cancer and
> a documented history of exposure of radiation.
>
> o Even for cancers which do not ultimately cause the
> death of the patient (only half of breast cancers, for
> example, are fatal), there will be concern about the
> question of possible radiation causality.
>
> o When, as often happens, questions of liability and
> possible compensation arise, it would appear
> unreasonable to demand that the question of possible
> radiation causation await the death of the patient for
> determination.

The Baseline Incidence of Cancer

   Cancer incidence rates for the U. S. are available in the
report of the Surveillance, Epidemiology, and End Results
(SEER) program of the National Cancer Institute.[1] This
report presents incidence (and mortality) data for 10 areas in
the United States, plus Puerto Rico. The combined population
of the 10 mainland areas (excluding Puerto Rico) in 1977 was
21.6 million, nearly 10 percent of the population of the United
States, and is broadly representative of the nation with
respect both to geography and race. The total number of
incident cases of cancer included in the report is 327,627 for
the years 1973 to 1977.

   Cancer incidence rates vary among geographic areas. Among
the 10 areas (excluding Puerto Rico) included in the SEER
cancer registration system for 1973-77, the age-adjusted
incidence rate varied between a high of 363.5 per 100,000
annually in the San Francisco-Oakland area and a low of 279.8
in Utah. That is, overall cancer rates were nearly 30 percent
higher in the San Francisco-Oakland area than in Utah.

   There is large variation among areas in incidence for some
types of cancer, less for others. For a few cancers of special
interest with respect to radiation, SEER shows high and low
age-standardized incidence rates per 100,000 among the 10 areas
as follows:

Site	High Rate	Low Rate	Ratio
Leukemia (except chronic lymphatic leukemia)	7.5 Iowa	6.4 New Orleans	1.17
Breast (Females)	96.0 San Francisco/ Oakland	70.6 Hawaii	1.36
Lung	63.4 New Orleans	23.5 Utah	2.70
Thyroid	8.2 Hawaii	3.0 Iowa	2.73

It has been suggested that the very low incidence rates for some cnacers in Utah (e.g., lung, esophagus, pancreas) result from the Mormon interdiction of smoking, consumption of alcoholic beverages, coffee, etc. Other variations, however, are unexplained, for example the high rates of thyroid disease in Hawaii or breast cancer in the San Franciso Bay area. The very high incidence rate for thyroid cancer in Hawaii appears to result from unusually high (and unexplained) rates in certain racial subgroups:

Thyroid Cancer Age-Standardized Incidence Rates per 100,000

	Male	Female
Hawaii - Total	6.2	10.5
White	3.7	6.8
Hawaiian	7.5	19.2
Filipino	7.9	17.1
Chinese	9.9	13.8
Japanese	6.0	7.0
U. S. - Total	2.5	5.5

Thyroid cancer incidence rates vary little among the 10 SEER areas (except for Hawaii), and are similar for whites and blacks. The principal factors associated with high rates are female sex and native Hawaiian, Filipino, or Chinese race.

The overall cancer incidence rates represented by the SEER All Areas rates, published by the National Cancer Institute[1] are used as the "baseline rates". Evidently, it would be desirable to take account explicitly of factors that affect cancer rates in an important way and the calculations are specific with respect to age and sex. Geography of residence is not considered, however, for two reasons. First, unlike age and sex which can be ascertained unequivocally, residences are changed from time to time and the relevant geography for many individuals is difficult to specify; second, incidence rates are not available for all geographical areas, only for the SEER areas.

In addition to age, sex, and geography of residence, race, as shown in the SEER data, appears to be an important factor with respect to some particular cancers. Environmental characteristics that may have great influence include benzene exposures in relation to leukemia, occupational factors with respect to many cancers, including asbestos-induced lung cancers or mesotheliomas, and, most important of all, cigarette smoking in relation to lung cancer.

Despite its importance with respect to some cancers, race is not taken into account explicitly. It might well be that a race-specific assessment would, in some sense, be more accurate, but a social issue intervenes. In the United States it would not be acceptable to have a system in which a person of one race might be compensated while a person of another race, with an identical history, would not be. Interestingly, in the U. S. the practice of insurance companies of taking sex into account when calculating annuity benefits has been successfully challenged in court, despite the well-known differences in average longevity between males and females. Social policy must condition any process that impinges upon the public.

The Risks of Radiation as a Cause of Cancer

The chance that a given dose of ionizing radiation will cause a cancer to occur at some later time is the probability that a cancer will occur that would not have occurred in that person, had the radiation not been received. Estimates of these risks, both lifetime, and on an annual basis, have been published by the BEIR Committee of the National Academy of Sciences[2] and by the United Nations Scientific Committee on the Effects of Atomic Radiation (UNSCEAR).[3] BEIR provides incidence risk estimates by site for low LET radiation (X- or gamma ray) only on the linear dose-response model, although so-called linear-quadratic risk estimates are also given for leukemia and for mortality from other cancers than leukemia. The linear estimates are based on the assumption that the risk is strictly proportional to the dose, independently of dose rate, and vanishes only when the dose is zero.

There has been great debate within each of the two groups that have been working on this problem concerning the proper risk coefficients. No human epidemiological data exist that have much to say about radiation cancer risks below acute doses of ten rads or so. In fact, the risk estimates are very largely derived from human experience following doses of 100 rads or more. Radiobiological theory and experimental results alike tell us that a linear-quadratic response curve is appropriate for most end-points, following acute exposure to low LET radiation. For present purposes, however, the quadratic portion of the curve need not concern us; the BEIR III "crossover" value, that is to say, the dose at which the linear and quadratic contributions to the risk are equal, is more than 100 rads as an organ dose. For occupational exposures or other non-medical exposures that might give rise to claims for compensation, acute organ doses as large as 10 rads are very rare. It follows, then, that because the doses are low, to use the linear-quadratic response curve is really to use only the linear portion of that curve. This corresponds to the use of a risk per rad factor only 0.4 times that obtained from the strictly linear response curve. This change can, alternatively, be thought of as a dose-rate reduction factor of 2.5. This is the approach, essentially, that has been adopted by the NIH Committee for all cancers except thyroid and breast cancer. The available data for those cancers show little or no evidence of the curvature that would be implied by a linear-quadratic response model.

The risk estimates provided by the BEIR Committee are what may be termed "absolute risk estimates". That is, they purport to measure the excess rate for all cancers or for particular cancers per million per unit exposure over a time period following exposure, 10 to 30 years. For some cancers the risk estimates depend upon age at exposure and they usually depend upon sex. They do not, however, depend upon the time from exposure except insofar as a minimum latent period is specified. Is this reasonable? The NIH Working Group has concluded not, for most cancers. Figure 1 is adopted from the data of Kato and Schull[4] and it can be seen that for a cohort aged 20-34 in 1945, by about 1959 the relative risk of death from cancer had reached the value two for survivors who had doses of 100 rads or more and thereafter varied somewhat but showed no evidence of a general trend either up or down; on the contrary, the absolute risk rose pretty sharply, more or less following the increase in baseline cancer rates with the increasing age of the cohort. Essentially the same pattern is shown by the cohort aged 35-49 at exposure (Figure 2): Apart from what appear to be random rises and falls which are, presumably, the result of sampling variation, the relative

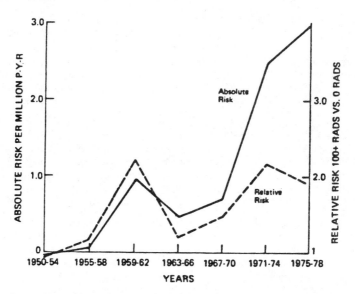

Figure 1: Absolute and Relative Risks of Death From Malignant
Neoplasms Except Leukemia - Ages 20-34 at Exposure,
1950-1978

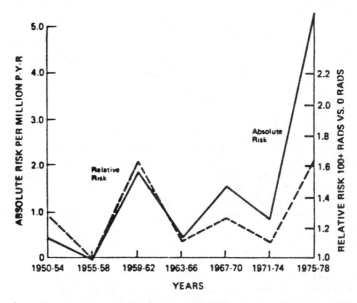

Figure 2: Absolute and Relative Risks of Death From Malignant
Neoplasms Except Leukemia - Ages 35-49 at Exposure,
1950-78

risks show little or no evidence of trend with the passage of time after 1959 while the absolute risks increase, especially in the 1975-1978 time period.

In contrast to the pattern for the solid tumors, leukemia and bone cancer are well known to follow a wave-like course in time, the rise beginning about two years after exposure, reaching a peak after perhaps 5 to 8 years, and then slowly declining. The Working Group decided to model this behavior by using a log-normal distribution. There is, of course, no theoretical basis for this: the log-normal distribution empirically seems to fit the data reasonably well as would, indeed, a number of other mathematical forms.

The relative risk time trend model which was adopted brought with it a bonus in that under this model, calculation of the PC is much simpler than under an absolute risk model. The relative risk model was, it should be emphasized, chosen not in order to achieve simplicity in calculation, but because it seemed to fit the observations better. Further, although one would not want to stress the point, it is possible to devise multi-stage models and postulate the place of radiation in them, that lead, if not to a relative risk time dependency, to something to which such a dependency would be a first approximation. Be that as it may, the relative risk model does vastly simplify calculations.

Figure 3 shows the formulas for the PC in the simplest case using the two models. In the absolute risk model "b" is the risk estimate expressed as the excess risk per million per rad, "D" is the dose and the baseline rate is the cancer rate, whether incidence or mortality, at the age of onset or of death. The risk "b" is, for most cancers, dependent upon the age at exposure.

In the Relative Risk model, "C" is the risk coefficient now expressed as the fractional increase per rad in the natural or baseline cancer rate, while "D", as before is the radiation dose to the organ concerned. As can be seen, the baseline cancer rate very conveniently cancels out of the formula so that, once the latent period has expired, the PC is independent of the age at onset or death. The risk coefficient, "C", will, of course, still depend upon the age at exposure, but the tasks of calculating and tabling the PC's become very much simplified.

An important issue which is raised almost immediately by every audience which is introduced to PC's concerns multiple causes. It will be asserted, for example, that cigarette smoking is a much more important cause of lung cancer than is

1. Absolute Risk

$$PC = \frac{b \times D}{b \times D + \text{Baseline (age)}} \ .$$

2. Relative Risk

$$PC = \frac{C \times D \times \text{Baseline (age)}}{c \times D \times \text{Baseline (age)} + \text{Baseline (age)}}$$

$$= \frac{C \times D}{C \times D + 1} \ .$$

Figure 3: Probability of Causation Under Absolute and Relative Risk Time Dependent Models

1. Multiplicative Interaction

$$PC = \frac{C \times D \times S \times \text{Baseline}}{C \times D \times S \times \text{Baseline} + S \times \text{Baseline}}$$

$$= \frac{C \times D}{C \times D + 1}$$

2. Additive Interaction

$$PC = \frac{(C \times D) \times \text{Baseline}}{(C \times D) \times \text{Baseline} + S \times \text{Baseline}}$$

$$= \frac{C \times D}{C \times D + S}$$

Figure 4: Interaction Models for the Probability of Causation

occupational exposure to ionizing radiation. How, then, it is
asked, can the cause be allocated if a regular cigarette smoker
who has been exposed, develops a lung cancer? The answer to
this question comes in two parts.

First, no attempt is made to allocate cause as between the
two factors. The problem is phrased conditionally: Given that
the person is a cigarette smoker, by how much was his lung
cancer risk increased by the radiation exposure, and what was
the ratio of that increase to his total cancer risk? The
problem we face is not to compare the risks imposed by the two
possible causes, but to assess the magnitude of the increase in
risk imposed by the exposure, given the person with whatever
characteristics he may have that are known and are pertinent,
such as age, sex, and cigarette smoking characteristics.

Second, having decided that it is desired, not to allocate
causation as between factors, but to condition one factor on
the level of the other, how is this to be done? To answer this
question we must first know how the two factors combine.
Although there are many possibilities, the simplest and most
obvious are multiplicative or additive interaction.

The formulas appropriate to these two models are shown in
Figure 4. It turns out, of course, that if the interaction is
multiplicative, then the PC is independent of the level of the
second factor, for which the relative risk is denoted by "S".
If, however, the interaction is additive, things are not quite
so simple: The coefficient "S" appears in the formula. "S"
is, of course, the relative risk appropriate to the level of
the second factor, taking the general population as the basis
of comparison. Actually to apply this formula it is necessary
to know the relative risks for each level of the second factor
and it must be assumed that these relative risks are
independent of age at onset of disease, or at least are nearly
independent.

Unfortunately, for few carcinogens apart from radiation, is
it possible to measure the level of exposure or to specify the
relative risk for each level. Still less is it known how such
carcinogens interact with radiation. The most important,
however, is cigarette smoking as a cause of lung cancer and for
that factor enough information is available. Smoking levels
are determinable and there is a wealth of data concerning
relative risks of various cancers, especially lung cancer, for
different levels of smoking. Information concerning the nature
of the radiation and smoking interaction is somewhat more
ambiguous: Whittemore and McMillen[5] concluded that, among
uranium miners, smoking and radon exposures were multiplicative, while Prentice et al.[6] found evidence favoring an

additive model and Blot et al.[7] concluded that multiplicative
interaction could be ruled out. These discrepancies are
puzzling, but the conditions of exposure studied by these
authors were quite different: chronic radiation by alpha
particles from radon daughters in one case and acute gamma
radiation in the other. In any event, the NIH Working Group
has decided to employ the additive interaction model for
cigarette smoking and lung cancer.

Many questions can - and have been - asked about the
Probability of Causation approach. One is frequently asked,
and appears to be the most important to such organizations in
the U. S. as the Office of Management and Budget, the
Department of Energy and insurance companies that underwrite
liability insurance for employers whose workers may be
occupationally exposed. That question has nothing to do with
the scientific merit of the approach or the quality of the data
which are necessary ingredients in the methodology; it is,
simply, "What will it cost? What will the consequences be?"
In a general way it can be answered that the most important
result of the application of the method will be to label the
majority of claims as lacking merit. This will not, however,
be true of all claims.

Table 1 shows the results of a few simple calculations,
using the methods of the NIH Working Group. It is evident that
although the doses that are hypothesized are not small, only
for the childhood case of leukemia is the PC quite large. The
PC for the adult case of chronic granulocytic leukemia is small
because of the very long interval between exposure and onset.
The difference between the PC's for the otherwise identical
cases of lung cancer reflect the effect of the smoking history
upon the calculation. It should be emphasized that the doses
used here are not external doses such as might be measured by a
personal dosimeter, but are doses to the <u>organ</u>, the stomach,
the bone marrow, etc.

Table 2 is more pertinent to the question of what would be
the effect of such a system with respect to occupational
exposures. The system of calculation used here is that which
was originally drafted by the NCRP Committee, and which has
since been superseded by the methodology of the NIH Working
Group. The PC's are a little larger than would be calculated
now because the dose-rate reduction factor is not used.

The question asked was "Suppose that one thousand men
became employed at age 20 and, at ages 20 through 40 received
doses to the marrow which varied from 0.5 rad to 2 rad
annually, the total being 24 rad over the employment history of
21 years. What would the consequences be?" Such a hypothetical

Table 1

Examples of PC Calculations

Type of cancer	Dose to organ (rad)	Sex	Age at exposure	Age at onset	Probability of causation (percent)
Stomach	10	F	25	50	8
Colon	5	F	45	58	0.2
Lung (non-smoker)	5	M	20	50	7
Lung (1 pack/day)	5	M	20	50	0.8
Leukemia (acute)	5	F	5	9	47
(Chronic granulo-cytic)	2	F	20	44	2

cohort can be followed for a lifetime using a lifetable to estimate survival, population incidence rates to estimate the number of baseline cases of leukemia to be expected in each quinquennium, and the number of excess, radiation induced cases, using the BEIR risk estimates (Table 2). The last column of the table shows, for each interval, the PC that would be calculated for a case of leukemia that arose in that interval. The PC's rise to as high as 60 percent with increasing length of employment (and increasing accumulated dose), then begin to fall after exposure has ended at age 40.

Although the PC's are fairly large in the middle adult years from say 25 to 55, the number of cases is small, whether baseline cases or induced cases. According to these calculations, there would be an excess of about one and one-half radiation-induced cases to add to slightly more than six cases to be expected at population rates.

Table 2

Leukemia (Except Chronic Lymphocytic) in 1,000 Workers
With Total Bone Marrow Dose of 24 Rads

Age	Number alive at start of interval	No. of Cases at population rate	Excess radiation cases	Probability of causation
20-24	1,000	.085	.011	11
25-29	991	.138	.083	38
30-34	981	.137	.176	56
35-39	971	.179	.237	57
40-44	959	.176	.267	60
45-49	939	.254	.266	51
50-54	909	.324	.227	41
55-59	864	.453	.149	25
60-64	798	.731	.070	9
65-69	704	.734	.020	3
70-74	588	.982	.001	–
75-79	447	1.104	–	–
80-84	294	.868	–	–
		6.165	1.507	

Table 3 exhibits the distribution of the cases by the PC.
Of the more than six baseline cases for only 1.7 would the PC
be as much as 10 percent, while 1.4 out of the 1.5 induced
cases would qualify at that level. In a word, although no
system can distinguish unequivocally between cases that have
been induced and those that have not, the 10 percent PC level
catches 94 percent of the induced cases but only 28 percent of
the baseline cases. A 50 percent PC level identifies 63
percent of the induced cases, but only 12 percent of the
baseline cases. Where the line should be drawn for
compensation purposes and how a compensation scheme should be
structured is a matter for public policy decision, not a
scientific issue. The point is, however, that even if the
compensation line were drawn at 10 percent, only a little over
3 cases, or 41 percent would qualify out of the more than 7
cases that might occur.

The system is far from perfect. Many of the numbers, such
as the risk estimates, that enter into the calculations are but
imperfectly known. The very shape of the dose-response curve
at the low dose levels that concern us is a subject of some
controversy. Our knowledge is, however, not so deficient that
we cannot say with some assurance that if a PC is evaluated at

0.2 percent or 0.8 percent, the chance is negligible that radiation caused the cancer in question. For larger values of the PC, exactness of calculation seems not so important; a PC of 30 percent or 40 or 50 say alike that there was a

Table 3

Expected Numbers of Compensable Cases of
Leukemia Corresponding to Different Levels of PC

Probability of causation	Baseline	Excess	Total
10	1.746	1.416	3.162
20	1.661	1.405	3.066
30	1.208	1.256	2.464
40	1.070	1.173	2.243
50	.746	.946	1.692

substantial chance that radiation was the cause of the injury and my personal opinion is that some degree of compensation would be warranted. The imprecision in the results of the calculation would, however, argue against an award system that tied the amount of compensation closely to the value of the PC.

REFERENCES

1. J. L. Young, Jr., C. L. Percy, and A. J. Asire, "Surveillance, Epidemiology, and End Results, Incidence and Mortality Data: 1973-77," National Cancer Institute, Bethesda, Maryland (1981).
2. Committee on the Biological Effects of Ionizing Radiation, "The Effects on Populations of Exposure to Low Levels of Ionizing Radiation: 1980," National Academy Press, Washington, D. C. (1980).
3. United Nations Scientific Committee on the Effects of Atomic Radiation, "Sources and Effects of Ionizing Radiation," New York (1977).
4. H. Kato and W. J. Schull, Studies of the Mortality of A-bomb Survivors. 7. Mortality, 1950-1978: Part I. Cancer Mortality, Radiat. Res. 90:395-432 (1982).
5. A. S. Whittemore and A. McMillan, Lung Cancer Mortality Among U. S. Uranium Miners: A Reappraisal, J. Natl. Cancer Inst. 71:489-499 (1983).
6. R. L. Prentice, Y. Yoshimoto, and M. W. Mason, Relationship of Cigarette Smoking and Radiation Exposure to Cancer Mortality in Hiroshima and Nagasaki, J. Natl. Cancer Inst. 70:611-622 (1983).
7. W. J. Blot, S. Akiba, and H. Kato, Ionizing Radiation and Lung Cancer: A Review Including Preliminary Results From a Case-Control Study Among A-Bomb Survivors, in: "Atomic Bomb Survivor Data: Utilization and Analysis," Ross L. Prentice and Donovan J. Thompson, eds., Society for Industrial and Applied Mathematics, Philadelphia, Pennsylvania (1984).

THE CARCINOGENIC EFFECTS OF DIAGNOSTIC AND THERAPEUTIC IRRADIATION

P. G. Smith

Department of Epidemiology
London School of Hygiene and Tropical Medicine
Keppel Street (Gower Street)
London WC1E 7HT

INTRODUCTION

STUDIES OF IRRADIATED POPULATIONS
Background radiation
In utero exposures
Radiologists
Therapeutic radiation exposure
    (a) Radiation induced menopause
    (b) Radiation treatment of cervix cancer
    (c) X-ray treatment of ankylosing spondylitis

RADIATION CARCINOGENESIS
Distribution of induction periods
Dose-response relationship
Age at exposure

FUTURE RESEARCH

This paper is a shortened version of a paper first published in
Cancer Risks and Prevention Eds M P Vessey and J A Muir Gray
Oxford University Press 1984

INTRODUCTION

Human exposure to ionizing radiations is ubiquitous. Current estimates of the carcinogenic risks associated with exposure, however, suggest that such radiations are responsible for only a relatively small proportion of all cancers. About two-thirds of the radiation dose received by the United Kingdom population is from cosmic radiation, from rocks and soil and from within the body. Most of the remaining one third is from medical procedures, both diagnostic and therapeutic. The amount contributed by nuclear fallout, occupational exposure and the disposal of radioactive wastes is about 1% of the total population exposure. The average per capita dose from all sources is of the order of 0.15 rems per year (Taylor and Webb, 1978). In the United Nations report on the effects of radiation (UNSCEAR 1977) it is estimated that exposure of one million persons to one rad of ionizing radiation will induce about 20 leukaemias and 100 fatal cancers of other sites. On this basis we might attribute to radiation exposure about 150 (5%) of the 3000 leukaemia deaths a year in England and Wales and 750 (0.6%) of the 120,000 deaths from other malignant disease. Jablon and Bailar (1980) conducted a detailed analysis of this kind for the United States and concluded that less than 3% of cancers may be attributed to radiation.

Although it seems that radiation is not a very powerful human carcinogen, it is among those that have been most extensively studied and one about which there is much public concern. The reasons for the latter may be at least threefold. Firstly, because of the association of radiation exposure with nuclear weapons. Secondly, because it seems likely that more individuals will be exposed to larger doses of radiation with the development of nuclear power as other energy sources are depleted. Thirdly, because the assumptions underlying the current estimates of the carcinogenic effects of low doses of radiation have been questioned by some workers.

In this paper some of the main epidemiological investigations upon which current estimates of radiation effects and risks are based are summarised and some of the difficulties of interpretation are discussed. More extensive discussions of these and other studies have been published by UNSCEAR (1977) and BEIR (1980). For the most part, attention is focussed in the present review on studies of persons exposed to radiation as a consequence of medical investigations or treatment.

STUDIES OF IRRADIATED POPULATIONS

Apart from nuclear warfare, most public health interest in the long-term effects of exposure to ionizing radiations is concentrated on the consequences for those exposed to low doses. In the normal course of events, high doses are likely to be received only by rare accident or in the treatment of malignant disease, for which the long-term hazards of radiotherapy are usually far outweighted by the immediate therapeutic benefits. Very large populations, however, are exposed to low doses of radiation as a consequence of their employment or through diagnostic radiology.

If the carcinogenic effects of radiation were such as to produce cancers of a type that were clearly distinguishable from those due to other causes, it would be relatively easy to identify small effects in populations exposed to very low doses. Unfortunately, this is not the case as tumours induced by radiation are presently indistinguishable from those due to other causes. It is necessary to search, therefore, for radiation effects superimposed on the background level of cancers due to all other causes. In such circumstances even if very large populations exposed to low doses (of size perhaps a million or more) are studied, the chance of detecting carcinogenic effects of the size of current risk estimates may be small (Land, 1980). For this reason many of the epidemiological investigations on radiation effects have been conducted on groups of persons exposed to doses of radiation larger than those that are of most public health concern. By study of such groups it was hoped that it would be easier to identify radiation effects, and that it would be possible to predict the effect of low doses based upon observations at higher doses. Such backwards extrapolation requires that assumptions are made about the form of dose-response relationships and it is this aspect that has proved perhaps more complicated than was initially anticipated.

Background radiation

To detect the carcinogenic effects of exposure to very low doses of radiation it is necessary to examine the disease experience of very large populations, if radiation risks are as low as have been estimated by international bodies (Land, 1980). An apparently attractive way of doing this is to study populations with different exposures to natural background radiation. Such exposures vary with altitude, with the geological composition of the earth and according to the materials from which dwellings are constructed. Studies which have tried to associate cancer mortality with variations in background radiation have not, however, demonstrated clear effects. Court Brown et al (1960a) examined mortality from leukaemia over an 18 year period in different parts of Scotland. Although it was found that inhabitants of the "granite city" of Aberdeen received a background radiation dose that was 20% higher than that of persons living in Edinburgh and also that the rate of leukaemia was higher in the former city, the authors considered that the overall variation in leukaemia risk between areas could not be attributed to background radiation. They concluded that in studying geographical variations in leukaemia rates it was insufficient to consider only variation in the background levels of radiation and it would be necessary to take into account social and economic factors that might relate to the risk of leukaemia or to the probability of its diagnosis.

It is perhaps for these reasons that similar studies of this kind, seeking to relate background radiation to an increased risk of cancer, have been unrewarding. The contribution of other factors, beside radiation, to cancer induction is so large that it is very difficult to rule out their confounding effects in relating geographic variations in mortality to background radiation exposures.

In-utero exposures

Evidence that in utero exposure to diagnostic radiation might lead to the development of childhood leukaemia and other cancers was first reported by Stewart and her colleagues in Oxford on the basis of a national case-control study of childhood cancers (Stewart et al, 1956; Stewart, Webb and Hewitt, 1958). These workers attempted to interview the parents of all children who had died of leukaemia or cancer before their tenth birthday in England and Wales during the years 1953 to 1955. By comparing the responses of the parents to questions about in utero radiation with those of the parents of selected control children they showed that in utero exposure to diagnostic x-rays appeared to increase the risk of childhood leukaemia and other cancers by about twofold. The findings of this study created considerable controversy and the causative nature of the association was questioned. Criticisms were directed especially at the retrospective method of enquiry used in the survey, as biased recall of radiation exposure by the parents of children who had died of cancers, relative to that of the parents of the control children, could not be excluded.

In an attempt to overcome this problem Court Brown et al (1960b) searched the radiological records of eight hospitals to compile a list of about 40,000 women who had received a diagnostic x-ray examination to the pelvis or abdomen during pregnancy in the period 1945 to 1956. By linking the names of the children in this cohort to a national leukaemia registry they were able to identify 9 who had died of leukaemia, against an expected number of 10.5 based upon national mortality rates. Thus the findings from this study appeared to offer no support to the observations of Stewart and her colleagues.

A study was conducted by MacMahon (1962) in the United States of over 700,000 children born between 1947 and 1954 in 37 maternity hospitals. Deaths from cancer among all the children in the period

1947 to 1960 were traced and the frequency of prenatal exposure to radiation among those who had died of cancer was contrasted with that of a 1% sample of all children who had been born in the same 37 hospitals. It was found that irradiated children had a mortality rate from both leukaemia and other cancers that was about 45% higher than that of non-irradiated children. This study was later extended to include a further 5 hospitals and also to include all deaths from cancer between 1947 and 1967 among children born in the 42 hospitals between 1947 and 1960 (Monson and MacMahon, 1984). No excess risk of leukaemia or other cancers was apparent among in utero-irradiated children after the age of 10 years. Before this age irradiated children had a 50% increased risk of death from leukaemia compared to non-irradiated children, similar to the finding in the initial study. The risk of death from a cancer other than leukaemia was only 30% higher in the irradiated group; lower than the 50% excess observed in the initial study. The findings with respect to leukaemia and solid tumours were not significantly different, however, and Monson and MacMahon (1984) attributed the apparent discrepancy to chance.

A number of other studies of this issue have been reported (UNSCEAR, 1977) and most are consistent (including that of Court Brown et al, 1960b) with an increased risk of leukaemia and other cancers among irradiated children of about 40%. A possible bias, which is hard to rule out in all of these studies, is that the increased cancer risk is related to the reason the women were irradiated rather than due to the x-ray exposure. Some evidence against this interpretation was provided by Stewart and her co-workers (Stewart and Kneale, 1968; Bithell and Stewart,1975), who analysed data on 8513 childhood cancer deaths in the period 1953 to 1967 and an equal number of matched control children. Overall, irradiated children had a 50% higher risk of cancer than those who had not been exposed to in utero radiation. Furthermore, the cancer risk was directly related to the number of times that x-ray exposure has occurred in the pregnancy. A steadily declining risk was found with year of birth and it was suggested that this was due, at least in part, to a reduction in both the number of exposures and the radiation dose for each exposure over the period of the study (Bithell and Stewart, 1975).

Further evidence favouring a causative interpretation of the association was given by Mole (1974). He noted that in the Oxford survey, 55% of twin pregnancies were investigated radiologically compared to only 10% of singletons but the risk of a subsequent tumour was similar in an irradiated twin and an irradiated single-ton. He argued that such a finding was unlikely unless the cancers were attributable to the radiation exposure.

Studies of the survivors of the atomic bomb (A-bomb) explosions, which have contributed much to our knowledge of the carcinogenic effects of radiation, have given results with respect to in utero radiation which appear to conflict with other epidemiological studies. Jablon and Kato (1970) found only one cancer death among children who had been in utero at the time of the atomic bomb explosions against about 0.4 expected on Japanese national rates. Assuming a linear dose-response relationship between radiation dose and cancer induction they argued that the small excess they observed was incompatible with the effect expected based on the estimates given by Stewart and Kneale (1970) from the Oxford survey. A possible explanation of this apparent discrepancy was offered by Mole (1974) who questioned the assumption of a linear dose-response relationship and showed that if a "cell-killing" effect of radiation was taken into account the findings from the A-bomb survivors appear to be not so discrepant from those of other studies. The argument that he advanced has relevance to studies among adults also and will be discussed in a later section.

Relative risks of the order of 1.5 in epidemiological studies often pose problems with respect to causal interpretations. While there is still room for some doubt that in utero radiation exposure does increase the risk of childhood cancers, the weight of the evidence would seem to favour a cause-effect interpretation. Furthermore, the available data suggest that the fetus may be especially sensitive to the carcinogenic effect of small doses of radiation. This was taken into account by UNSCEAR (1977) who estimated that the risk of a fatal malignancy might be in the region of 200 to 250 per million exposures of 1 rad, about twice as high as the risk estimated for adults.

Radiologists

Radiologists have been studied for longer than any other defined population to assess the late effects of exposure to ionizing radiations received as a consequence of their occupation.

In the mid 1950s there were reports that the average age at death of American radiologists was about 5 years less than that of American physicians who were not routinely exposed to radiation. It was suggested that radiation was having a non-specific life-shortening effect causing the radiologists to "age" at an increased rate due to the accumulation of genetic damage in the somatic tissues. Comparisons of average ages at death usually have to be regarded with some caution, especially in situations in which persons may enter the compared groups at different ages and also leave for reasons other than death. Nevertheless, there was clear evidence that the deaths of some early radiologists were directly attributable to their exposure to radiation sources (for example, due to cancers of the skin of the hand) and in 1956 Court Brown and Doll (1958) initiated a study of the mortality experience of 1300 doctors who had been members of the two major British radiological societies between 1897 and 1954.

In the early days of radiology the potential hazards of radiation exposure were not appreciated and precautions against exposure were either minimal or non-existent. It was only around 1920, following recommendations from the X-ray and Radium Protection Committee, that protective measures became widespread in the United Kingdom. Thus many of those who practised radiology before 1921 are likely to have accumulated exposure to very high radiation doses. In this group there was evidence of a substantial excess of cancer (Smith and Doll, 1981). The sites for which the excesses were most apparent were for leukaemia (4 deaths against 0.65 expected) and cancers of the skin (6 deaths against 0.77 expected) and there were also significant excesses of cancers of the lung and pancreas. Among those who joined the societies after 1920 there was no overall excess of cancer deaths but there was a statistically significant increase in the ratio of observed to expected deaths with increasing length of follow-up. Thus it appears that a cancer risk may be emerging as the follow-up time of this group increases.

Unfortunately, it has proved impossible to make good estimates of the doses which the men in this study are likely to have received. Some of those who joined the societies before 1921 may have accumulated, over a period of years, whole body doses of over 1000 rads and even many of those who joined later may have accumulated whole body doses of the order of 100 to 500 rads (Smith and Doll, 1981). The uncertainties about individual radiation doses limit the usefulness of this population in quantifying the effects of repeated exposure to low doses of radiation.

Studies of US radiologists have also shown excess cancer mortality rates compared to physicians in other specialities (Seltzer and Sartwell, 1959; 1965; Matanoski et al, 1975a; b; 1981) but for this group also it has not been possible to relate the excess mortality to radiation dose other than through the presumed reductions in doses to which radiologists have been exposed in more recent years.

A contrasting finding in the US studies has been an apparent increased risk of death from causes other than cancer. This has been interpreted as being consistent with a non-specific ageing effect of radiation, as originally postulated on the basis of the age at death comparisons. There is, however, little support for this theory of radiation action from other studies on human populations. British radiologists, even those who entered the profession before 1921, had a mortality rate from all causes other than cancer which was less than that of other doctors or other men in social class 1. Furthermore, no life shortening effect, other than through the induction of cancer,has been found among survivors of the Atomic bomb explosions (Beebe et al,1978a; Kato et al, 1982). Nor is such an effect apparent among patients irradiated for ankylosing spondylitis (Radford et al, 1977; Smith et al, 1977) or for the induction of an artificial menopause (Smith and Doll, 1976).

Therapeutic radiation exposures

Before the long-term hazards of radiation exposure were appreciated the use of relatively high doses of radiation in the treatment of benign disease was not uncommon. X-ray therapy was used, for example, to reduce enlarged thymus glands (Hempelmann et al, 1975) and for the treatment of ringworm of the scalp (Ron and Modan, 1980) and in both of these series excesses of thyroid cancers were reported. There were also small excesses of leukaemias, though this was not significant in the latter series. Radioactive isotopes have also been widely used in the investigation and treatment of benign conditions (see Boice and Land (1982) for a recent brief review of the results of studies on these groups).

Below we discuss three studies on patients treated with radiotherapy that have, in some respects, produced apparently conflicting results.

(a) Radiation-induced menopause   From the 1930s onwards x-irradiation of the ovaries was a commonly used method to induce an artificial menopause among women with benign menopausal bleeding. Court Brown suggested that it would be of considerable interest to study the mortality experience of women so treated. About 2000 women were identified who had had a radiation-induced menopause at three Scottish radiotherapy centres between 1940 and 1960 and their subsequent mortality experience was contrasted with that of the general population of Scotland (Doll and Smith, 1968; Smith and Doll 1976). By the early 1970s 25% of the women had died and there had been 7 deaths from leukaemia (against 2.7 expected on the basis of general population rates, p < 0.03). Deaths from cancers other than leukaemia were divided into those originating in sites that would have been directly in the radiation treatment beams (mainly intestines, rectum, uterus, ovary and bladder) and those in other sites. There was a statistically significant excess of deaths from cancers of the pelvic sites combined but no excess of other cancers. The excess of cancers in the irradiated sites first became apparent 5 to 9 years after treatment and an excess cancer risk persisted beyond 20 years after treatment. These findings were in line with other studies on similar groups of women in the United Kingdom and in the United

States (Smith, 1977). No "control" series treated by means other than radiation has been studied and it has not been possible to exclude the possibility that any increased risk of malignancy is associated with the presenting condition and not the radiation exposure. Evidence against this interpetation is provided by the finding that excess risk was confined to those sites in the radiation fields and that the increased risk was not confined to genital sites. It was estimated that the excess risk of leukaemia (per rad) was very similar to that observed among the atomic bomb survivors and among patients with ankylosing spondylitis treated with radiotherapy (Smith and Doll, 1976).

(b) Radiation treatment of cervix cancer   Cervix cancer is usually treated by the insertion of radium or by high doses of x-rays directed at the cancer or by both of these methods. Survival following treatment is relatively good and it seemed that a population of such women would be well suited to study the leukaemogenic effects of radiation exposure. There was some surprise therefore when no excess of leukaemia cases was found in a study of over 70,000 women treated in this way (16 observed against about 16 expected) (Simon et al, 1960). It was thought that inadequate follow-up of patients in this study may have been responsible for the failure to find the expected excess of leukaemia deaths, but the finding was confirmed in a recent collaborative study of the follow-up of over 80,000 women treated with radiotherapy for cancer of the cervix in one or other of eight countries (Boice et al, 1984). Altogether there were 77 cases of leukaemia arising in these women against about 66 cases expected on the basis of national leukaemia incidence rates.

Using the radiation risk estimates given by UNSCEAR (1977) it would be predicted that in the study of Boice et al (1984) there would have been several hundred leukaemias induced as a result of the radiation doses received, yet the actual leukaemia excess was only 11 cases. Thus it is clear that the assumption of a linear relationship between the induction of leukaemia and radiation dose is invalid, at least in so far as very high radiation doses are concerned. Discussion as to the possible reasons for this finding among the cervix cancer patients will be deferred until the section on dose-response relationships.

(c) X-ray treatment of ankylosing spondylitis   The study initiated by Court Brown and Doll of the mortality experience of patients given radiotherapy for ankylosing spondylitis was one of the first to be set up to assess the carcinogenic hazards of radiation exposure and it has also been among the most informative. There are several reasons for this. Firstly, the group of patients followed was large, over 14,000. Secondly, there has been a long period of follow-up of the irradiated population. Thirdly, reasonably high radiation doses were used in the treatment of this benign condition so that the radiation effects have been correspondingly large.

Starting in August 1955, an attempt was made to identify all of the patients who had been treated with x-rays for ankylosing spondylitis between 1935 and 1954 in 81 radiotherapy centres distributed throughout the United Kingdom. Over 13,000 such patients were identified.

An initial report dealt with the mortality from leukaemia up until 1956 (Court Brown and Doll, 1957) and a later report extended the follow-up to 1960 and considered deaths from other causes (Court Brown and Doll, 1965).

From these first two reports it was clear that the patients had suffered a substantially increased risk of leukaemia and aplastic anaemia (67 deaths against 6.0 expected) and of cancer (285 deaths against 194.5 expected). Furthermore, the excess cancer mortality rate was largely confined to those sites that were likely to have been directly in the radiation beams. Other sites, designated "lightly irradiated" as they may have received some radiation exposure due to scatter from the main beams, showed only a slight and non-significant excess (60 deaths against 52.4 expected). It was also found that the patients suffered an excess of mortality from causes other than cancer. About 10% of the deaths were attributed to spondylitis itself or to a closely allied condition but, in addition there was substantial excess mortality from a variety of other conditions not all of which had previously been thought to be associated with the presenting condition (Court Brown and Doll, 1965).

Support for the conclusion that the excess cancer risk was attributable to the radiation exposure but that the increased mortality from other causes was associated with the underlying condition was provided by a follow-up study of about 1000 patients with ankylosing spondylitis who had been identified at the time of the original survey but who, for various reasons, had not received radiation therapy. There was no evidence of an excess risk of leukaemia (0 deaths against 0.44 expected) or of other cancers (18 deaths against 17.21 expected) (Smith et al, 1977). The size of this non-irradiated group was small and only 80% were completely traced. It is not possible to rule out completely the possibility that these patients were at increased risk of cancer but the findings for leukaemia, at least, were significantly different from those for irradiated patients. For causes of death other than cancer the experience of this group of patients was very similar to that of the irradiated patients. It thus seems that patients with ankylosing spondylitis were at substantially increased risk of death from a variety of different causes, compared to the general population, but that except for cancer and aplastic anaemia, this risk was unrelated to the radiation treatment (Radford et al, 1977).

Many of the patients who were included in the studies of leukaemia (Court Brown and Doll, 1957) and other cancers (Court Brown and Doll, 1965) had been treated with x-rays for their spondylitis on more than one occasion. This introduced a complication into the interpretation of the late effects of the radiation treatment on mortality as it was not clear to what extent the second and subsequent treatment courses were responsible for the excess of deaths that persisted many years after the first radiation treatment. To overcome this problem in recent analyses, patients who received more than one course of treatment have been excluded from consideration shortly after receiving their second course. By thus confining the analysis to the mortality of patients following a single treatment course it has been possible to examine how the excess of leukaemia and other cancer deaths varies with time since exposure, age at exposure, and, for leukaemia, with radiation dose (Smith and Doll, 1982). The results of these analyses will be discussed in the following section.

RADIATION CARCINOGENESIS

There is abundant evidence that exposure to ionizing radiations increases the risk of leukaemia and other cancers and this relationship is beyond serious dispute. Certain important aspects of the association, however, are less clear. These include: the evolution and duration of risk following exposure, the magnitude of the risk following exposure to different types and doses of radiation and the way in which radiation interacts with other causes of cancer to affect risk. Some of these issues are discussed below.

Distribution of induction periods

The way in which the risk of a radiation-induced cancer varies with the time since exposure is easiest to look at in populations in which only one exposure of short duration has occurred. Two of the groups best suited in this respect are the atomic bomb survivors and patients with ankylosing spondylitis following a single treatment course. Both of these groups are large and substantial numbers of radiation-induced cancers have occurred. Neither group, unfortunately, is well suited to examine the risk in the period immediately following exposure. The A-bomb cohort was not defined until 1950 and thus does not include deaths from cancers other than leukaemia occurring in the first five years after the explosion of the bombs. Patients treated for ankylosing spondylitis may include some persons who, at the time of the first treatment, had a cancer that was causing symptoms that were incorrectly ascribed to spondylitis and which therefore provoked the radiation treatment.

In both the spondylitic population and the A-bomb survivors the induced leukaemias appeared, on average, considerably before other cancers. Figure 1 shows the change in the risk of a radiation induced leukaemia with time since exposure. For the spondylitics "expected" numbers of leukaemia deaths have been calculated on the basis of the general population death rates (Smith and Doll, 1982) whereas, in the most recent publication of data on the A-bomb survivors, the leukaemia induction rates have been derived by fitting linear dose-response relationships to those estimated to have received different doses of radiation (Kato and Schull, 1982). These differences limit the comparisons that may be made between the two sets of curves but the way in which the leukaemia risk changes with time since exposure may be compared for the two groups. Graphs are shown for both relative risk and excess risk. In the spondylitics the leukaemia risk is greatest 3 to 5 years after exposure and subsequently declines such that by 20 years there is no evidence of an excess risk. It should be noted, however, that the total number of leukaemia deaths is small and the follow-up of the population beyond 20 years is not yet extensive (Smith and Doll, 1982). The apparent secondary peak of leukaemias 15 to 17 years after exposure is based on only 4 cases and is probably an artifact.

No data are given by Kato and Schull (1982) for the first five years after exposure among the A-bomb survivors but the greatest measured risk is in the period immediately following this, 5 to 9 years after exposure. Subsequently the excess risk declines in a fairly regular manner and there is only a small excess mortality 25 or more years after exposure. Thus it seems reasonable to conclude from these results, firstly, that most radiation induced leukaemias occur by 10 to 15 years after exposure and, secondly, beyond 20 or 25 years the risk associated with radiation may be near zero. The veracity of this latter conclusion should become apparent with further follow-up of both populations.

The evolution of the risk of radiation-induced cancers, other than leukaemia, following exposure shows a different pattern from that of leukaemia, both among the ankylosing spondylitics and the A-bomb survivors. This is shown in Figure 2. The numbers of induced cancers are, in general, too small to permit detailed examination of the changes in risk with time since exposure for individual cancer sites. Thus for the A-bomb survivors the graphs shown are for all cancers combined (excluding leukaemia). For the spondylitics, data for cancers of all sites that were likely to have been directly in the radiation beams ("heavily irradiated" sites) have been combined. The excess risk among the spondylitics in the first few years after treatment is difficult to interpret, for reasons already discussed, and may be an artifact. A notable increase in both relative and excess risk occurs between

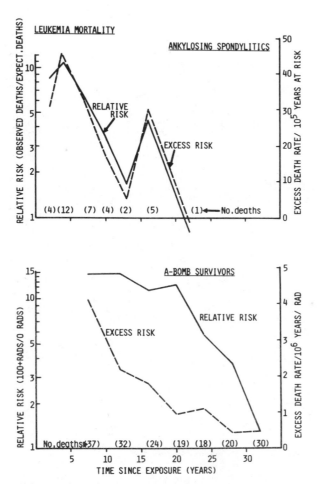

Figure 1. Risk of radiation induced leukaemia deaths at different times after exposure in ankylosing spondylitics and A-bomb survivors. Derived from Smith and Doll (1982) and Kato and Schull (1982)

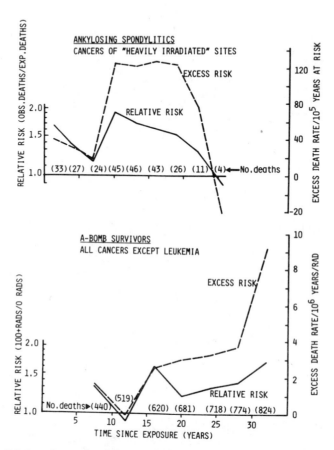

Figure 2. Risk of radiation induced cancer deaths (other than leukaemia) at different times after exposure in ankylosing spondylitics and A-bomb survivors. Derived from Smith and Doll (1982) and Kato and Schull (1982)

9 and 11 years after exposure and the excess risk remains at an approximately constant level thereafter until about 20 years after exposure. The subsequent decline, though graphically dramatic, is based on a comparison of only small numbers of observed and expected cases and is not statistically significant. The apparent decline in the relative risk in the period 10 or more years after first treatment is also not statistically significant.

Among the A-bomb survivors the excess risk 5 to 9 years after exposure is just significant (p = 0.02) but there is no risk apparent in the following five years and only 15 or more years after exposure is the increased risk highly significant. Subsequently the relative risk remains approximately constant with a tendency to increase 30 years after exposure. This disturbing trend is even more striking for the excess risk, the highest risk of an induced cancer being 30 or more years after exposure. This last point shown on this graph is based on reasonable numbers of deaths and may indicate a true increase in the risk at very long intervals after exposure (Kato and Schull, 1982).

Consideration of changes in the risk of radiation-induced cancers with time since exposure must be examined in conjunction with the ages at which the exposures occurred. In interpreting the data on the A-bomb survivors it is important to take into account the observation that those irradiated under the age of 10 years have a higher relative risk of a radiation-induced cancer than those exposed at a later age. This is illustrated in Table 1 which is taken from Kato and Schull (1982) and also in Figure 4. The increase in the excess risk of cancer among the A-bomb survivors, shown in Figure 2, is due, at least in part, to those who appear to be at high relative risk of a radiation-induced cancer reaching ages at which the "natural" rate of cancer is becoming high.

It may be concluded that the risk of a radiation-induced cancer, other than leukaemia, may be small in the first 10 years following exposure but, subsequently, the risk remains elevated until at least 20 years after exposure and possibly for the rest of life. Further follow-up will be necessary to determine whether or not the excess cancer rate increases at very long periods after exposure. This has not been observed in the spondylitics (in fact at present the reverse appears to be the case) but, currently, the person-years of experience beyond 20 years is small in this series.

Dose-response relationships

Most public health interest centres on the likely effect of low doses of radiation as it is to these which a substantial proportion of the population may be exposed. The spondylitics were, in general, exposed to large doses of radiation as were many of the A-bomb survivors, though most of the latter group received doses of less

Table 1: Relative Risk of Death from a Cancer other than Leukaemia, Among Atomic Bomb Survivors by Age at Irradiation and Age At Death.
(The numbers shown in the body of the table are the ratios of the death rates among those exposed to more than 100 rads compared to those not exposed (Kato and Schull, 1982))

Age at exposure (years) (in 1945)	Age at death (years)					
	<30	30-39	40-49	50-59	60-69	70+
< 10	15.1	5.0	6.8	–	–	–
10-19	1.0	2.5	2.4	8.2	–	–
20-24	–	1.8	1.9	2.0	1.6	–
35-49	–	–	1.2	1.1	1.3	1.4
50+	–	–	–	2.2	1.0	1.4

than 10 rads. There are clear advantages in studying a group in which exposure has been high as effects of a larger magnitude are to be expected. Problems arise when attempts are made to extrapolate from the observations to estimate the effects of exposure to very low doses. The simplest assumption to make is that effects are linearly related to dose and to extrapolate backwards on this basis. This has been the general approach adopted for many of the analyses of data from studies of the A-bomb survivors. For leukaemia, the cause of death for which the radiation induced excess is most apparent, this form of dose-response relationship fits the data quite well though it is a better fit for the Hiroshima data than for the Nagasaki data and also the leukaemia risk, for a specified dose, seems to be higher in Hiroshima than Nagasaki. In part this difference may be due to the different relative contributions of neutron and gamma radiation in the two cities, but the original dosimetry on the A-bomb survivors has been questioned (Loewe and Mendelsohn, 1981) and the reassessment of the effects of the different kinds of radiation must await the revised dosimetry.

If the data from the two cities are combined and linear dose-response curves are fitted to the leukaemia excess mortality the estimate of the induction rate is 1.9 leukaemia deaths per million person years at risk per rad and for other cancers the rate is 2.2 per million person years at risk per rad (Beebe et al, 1978b).

For the spondylitics, organ dose estimates are not yet available, except for the bone marrow. Estimates of the mean bone marrow dose of radiation have been made for patients dying of leukaemia and

for a random sample of all patients and these have been used to
relate the excess leukaemia risk to radiation dose. Details of the
procedures used are given in Smith and Doll (1982) and Figure 3 is
taken from that paper.

The greatest risk of leukaemia induction is in those patients
with a mean marrow dose of 100 to 200 rads. At high doses the risk
appears to be reduced. The data are not well fitted by a linear
dose-response curve passing through the origin (line 1 in Figure 3)
and, indeed, the assumption that the excess risk is unrelated to
dose fits the data better (line 0 in Figure 3). This surprising
finding was not apparent in the original analyses (Court Brown and
Doll, 1957) when patients receiving multiple courses of x-ray
treatment were included and marrow dose estimates from the different
courses were simply added. In that analysis a linear dose-response
relationship, passing through the origin, appeared reasonable.
The reasons for these differences are not clear but it is possible
that the effect of two or more courses of radiation may be greater
than the same amount of radiation given in a single course.

Evidence that a simple linear dose-response relationship for
the induction of leukaemia may be incorrect was provided by the
finding of little or no excess risk of leukaemia among women
irradiated for the treatment of cervix cancer. Women given a
radiation-induced menopause received a substantially smaller dose
to the bone marrow and yet showed a statistically significant
excess mortality for leukaemia. It was suggested that patients
irradiated for cervix cancer may not be at greatly increased risk
of leukaemia because the radiation treatment is given in such a
way that some of the bone marrow received a very high dose of
radiation, sufficient to sterilise the marrow cells in the vicinity
of the cervix, and that the dose to the marrow falls off rapidly
with distance from the cervix such that the mean dose to surviving
cells may be quite small. Thus the "effective" dose for leukaemia
induction is small (Hutchison,1968; Mole 1973; Boice et al, 1984).

In the treatment of ankylosing sponylitis, usually only the
spine and sacroiliac joints were irradiated but the doses shown in
Figure 3 relate to the mean marrow dose. The dose to cells directly
in the radiation field may have been higher than the mean dose by
a factor of two or more and many of these cells may have received
a dose large enough to sterilise them.

Dose-response curves for cancer induction that take account of
the cell sterilising effect of radiation have been discussed by
Gray (1965), Mole (1975) and others. Mole and his colleagues have
also developed a mouse system for the induction of leukaemia by
x-rays in CBA mice in which the leukaemia induction data is well
fitted by a mathematical model assuming an exponential cell-sterilisation effect, and a leukaemia induction rate among non-sterilised

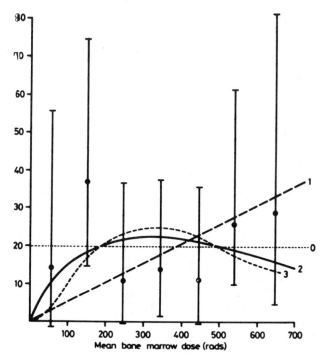

Figure 3. Excess death rate from leukaemia among ankylosing
spondylitics according to mean bone marrow radiation
dose. Curves are based on maximum likelihood fit of
the following models:

(0)   ER = b; b = 19.6 x 10^{-5} (1) ER = bD; b = 0.52 x 10^{-6}

(2) ER = $bDe^{-\lambda D}$; b = 2.02 x 10^{-6}, λ = 0.33 x 10^{-2}

(3) ER = $bD^2e^{-\lambda D}$; b = .018 x 10^{-6}, λ = .63 x 10^{-2},

where ER is the excess leukaemia death rate, D is the
mean bone marrow dose and b and λ are constants estimated by the method of maximum likelihood (from Smith
and Doll (1982) reproduced by kind permission of the
editor of the British Medical Journal)

cells proportional to the square of the radiation dose (Major and Mole, 1978; Mole et al, 1983). We have fitted models of this general form to the data shown in Figure 3. Line 2 shows the best fit of a curve predicting the excess death rates as

$$aDe^{-bD}$$

where D is the mean marrow dose and a and b are constants which are estimated. Line 3 fits a model of the form

$$aD^2e^{-bD},$$

which does not fit quite as well. Unfortunately, the confidence bands on the leukaemia excess risk at each dose point are sufficiently large that a wide range of different possible models would fit the data. It should be noted also that it is not strictly appropriate to fit models of this form for this data set. As only part of the marrow is irradiated, and the fraction varies from patient to patient, different portions of the marrow will receive different doses and this should be taken into account in the model fitting procedure. The necessary data relating to the dose to different parts of the marrow for each patient are not yet available, however.

A further complication in interpreting these data derives from the fact that a radiation treatment course for ankylosing spondylitis may have been spread over a month or more. In calculating the marrow dose we simply added together the contributions from the different fractions. It is well established that the cell killing effect of radiation is modified by fractionation of the radiation dose and it has been suggested that the same may be true for leukaemia induction. Using the same mouse model as discussed above, Mole and Major (1983) have demonstrated recently that with fractionated exposure a dose-response curve is obtained remarkably similar to that which has been observed for the spondylitics. The relevance of the mouse model for human data is unclear but at least, it suggests that extrapolating from the effects of high radiation doses given at high dose rates to predict the effects of low doses at low dose rates may be a more complicated procedure than was perhaps initially anticipated!

Age at exposure

Several workers have advanced the hypothesis that individuals may vary in their susceptibility to a radiation-induced cancer. Bross and Natarajan (1972) in particular, have suggested, with respect to in utero radiation exposure that some fetuses may be many times more susceptible than others to radiation carcinogenesis. Whilst this is a plausible theory the evidence advanced to support the argument has been unconvincing. There is, however, good evidence that age at exposure is related to radiation risk. We have mentioned earlier that the fetus seems to be more sensitive to radiation than are adults (UNSCEAR, 1977) and in Figures 4 and 5 the induction rates of leukaemia and other cancers are compared among patients with ankylosing spondylitis and the A-bomb survivors according to their ages at the time of the radiation exposure.

Among the spondylitics, there is no evidence that the <u>relative</u> risk of leukaemia varies significantly with age at exposure but the excess risks show a steep and, statistically, highly significant increase as the age at exposure increases.

There were no young children among the spondylitics but among the A-bomb survivors there is evidence that children may be especially susceptible to leukaemia induction (at least as measured by the relative risk). The excess risk among children is similar to that among adults up to the age of 50 years and it rises slightly after this. The increase in the excess risk with age is much steeper among the spondylitics than in the A-bomb survivors. Doll (1970) noted that the incidence of leukaemia among non-irradiated persons also increased much more steeply with age in Britain than in Japan. This suggests that, among adults at least, radiation may be interacting in a multiplicative way with other factors which induce leukaemia.

For cancers other than leukaemia the situations appears to be similar (Figure 5 and Table 1). In both population groups shown the excess risk increases regularly with age at exposure among adults. The relative risk among those who were children at the time of the A-bomb explosions is especially high. In the spondylitics the relative risk of a radiation-induced cancer shows no significant variation with age but the excess risk for those irradiated at age 55 years or more is over 10 times higher than that for persons irradiated at ages under 35 years. These observations also suggest, as for leukaemia, that radiation interacts in a way that may be approximately multiplicative with other factors which induce cancer. Of relevance in this respect also is the observation that for most individual cancers the radiation risk is approximately proportional to the expected death rate from the cancer in the absence of radiation (Smith and Doll, 1972; Kato and Schull, 1982). These conclusions must be tentative, however, as it remains to be seen how the risk of radiation-induced cancers will evolve in later life among persons irradiated at a young age. There is some evidence also that the effect of age at irradiation is not the same for all cancers. For example, among the A-bomb survivors, McGregor et al (1977) found that the risk of radiation-induced breast cancer was highest among those exposed at ages 10 to 19 years and showed a significant decrease associated with exposure at older ages. More recent observations on the A-bomb survivors indicate that those exposed under the age of 10 years are also at increased risk of breast cancer. At present the radiation-associated <u>excess</u> risk of breast cancer among those irradiated as young children is lower than

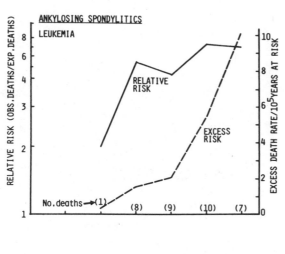

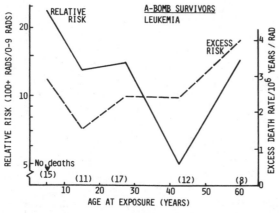

Figure 4. Risk of radiation induced leukaemia deaths at different
ages at exposure in ankylosing spondylitics and A-bomb
survivors. Derived from Smith and Doll (1982) and
Beebe et al (1977)

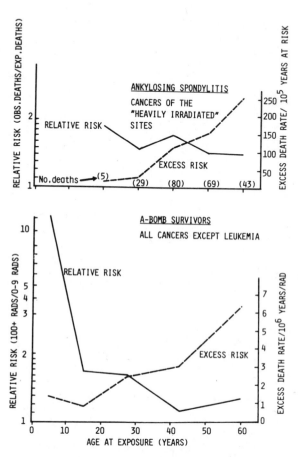

Figure 5. Risk of radiation induced cancer deaths other than leukaemia at different ages at exposure in ankylosing spondylitics and A-bomb survivors. Derived from Smith and Doll (1982) and Beebe et al (1977)

that of those aged 10 to 19 years at the time of the explosions. The relative risk of breast cancer is higher, however, among those irradiated in the first decade of life (Tokunaga et al 1984). Thus it is possible, with further follow-up of the population, that those irradiated at the youngest ages may be at greatest absolute risk of a radiation-induced breast cancer.

FUTURE RESEARCH

Ionizing radiations are one of the most well studied of carcinogens yet there is still considerable controversy regarding the magnitude of their effect in the induction of cancer at low doses. This is perhaps not surprising as they are a relatively weak carcinogen and it seems likely that they are responsible for only a small proportion of all human cancers. Thus to separate out their effects from those of other, and often more powerful, carcinogenic agents poses considerable difficulties. This is especially likely to be the case when populations whose members have been exposed to very low levels of radiation are studied. It is perhaps for these reasons that studies of cancer mortality in geographical areas with different levels of background radiation have been unrewarding. Most public health interest in the carcinogenic effects of radiation with respect to populations who might have a low, but higher than average, exposure as a consequence of their occupation or through exposure to the products of nuclear industries or to diagnostic radiation. The risk estimates on which existing international exposure standards are based would suggest that exposure at the limit of recommended levels are likely to produce only a small increase in an individual's cancer risk - of a magnitude that would be very difficult to detect even in large epidemiological studies (Land 1980). Nevertheless, we have seen above that there are still several important areas of uncertainty that should encourage caution in deducing the effects of low level exposure from effects seen in special population groups exposed to high radiation doses.

There are theoretical and experimental grounds for believing that the dose-response curve for x-ray induction of cancer is not simply linear but should include a quadratic component and take account of cell sterilisation. If this is the case, it has been assumed that fitting linear dose-respone curves may lead to overestimates of the effects of low level exposure (ICRP 1977), Whilst it seems unlikely that the carcinogenic effects of low levels of radiation have been seriously underestimated this possibility cannot be completely excluded and, therefore, it will be important to monitor carefully the experience of those whose employment involves radiation exposure. Fortunately many of those in this position have worn film badges which enable reasonable estimates to be made of the magnitude of exposure and it should thus be possible to relate cancer risk to dose. Studies of this kind have been conducted of US atomic energy workers and studies of similar UK populations are under way. The confidence intervals on any estimates of risk obtained from these studies will be wide but they should, at least, provide information on whether or not the current estimates of risk (based on extrapolation from populations exposed to high doses) are out by an order of magnitude.

The choice of an appropriate dose-response curve for extrapolation is still a matter of considerable controversy and uncertainty (BEIR, 1980) and this is an area where more work is needed. Unfortunately the way forward is not entirely clear. It is likely that the revised dose estimates for the A-bomb survivors that are now being derived will lead to changes in the risk estimates based on this population. They may also lead to a reassessment of the relative carcinogenic effects of gamma and neutron radiation. The basic methods by which dose estimates for this population are derived are, however, necessarily crude and this may frustrate attempts to elucidate the detailed shape of dose-response relationships. The estimation of the radiation dose to the spondylitic patients is, in principle, easier as reasonably good data are available on the treatment schedules employed for a sample of patients. Interpretation is complicated, however, as organs, including the bone marrow, were not uniformly irradiated and, furthermore, the radiation exposure may have been given over a period of a month or more. Mole and his colleagues have suggested, and also shown in their mouse model, that it may be important to take account of both of these factors in constructing dose-response relationships, although the way in which this should be done, especially with respect to fractionation, is unclear. By taking account of the dose-distribution to different parts of the marrow it should be possible to fit more appropriate models, incorporating cell-sterilisation effects, of the form illustrated in Figure 3.

At present efforts are being made to extend the follow-up of spondylitis patients who received more than one course of radiotherapy. It is likely that comparison of the cancer risks to such patients with the risks to patients following a single treatment course will enable the effects of exposures separated in time to be estimated. This is of interest as, for example, in situations of occupational exposure, radiation doses to workers are likely to be accumulated in this way, though at lower doses. There may be considerable difficulties, however, in extrapolating the effects seen at the high doses received by patients with spondylitis to predict effects at much lower dose levels.

Studies of the way in which radiation interacts with other carcinogens are of considerable scientific and public health interest. The finding that the excess of risk of leukaemia and other cancers following radiation exposure varies according to the age at exposure strongly suggests that the effects of radiation are not independent of other carcinogenic factors. Unfortunately in few of the published studies of population groups exposed to moderate doses of radiation is there any information on exposure to other potential carcinogens. For example, among the spondylitics deaths from lung cancer are a high proportion of all deaths from cancers of "heavily irradiated" sites. There are, however, no data available on the smoking habits of the patients in this series so that it is possible neither to assess how much of the excess risk of lung cancer is due to differences in smoking habits from those of the general population nor to determine how rates of radiation-induced lung cancer vary with smoking habits. Whittlemore and McMillan (1983) analysed data on the mortality of uranium miners from lung cancer in relation to both their smoking habits and estimated radiation exposure. They found that a model in which the risk associated with exposure to both factors was estimated by a multiplication of the risks associated with each factor alone gave a satisfactory fit to the data whereas an additive model did not. Prentice et al (1983) could not distinguish between the two types of model in their analysis of data on lung cancer mortality and smoking habits among survivors of the atomic bomb explosions. For smoking related cancers of other sites, however, these authors found that the joint effects of smoking and radiation exposure were not only less than multiplicative but, for some cancer sites, there was some evidence that the joint effects were less than additive.

Although the risk of a radiation-induced leukaemia appears to decline by 10 years after exposure, and may be near zero more than 20 years after exposure, the risk of other radiation-induced cancers remains relatively high in this period. In order to estimate the total number of cancers induced by a given radiation exposure it will be necessary to follow the members of exposed populations for many decades and probably throughout life. It is possible that the induced cancer risk will persist throughout life or it may even increase in later years. Among the A-bomb survivors the relative risk of a cancer other than leukaemia among those estimated to have received more than 100 rads, compared to those not irradiated, is greatest among those irradiated at the youngest ages. If these relative risks remain constant throughout life, the absolute risk of a radiation-associated cancer will increase as the follow-up time increases. There is a disturbing suggestion of such a trend in recent data from the A-bomb survivors (Figure 2 and Kato and Schull, 1982). It is especially important to continue to follow population groups that have already been under study for several decades (eg the A-bomb survivors and patients with anky-losing spondylitis) as there is presently little information on radiation effects 30 or more years after exposure.

ACKNOWLEDGEMENTS

I am grateful to Gilbert Beebe and John Boice for their comments on an earlier version of this paper.

REFERENCES

Beebe, G.W., Kato, H., and Land, C.E., 1977, Mortality experience
of atomic bomb survivors 1950-74, Radiation Effects Research
Foundation, Life span Study Report 8, Technical Report
RERF TF 1-77.

Beebe, G.W., Land, C.E., and Kato, H., 1978a, The hypothesis of
radiation-accelerated aging and the mortality of Japanese
A-bomb victims, in: "Late Biological Effects of Ionizing
Radiation", Vol 1, International Atomic Energy Agency,
Vienna.

Beebe, G.W., Kato, H., and Land, C.E., 1978b, Studies of the
mortality of A-bomb survivors. 6. Mortality and radiation
dose, 1950-74, Radiat.Res., 75: 138-201.

BEIR, 1980, The effects on populations of exposure to low levels
of ionizing radiation: 1980. Committee on the Biological
Effects of Ionizing Radiations. National Research Council.
National Academy Press, Washington D.C.

Bithell, J., and Stewart, A., 1975, Prenatal irradiation and childhood malignancy: a review of British data from the Oxford
survey, Brit. J. Cancer, 31: 271-307.

Boice, J.D., Hutchison, G.B.,1980, Leukemia following radiotherapy
for cervical cancer. 10 year follow up of an international
study, J. Natl. Cancer Inst., 65: 115-129.

Boice, J.D. Jr., and Land, C.E., 1982, Ionizing radiation, in,
"Cancer Epidemiology and Prevention", D. Schottenfeld, and
J.F. Fraumeni, Jr., eds., W.B Saunders Co, Philadelphia.

Boice, J.D., Day, N.E., and 34 others, 1984, Cancer risk following
radiotherapy of cervical cancer: a preliminary report, in:
"Radiation Carcinogenesis: Epidemiology and Biological
Significance", J.D. Boice, and J.F. Fraumeni, eds., Raven
Press, New York.

Bross, I.D.J., and Natarajan, N., 1982, Leukemia from low-level
radiation. Identification of susceptible children, New
Eng. J. Med., 287: 107-110.

Court Brown, W.M., and Doll, R., 1957, Leukaemia and aplastic
anaemia in patients irradiated for ankylosing spondylitis,
Special Report Series, Medical Research Council, No. 295,
HMSO, London.

Court Brown, W.M., Doll, R., 1958, Expectation of life and mortality
from cancer among British radiologists, Brit.Med.J.,2: 181-187.

Court Brown, W.M., Spiers, F.W., Doll, R., Duffy, B.J., and McHugh,
M.J., 1960a, Geographical variation in leukaemia mortality
in relation to background radiation and other factors,
Brit.Med. J., 1: 1753-1759.

Court Brown, W.M., Doll, R., and Hill, A.B., 1960b, Incidence of
leukaemia after exposure to diagnostic radiation in utero,
Brit. Med. J., 4: 1539-1545.

Court Brown, W.M., and Doll, R., 1965, Mortality from cancer and
other causes after radiotherapy for ankylosing spondylitis,
Brit.Med. J., 2: 1327-1332.

Doll, R., and Smith, P.G., 1968, The long term effects of x-irradiation in patients treated for metropathia haemorrhagia, Brit. J. Radiol., 41: 362-368.

Doll, R., 1970, Cancer and aging: the epidemiologic evidence, in: "10th International Cancer Congress. Oncology 1970", Year Book Medical Pub. Inc., Chicago.

Gray, L.H., 1965, Radiation biology and cancer, in: "Cellular Radiation Biology", Williams and Wilkins, Baltimore.

Hempelmann, L.H., Hall, W.J., Phillips, M., Cooper, R.A., and Ames., W.R., 1975, Neoplasms in persons treated with x-rays in infancy: fourth survey in 20 years, J. Natl. Cancer Inst., 55: 519-530.

Hutchison, G.B., 1968, Leukemia in patients with cancer of the cervix treated with radiation. A report covering the first 5 years of an international study, J. Natl. Cancer Inst., 40: 951-982.

ICRP, 1977, Recommendations of the International Commission on Radiological Protection, in: "ICRP Publications 26", Pergamon Press, Oxford.

Ichimaru, T.M., Ishimaru, T., Belsky, J.L., 1978, Incidence of leukaemia in atomic bomb survivors belonging to a fixed cohort in Hiroshima and Nagasaki, 1950-71, J. Radiat. Res., 19: 262-282.

Jablon, S., and Kato, H., 1970, Childhood cancer in relation to prenatal exposure to atomic bomb radiation, Lancet, 2: 1000-1003.

Jablon, S., and Bailar, J.C., 1980, The contribution of ionizing radiation to cancer mortality in the United States, Preventive Med. , 9: 219-226.

Kato, H., Brown, C.C. Hoel, D.G., and Schull, W.J., 1982, Studies of the mortality of A-bomb survivors, Report 7. Mortality 1950-1978: Part II Mortality from causes other than cancer and mortality in early entrants. Radiat. Res., 91: 243-264.

Kato, H., and Schull, W.J., 1982, Studies of the mortality of A-bomb survivors 7. Mortality, 1950-1978, Part 1, Cancer mortality, Radiat. Res., 90: 395-432.

Land, C., 1980, Estimating cancer risks from low doses of ionizing radiation, Science, 209: 1197-1203.

Loewe, W.E., and Mendelsohn, E., 1981, Revised dose estimates at Hiroshima and Nagasaki, Health Phys., 41: 663-666

MacMahon, B., 1962, Prenatal x-ray exposure and childhood cancer, J. Natl. Cancer Inst., 5: 1173-1191.

Major, I.R., and Mole, R.H., 1978, Myeloid leukaemia in x-ray irradiated CBA mice, Nature, 272: 455-456.

Matanoski, G.M., Seltser, R., Sartwell, P.E., Diamond, E.L., and Elliott, E.E., 1975a, The current mortality rates of radiologists and other physician specialists: deaths from all causes and from cancer. Am. J. Epidem., 101: 188-198.

Matanoski, G.M., Seltser, R., Sartwell, P.E., Diamond, E.L., and Elliott, E.E., 1975b, The current mortality rates of radiologists and other physician specialists: specific cause of death, Am. J. Epidem., 101: 199-201.

Matanoski, G.M., 1981, Risk of cancer associated with occupational exposure in radiologists and other radiation workers, in: "Cancer: achievements, challenge and prospectives for the 1980s", J.H. Burchenal, and H.F. Oettgen, eds., Grune and Stratton, New York.

McGregor, D.H., Land, C.E., Choi, K., Tokuokas, S., Liu, P.I., Wakabayashi, T., and Beebe, G.W., 1977, Breast cancer incidence among atomic bomb survivors Hiroshima and Nagasaki, 1950-1969. J. Natl. Cancer Inst. 59: 799-811.

Mole,R., 1973, Late effects of radiation: carcinogenesis, Brit. Med. Bull., 29: 78-83.

Mole, R.H., 1974, Antenatal irradiation and childhood cancer: causation or coincidence? Brit. J. Cancer, 30: 199-208.

Mole, R.H., 1975, Ionizing radiation as a carcinogen: practical questions and academic pursuits, Brit. J. Radiol. 48: 157-169.

Mole, R.H., and Major, I.R., 1983, Myeloid leukaemia frequency after protracted exposure to ionizing radiation: experimental confirmation of the flat dose response found in ankylosing spondylitis after a single treatment course with x-rays, Leuk. Res., 7: 295-300.

Mole, R.H., Papworth, D.C., and Corp, M.J., 1983, The dose-response for x-ray induction of myeloid leukaemia in male CBA/H mice, Brit. J. Cancer, 47: 285-291.

Monson, R.R., and MacMahon, B., 1984, Prenatal x-ray exposure and cancer in children, in: "Radiation Carcinogenesis: Epidemiology and Biological Significance", J.D. Boice and J.F. Fraumeni, eds., Raven Press, New York.

Prentice, R.L., Yoshimoto, Y., and Mason, M.W., 1983, Relationship of cigarette smoking and radiation exposure to cancer mortality in Hiroshima and Nagasaki, J. Natl. Cancer Inst., 70: 611-622.

Radford, E.P., Doll, R., and Smith, P.G., 1977, Mortality among patients with ankylosing spondylitis not given x-ray therapy, New Engl. J. Med., 297: 572-576.

Ron , E., and Modan, B., 1980, Benign and malignant thyroid neoplasms after childhood irradiation for tinea capitis, J. Natl. Cancer Inst.,65: 7-11.

Seltser, R., and Sartwell, P.E., 1959, The application of cohort analysis to the study of ionizing radiation and longevity in physicians, Amer. J. Pub. Hlth., 49: 1610-1620.

Seltser, R., and Sartwell, P.E., 1965, The influence of occupational exposure to radiation on the mortality of American radiologists and other medical specialists, Am. J. Epidem., 81: 2-22.

Simon, N., Brucer, M., and Hayes, R., 1960, Radiation and leukaemia in cancer of the cervix, Radiology, 74: 905-911.

Smith, P.G., and Doll, R., 1976, Late effects of x irradiation in patients treated for metropathia haemorrhagica, Brit. J. Radiol., 49: 224-232.

Smith, P.G., 1977, Leukaemia and other cancers following radiation treatment of pelvic disease, Cancer, 39: 1901-1905.

Smith, P.G., Doll, R., and Radford, E.P., 1977, Cancer mortality among patients with ankylosing spondylitis not given x-ray therapy, Brit. J. Radiol., 50: 728-734.

Smith, P.G., and Doll, R., 1981, Mortality from cancer and all causes among British radiologists, Brit. J. Radiol., 54: 187-194.

Smith, P.G., and Doll, R., 1982, Mortality among patients with ankylosing spondylitis after a single treatment course with x rays, Brit. Med. J., 284: 449-460.

Stewart, A., Webb, A., Giles, D., and Hewitt, D., 1956, Malignant disease in childhood and diagnostic irradiation in utero, Lancet, 2: 447.

Stewart, A., Webb, J., and Hewitt, D., 1958, A survey of childhood malignancies, Brit. Med. J., 1: 1495-1508.

Stewart, A., and Kneale, G.W., 1968, Changes in the cancer risk associated with obstetric radiography, Lancet, 1: 104-107.

Stewart, A.M., and Kneale, G.W., 1970, Radiation dose effects in relation to obstetric x-rays and childhood cancers, Lancet, 1: 1185-1188.

Taylor, F.E., and Webb, G.A.M., 1978, Radiation exposure of the UK population, National Radiological Protection Board Report NRPB-R77.

Tokunaga, M., Land, C.E., Yamamoto, T., Asano, M., Tokuoka, S., Ezaki, H., Nishimore, I., and Fujikura, T., 1984, Breast cancer among atomic bomb survivors, in: "Radiation Carcinogenesis: Epidemiology and Biological Significance", J.D. Boice, and J.F. Fraumeni, eds., Raven Press, New York.

UNSCEAR, 1977, Sources and effects of ionizing radiation. United Nations Scientific Committee on the Effects of Atomic Radiation, United Nations, New York.

Whittlemore, A., McMillan, A., 1983, Lung cancer mortality among US uranium miners: a reappraisal, J. Natl, Cancer Inst., 70: 489-499.

DOSE-RESPONSE IN RADIATION CARCINOGENESIS:

ANIMAL STUDIES

David G. Hoel

Radiation Effects Research Foundation
Hiroshima, Japan

INTRODUCTION

The Oak Ridge National Laboratories (ORNL) have, over the
years, conducted a large number of experiments involving several
types of ionizing radiation. These studies were conducted on
experimental mice irradiated at a young age, and followed for the
remainder of their natural lifetime. The exposures involved
neutrons, gamma irradiation or x-rays. These exposures were
administered either at high dose-rates in which the entire
exposure was completed in a matter of minutes, or at low-dose
rates, some of which continued for a matter of months.

A variety of neoplasms were induced by the irradiation, and
these included primarily neoplasms of the reticular tissue,
including myeloid leukemia, and thymic lymphoma with reductions
in reticulum cell sarcomas. Further, a number of solid tumors
also were observed to be induced by ionizing radiation. These
included mammary, pulmonary, ovarian, pituitary and Harderian
gland tumors. The experiments have provided much insight into
questions of dose-response, strain and sex variability, and
dose-rate effects in mice. Hopefully, the findings have a basic
biological relevance and in their extrapolated form are useful in
the analysis of human data. For example, it is observed that for
many of the neoplasms in mice, a lower dose-rate for a given
total dose of low linear-energy-transfer (LET) radiation reduces
tumor incidence. Since there is a lack of human data at low
dose-rates, one would like to incorporate the findings in the
mouse into risk estimates for humans potentially exposed to low
dose-rate exposures.

In this paper we will attempt to briefly describe some of the long-term animal studies and describe the importance of the findings to human risk estimation. As always, the animal studies provide much-needed scientific information on the mechanisms of carcinogenesis. However, the issue of species extrapolation as it is used in human risk assessment remains a controversial issue, and lies mostly in the realm of judgment.

DOSE RESPONSE

The first large series of animal studies was conducted by Upton and co-workers at ORNL during the 1950's and 1960's. These studies were carried out on the RF mouse, which has a high natural incidence of tumors. Of particular interest were the findings of myeloid leukemia in the male mouse. The data, which we have reproduced in Figure 1, is a classic example of two general findings in mouse radiation studies. The first observation is that at high doses, the incidence of tumors drops, and for this particular study, this was the case for doses over 300 rads. An explanation for this phenomenon is that cell-killing or cell-inactivation caused by the high radiation doses competes with those cells which are initiated by the radiation. This, in fact, has led to the inclusion of an exponential cell-killing term in some statistical models for dose-response functions. For example, investigators have used the equation

$$(\alpha_1 d + \alpha_2 d^2)\exp(-\beta_1 d - \beta_2 d^2) \tag{1}$$

to describe tumor incidence for an administered dose d. The model is basically a linear-quadratic dose response with an exponential cell-killing term, which itself is linear-quadratic. For various

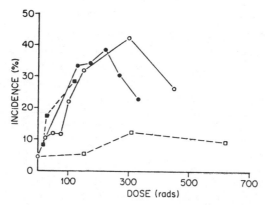

Figure 1. Myeloid Leukemia in Male RF Mice. Circles indicate single exposure and squares represent daily exposures. Open symbols denote gamma-rays and x-rays; solid symbols, neutrons. (Reprinted from Upton et al. with author's permission.)

data sets, some of these parameters will be taken to be zero. It should be mentioned that for the particular study of Upton's, there is some confusion concerning the amount of incidence reduction in myeloid leukemia over 300 rads. In a paper (Upton et al., 1958), the high-dose myeloid leukemia incidence data were statistically adjusted for intercurrent mortality resulting in no decreased incidence at 450 rads.

Recently, Mole et al. (1983) have reported similar findings on myeloid leukemia with regard to high dose-rate x-ray exposures to male CBA mice which have a very low spontaneous rate of myeloid leukemia. Their studies included exposures up to 600 rads, and they found a definite plateauing and subsequent decrease in myeloid leukemia for doses over 300 rads. Their preferred fit to the data was a quadratic dose-response function with a linear exponential cell-killing term. Mole (1984) also described some fractionated dose experiments which established the inactivation effects of ionizing radiation at high doses. In particular, he administered an optimal dose of 300 rads followed by a subsequent dose of 600 rads. If this second dose were given any time between a few hours and eight months after the initial exposure of 300 rads, the incidence of myeloid leukemia was reduced from about twenty percent to five percent or less. However, if the second dose were given twelve or sixteen months after the initial dose, then the incidence was only reduced to about sixteen percent. The earliest cases of myeloid leukemia occurred at about 8-10 months with 20 months being the median time.

A second series of lifetime mouse studies were conducted at ORNL by Ullrich and Storer (1979). In this series, approximately 16,000 female and 2,000 male RFM mice were exposed to gamma irradiation at a high dose-rate of 45 rads per minute. In the following table, the number of exposed animals at the various doses is shown. As with the studies by Upton et al. (1970), Ullrich and Storer observed a dose-response relationship for a variety of reticular cell neoplasms and solid tumors.

The data of Ullrich and Storer for gamma exposures have subsequently been analyzed by Prentice et al. (1982). They have used sophisticated statistical techniques incorporating relative risk modelling. They examined both general survival and dose-temporal patterns for the primary cancer types; namely, thymic lymphoma, myeloid leukemia, reticulum cell sarcoma, ovarian tumors, and pulmonary tumors. In analyzing the general survival patterns, Prentice found that the relative risk was significant for the female mice at all doses, including 10 rads. The log-relative risk model they used included a term in log-time, which they found to be negative at all dose levels except at 10 and 25 rads in females. This finding showed that the constant

relative risk model was not appropriate for effects on general
survival, and may be explained in part by the radiation effects
on a number of the reticular tissue neoplasms, some of which
occur at early ages.

Table 1.   Radiation Doses and Sample Sizes of RFM Mice

Dose	0	10	25	50	100	150	200	300
Females	4014	2827	985	1143	1100	1043	333	4133
Males	430	256	94	247	230	204	0	571

For modelling the specific tumor types, Prentice assumed the
log-relative risk to be of the form

$$\beta_1 d + \beta_2 d^2 + \beta_3 d \log t \tag{2}$$

which allowed for an interaction between dose and time, resulting
in a non-constant relative risk at a given dose level.   For all of
the tumors studied, the coefficient of the linear term β_1 was
positive.   This includes the reticulum cell sarcomas which were
shown to have a decreasing incidence with dose in the analysis
carried out by Ullrich and Storer.   The apparent contradiction is
probably due to the fact that reticulum cell sarcomas are late-
occurring tumors, and adjustments for intercurrent mortality are
needed.   Further, there is a question in the analysis as to
whether it is better to consider animals with a reticulum cell
sarcoma present at death or animals whose only tumor at death is
a reticulum cell sarcoma (see Prentice et al. for further
discussion).   Nonetheless, this illustrates the importance of the
choice of statistical methods applied to survival studies so that
proper interpretation of the data is made.

For the female mice, the quadratic dose term β_2 was negative at
all of the sites analyzed by Prentice.   For the males, it was also
negative except for pulmonary tumors and reticulum cell sarcomas,
where it was not significantly different from zero in the first
case and it was positive in the latter.   This curvature in the
relative risk model could be interpreted as being related to the
incorporation of cell-inactivation effects, which was discussed
with regard to the myeloid leukemia studies.   Using these
statistical methods, Prentice has shown that there seems generally
to be a negative curvature in the dose response model for a very
wide variety of tumor sites.   A final observation is that this data
did not include exposures at the 450-600 rad level.   Thus, direct

comparisons with the Upton and Mole data for myeloid leukemia cell-inactivation are not possible.

The third parameter β_3 in the model used by Prentice was found to be negative for all of the tumor types in both sexes for which the data were analyzed. This is an important finding, in that the radiation effects are shown not to be appropriately described by a simple relative risk model. The effects of the radiation decrease with time, the degree of which depends upon the tumor type. This is a finding which is consistent with what is predicted by a two-stage model of carcinogenesis (see Moolgavkar and Knudson, 1981).

DOSE RATE EFFECTS

One of the most significant results from the experimental studies on mice has been the observation that tumor incidence may be reduced when exposures are administered at low dose-rates. Since radiation risk estimation is often concerned with low dose-rate occupational or environmental exposures, the dose-rate issue is of great practical importance.

The ORNL studies by Upton, Ullrich and Storer were directed at the issue of dose-rate effects for both x-ray and gamma radiation and also the effects of neutrons. Upton's experiments were conducted on both male and female RF mice, whereas Ullrich and Storer experimented with RFM and BALB/c strains of female mice. Referring again to Figure 1 of Upton's results on myeloid leukemia, we see that for x-ray exposures there was very little increase in myeloid leukemia at low dose-rate exposures. For neutrons, however, the low and high dose-rate exposures produced similar increases in the incidence of myeloid leukemia. This is one of the most striking examples of a dose-rate effect in experimental studies on irradiated mice. Upton found similar results in the RF female mouse, however the results were not nearly as impressive due to smaller sample sizes and the fact that radiation had much less of an impact on myeloid leukemias in the female mice.

An extensive review of dose-rate studies is given in a National Council on Radiation Protection and Measurements (NCRP) Report 64 (1980). In their review, they attempted to estimate a dose-rate effectiveness factor (DREF) based on experimental studies. This effectiveness factor is essentially the ratio of the slopes of the high and low dose-rate dose response functions. The NCRP report calculated DREF values for the primary cancer types in the mice studies. These included myeloid leukemia, thymic lymphoma, ovarian tumors, thyroid tumors, mammary tumors, and so on. The values they observed, primarily from the ORNL studies, ranged between 2 and 6. In the summary of this experimental data, there are examples which are not included and

do not show much of a dose-rate effect. For example, Ullrich and
Storer found a strong dose-rate effect for the RFM female mouse
(DREF = 6.4). The BALB/c mouse, on the other hand, has a low
spontaneous rate of reticular cell tumors, which are relatively
unaffected by radiation. Upton's studies on the RF mouse did not
show a very strong dose-rate effect in either the male or female
mouse for thymic lymphoma. Tables 2 and 3 provide some detail
with a few values added to the NCRP analysis. For example, Table
3 shows little or no dose-rate effect for neutrons.

Recently, Mole and Major (1983) have considered the effects
on the incidence of myeloid leukemia after protracted gamma
radiation exposures to the CBA mouse. They exposed male mice at
doses 150, 300 and 450 rads either at a high dose-rate, or
continuously at a low dose-rate for one month, or in a series of
twenty consecutive high dose-rate exposures given once a day. In
this study they observed two interesting phenomena. First, both
the continuous and protracted exposure groups had a low constant
dose-response curve, which was considerably below the high dose-
rate frequencies (see Table 4). Mole (1984) observes that this
flat dose-response is remarkably similar to what is observed
with fatal leukemias in patients x-ray treated for ankylosing
spondylitis. There is not a good explanation for this
observation, but clearly it is important to both understanding
the mechanism of radiation-induced carcinogenesis and performing
quantitative risk estimation. Secondly, the protracted doses
which were administered at a high dose-rate produced the same
effects as the continual low dose-rate exposures. This suggests
the presence of repair mechanisms in addition to cell
inactivation.

The degree of impact of dose-rate on tumor incidence varies
with both strain, sex and tumor type. This certainly is not
surprising. From these experiments, though, we discern that
there is a general dose-rate effect for low LET radiation. Low
dose-rate exposures of gamma and x-rays do not seem to affect the
tumor incidence as much as high dose-rate exposures at equivalent
dose levels. The data are somewhat limited, however, which makes
it difficult to quantitatively adjust for dose-rate effects with
much confidence. It is presumed that the same effects apply to
some degree in man. This, however, is speculative since there is
no equivalent data for humans to support this extrapolation.

Table 2. Dose-rate Effectiveness Factors[†]
for Gamma and X-Ray Exposures

	Ullrich & Storer		Upton	
	RFM female	BALB/c female	RF male	RF female
Myeloid leukemia	*	**	6.7	2.3
Thymic lymphoma	6.4	**	1 to 2	1.3
Ovarian tumor	4.6	6.7		* to 1
Pituitary tumor	5.4			**
Harderian tumor	3.3		**	
Pulmonary adeno-carcinoma		2.8		
Mammary adeno-carcinoma		1.9		

[†]Adapted from Table 9.3 of NCRP Report 64.

*No apparent radiation effect at low dose-rate.

**No reported radiation effect or decreased incidence.

Table 3. Dose-Rate Effectiveness Factors
for Neutron Exposures

	Ullrich & Storer		Upton	
	RFM female	BALB/c female	RF male	RF female
Myeloid leukemia	**	**	1	0.9
Thymic lymphoma	1	1	1	0.7
Ovarian tumor	2 to 6	*		**
Pituitary tumor	1 to 2	**	**	
Pulmonary adenoma	1	***	****	****
Mammary adenoma	1	***		**

*Same pattern as with gamma exposures. High incidence after
small acute exposures, followed by gradual decrease.
Shallow dose-response for low dose-rate exposures.

**No reported radiation effect or decreased incidence.

***Large DREF values at doses less than 25 rads. Above 100
rads, DREF is less than 1. These results are for
adenocarcinomas.

****Radiation exposure reduced the incidence of pulmonary
adenoma. Low dose-rate exposures resulted in less of a
decrease.

Table 4. Acute Myeloid Leukemia in Male CBA Mice
After Exposures to Gamma Irradiation*

(rads)	low dose-rate[1]		high dose-rate[2] 20 fractions		high dose-rate single exposure	
	mice	cases (%)	mice	cases (%)	mice	cases (%)
150	71	3(4)	72	4(6)	99	11(11)
300	66	4(6)	65	4(6)	83	14(17)
450	66	4(6)	65	3(5)	104	26(25)

[1] 4-11 mrads per minute for 28 days' continuous exposure

[2] 25 rads per minute 5 days weekly for 4 weeks

*data from Mole and Major (1983)

MODELS

A variety of mathematical models have been developed for
describing the relationship between tumor incidence and
administered dose of a carcinogen. These models are mathematical
descriptions of very simple abstractions of hypothetical biological
mechanisms of carcinogenesis. The need for such models is
especially important when one attempts to predict biological
responses outside the experimental region. This is in fact the
basis of quantitative risk assessment.

The most common model used for describing genetic and
carcinogenic effects of ionizing radiation is the linear-quadratic
dose response function. This model assumes that cellular lesions
which result in either a genetic effect or carcinogenesis are the
result of at least two sublesions. The model also assumes that
repair processes are present. Thus, at low-dose or low-dose-rate
exposures the complete lesion will be necessarily caused by a
single ionizing track. This results in low-dose linearity without
a threshold. At high doses, two hits by separate ionizing tracks
have a reasonable probability of occurring prior to repair of
either of the two sublesions. Thus, a quadratic component is added
to the linear dose response function. This model has the ability
of being able to explain the reduced incidence of lesions when low
dose-rate exposures occur. This assumes sparsely ionizing
radiation, such as with gamma and x-ray. With the high density
tracks which occur with either alpha particles or neutrons, a
single track is sufficient for creating the entire lesion; hence

the dose response is linear and dose-rate effects are not relevant. This model coupled with exponential cell-killing is appealing because of its simplicity and its ability to describe much of the experimental data in both genetics and carcinogenesis.

Similar models based on microdosimetry have recently been proposed. For example, Mole (1984) considers what is called a diplosyncytic hypothesis for radiation-induced carconogenesis. Basically this model requires two adjacent cells to be genetically altered in order to produce a malignant clone. Mathematically, Mole uses the model

$$(c+aD^n)\exp(-\lambda D) \tag{3}$$

where c is the background incidence, and n is 1 for neutrons and 2 for x-ray or gamma radiation. He found that this model described the effects of acute myeloid leukemia in irradiated mice and suggests that it may also apply to mammary tumors in irradiated rats. It should be noted that the expression can be less than the background rate c under appropriate conditions. In other words, the model specifies that a small amount of radiation may in some circumstances be protective.

Models which incorporate time have recently been generally used for risk assessment in carcinogenesis. In particular, the multistage model has been used extensively in risk estimation. This model assumes that carcinogenesis is of single cell origin and the initial malignant cell is the result of a finite series of mutational changes. For this model, Whittemore (1977) has given the mathematical expressions for tumor incidence as a function of dose-rate and time after a single short-term exposure. The excess relative risk as a function of time-since-exposure is of the form

$$t^{k-j-1}x^{j-1}/(x+t)^{k-1} \tag{4}$$

where k is the number of stages in the multistage model, j is the stage affected by radiation, x is the age-at-exposure, and t is the time since exposure. This expression (4) shows that the relative risk will increase and then decrease in time, which is in agreement with the previously discussed analysis carried out by Prentice. This assumes that the radiation affects a single stage in the multistage model. Thus, the incidence rate is typically taken to be proportional to dose.

Finally, Moolgavkar and Knudson (1981) have developed a two-stage mutational model for carcinogenesis. This model assumes that a normal stem cell can be mutated to form a intermediate cell which can undergo a further mutation and become a malignant cell. The model incorporates both cell division and differentiation or death, and has been applied to a number of data sets, both experimental and epidemiological with good success. As with the multistage model, this two-stage model predicts a rapid increase in relative risk, followed by a gradual decline. Moolgavkar and Knudson have, by assuming that radiation can affect both stages, been able to predict some of the age-at-exposure effects that are seen in epidemiological studies. With regard to dependency on dose, the model predicts linearity in dose if only the first cell transition rate is assumed to be linear in dose. If, however, the division rate of an intermediary mutated cell is proportional to dose, then the incidence rate will not be a linear function of dose.

CONCLUSIONS

There is a wealth of both experimental and epidemiological data on carcinogenic effects of ionizing radiation. We have discussed but very little of this data. However, the lifetime animal studies conducted at ORNL provide us with considerable knowledge concerning both dose and temporal effects of ionizing radiation. What we see is a very complex process which differs by strain, organ site, dose-rate, and radiation type. The assumptions concerning these factors will continue to be debated in radiation risk assessment, but there are immediate improvements which can be made. What is needed is more systematic analyses using some of the newly developed statistical methods and mathematical models of the existing epidemiological and experimental data bases.

REFERENCES

Mole, R., 1984, Dose-response relationships, in: "Radiation Carcinogenesis: Epidemiology and Biological Significance," J. Boice and J. Fraumeni, ed., Raven Press, New York.

Mole, R., and Major, I, 1983, Myeloid leukemia frequency after protracted exposure to ionizing radiation: Experimental confirmation of the flat dose-response found in ankylosing spondylitis after a single treatment course with x-rays, Leuk. Res. 7:295.

Mole, R., Papworth, D., and Corp., M., 1983, The dose-response for x-ray induction of myeloid leukemia in male CBA/H mice, Br. J. Cancer 47:285.

Moolgavkar, S., and Knudson, A., 1981, Mutation and cancer: A model for human carcinogenesis, JNCI, 66(6):1037.

National Council on Radiation Protection and Measurements, 1980, Influence of dose and its distribution in time on dose-response relationships for low-LET radiations, National Council on Radiation Protection and Measurements Report 64.

Prentice, R., Peterson, A., and Marek, P., 1982, Dose mortality relationships in RFM mice following cs-ray irradiation, Radiation Res. 90:57.

Ullrich, R., Jernigan, M., Cosgrove, F., Satterfield, L., Bowles, J., and Storer, J., 1976, The influence of dose and dose rate on the incidence of neoplastic disease in RFM mice after neutron irradiation, Radiation Res., 68:115.

Ullrich, R., Jernigan, M., and Storer, J., 1977, neutron carcinogenesis: dose and dose-rate effects in BALB/c mice. Radiation Res., 72:487.

Ullrich, R., and Storer, J., 1979, Influence of irradiation on the development of neoplastic disease in mice I. Reticular tissue tumors, Radiation Res., 80:303.

Ullrich, R., and Storer, J., 1979, Influence of irradiation on the development of neoplastic disease in mice II. Solid tumors, Radiation Res., 80:317.

Ullrich, R., and Storer, J., 1979, Influence of irradiation on the development of neoplastic disease in mice III. Dose-rate effects, Radiation Res., 80:325.

Upton, A., Randolph, M., and Conklin, J., 1970, Late effects of fast neutrons and gamma-rays in mice as influenced by the dose-rate of irradiation: Induction of neoplasia, Radiation Res. 41:467.

Upton, A., Wolff, F., Furth, J., and Kimball, A., 1958, A Comparison of the Induction of Myeloid and Lymphoid Leukemias in X-Radiated RF Mice, Cancer Res. 18:842.

Whittemore, A., 1977, The age distribution of human cancer for carcinogenic exposure of varying intensity, Am. J. Epidemiol., 106(5):418.

DOSE-RESPONSE IN RADIATION CARCINOGENESIS:

HUMAN STUDIES

David G. Hoel and Dale L. Preston

Radiation Effects Research Foundation
Hiroshima, Japan

INTRODUCTION

Estimation of cancer risk to man resulting from exposure to ionizing radiation continues to be a difficult problem. The primary data for risk estimates are based on the atomic bomb survivors in Japan and a number of populations who have been exposed to radiation in medical therapy. The Japanese data have provided the best material for risk quantification purposes. This is due to the very large number of exposed individuals, the quality of the exposure information, and the prospective nature of the work. In this paper, we shall explore a few of the epidemiological models used for quantifying risk and apply them to some of the Japanese cancer data. Basing analyses on the Japanese data allows one to examine some of the temporal patterns of cancer effects after a single high dose-rate exposure to gamma radiation. Further, information concerning age susceptibility and dose response is available for analysis. However, many questions that are critical to risk estimation are not answerable by the Japanese data. These issues include dose-rate and population susceptibility. Potentially, either of these concerns can greatly alter any risk estimate made for low dose-rate exposures applied to populations with cancer incidence patterns which differ from those of the Japanese. Nevertheless, the Japanese data provide critical information on the cancer effects resulting from high dose rate exposures. To address the issues of dose-rate and population susceptibility, one would need to obtain data from other exposed populations and incorporate relevant laboratory findings on radiation carcinogenesis.

LEUKEMIA

The study of radiation-induced leukemias clearly indicates
that the temporal patterns for excess risk are quite different
from other cancers. It is generally believed that the excess
risk for non-leukemia cancers is approximately described by a
relative risk model with a latency period of about ten years or
more. Leukemia, on the other hand, has a short latency of about
two years and a greatly diminished excess risk after twenty
years. Studies of the atomic bomb survivors indicate that the
dose response depends upon age-at-exposure and histological type
of leukemia. Because of the small number of cases, the most
detailed histological grouping suitable for statistical analysis
is acute leukemias and chronic granulocytic leukemia. Chronic
lymphocytic leukemia is not believed to be radiation-induced.

For a graphical summary of the temporal patterns in the
excess risk for both acute leukemia and chronic granulocytic
leukemia (CGL), we used the Japanese data of Ichimaru et al.
(1981). Within each age-at-exposure group a log-normal
distribution was used to describe the excess incidence rate over
time-since-exposure. The choice of the log-normal distribution
was quite arbitrary but seemed to fit the data reasonably well.
Figures 1 and 2 illustrate both the age-at-exposure dependence
and the differences between acute leukemia and CGL.

The atomic bomb follow-up studies and resultant data began
five years after exposure. This presents a serious problem
because data from studies such as those of patients receiving
therapeutic x-ray exposures for ankylosing spondylitis indicate a
substantial risk of leukemia within the first five years after
first exposure. Table 1 shows that the excess cases are about
evenly divided between the post exposure period of less than 5.5
years and the period greater than 5.5 years. Further, the excess
rate for 2-5 years post exposure is equal to or somewhat greater
than the rate for 5-10 years post exposure. In Figures 1 and 2
it was assumed that the yearly rate for 2-5 years post exposure
was 50% of the yearly rate for the period 5-10 years post
exposure for each age group and histological leukemia type.
Also, it should be mentioned that the mix of histological types
for the two studies was about the same, with approximately 80%
acute leukemias. The use of 50% instead of 100%, say, was for
improved fits of the data to the log-normal distribution.

Table 1. Leukemia Deaths Among Ankylosing Spondylitis Patients[1]

| | Time Since Treatment in Years | | | | |
	0-1.5	1.5-2.5	2.5-5.5	5.5-10.5	10.5-
Observed	0	3	10	8	7
Expected	0.64	0.36	0.89	1.47	3.11
PY at risk	20,914	11,520	23,956	31,011	46,473
Excess death rate per 100,000	-3.1	22.9	38.0	21.1	8.4

[1] Data is from Smith and Doll (1982)

The fitted log-normal distributions (due to D. Shore) of Figures 1 and 2 provide a little more information. Specifically, the temporal pattern of excess risk for acute leukemia data is well described by a single log-normal distribution whose mean varies linearly with age-at-exposure [i.e. log (T-2) is normal with mean 1.2 + 0.05 x age-at-exposure and variance 0.72]. Chronic granulocytic leukemia, on the other hand, does not seem to vary with age-at-exposure [i.e. log (T-2) is normal with mean 2.68 and variance 1.52].

Pierce et al. (1983) used a much more sophisticated modelling approach to the problem. They studied the incidence of acute leukemia in the atomic bomb survivor cohorts using a hazard rate modelling procedure for grouped data. For these analyses the data are cross-classified on city, sex, age-at-exposure, dose, and time-since-exposure. For each cell in this cross-classification, the number of cases and the person-years at risk are computed. These values together with representative values for age-at-esposure (e), dose (d), and time-since-exposure (t), as well as indicators for city (c), and sex (s) serve as the basic input data for the statistical analyses. As needed, these class marks, or functions of them such as attained age (a=t+e), are used as covariates in models of the mortality rates.

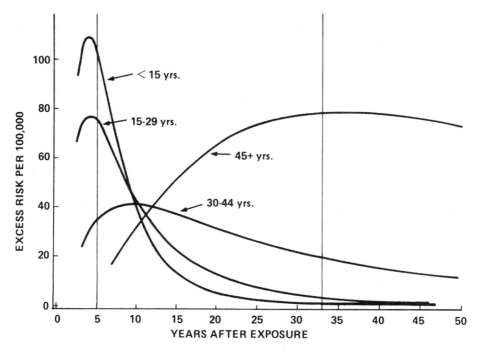

Figure 1.   Log-normal fit for acute leukemia by ATB group.

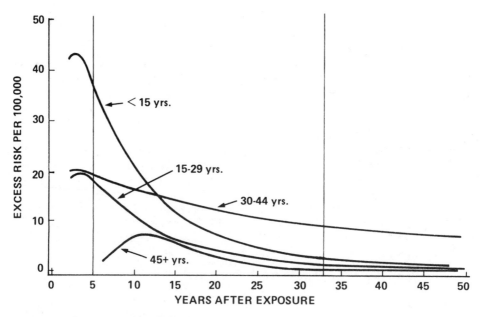

Figure 2.   Log-normal fit for chronic granulocytic leukemia by
ATB group.

As has been noted by Holford (1976) and others, if one assumes that the hazard (rate) function is constant within each of the time intervals, then the log-likelihood for the full data is formally equivalent to the likelihood which would arise if the number of deaths in each cell in the cross-classification were independent Poisson random variables with means equal to the number of person-years (PY) in the cell times the rate (λ). In the analyses described here, parametric or semiparametric models for the rate function have been specified. Straightforward extensions of linear Poisson regression methods are then used for parameter estimation and hypothesis testing in these models.

For the purposes of rate function modelling, it is especially convenient to make use of interactive computer programs. For many models of interest, much can be done with standard Poisson regression programs, especially GLIM (Baker and Nelder, 1979).

Rate models of interest in radiation effects studies include both relative and excess risk models. In relative risk models, the relative risk can be either multiplicative,

$$\lambda(t;z,d) = \rho(t;z)\exp(\nu(z,d))$$

or additive,

$$\lambda(t;z,d) = \rho(t;z)[1+\nu(z,d)].$$

It is often of interest to work with models in which the excess risk is modelled directly. One particularly useful class of excess risk models has the form

$$\lambda(t;z,d) = \rho(t;z)+f(d)\exp[\nu(z,t)]. \tag{1}$$

This model is a generalization of the classical additive model often seen in the literature on radiation effects. The major difference being that the radiogenic excess risk is allowed to depend upon attained age or time-since-exposure. Analogues of linear, quadratic, and linear-quadratic models for the dose effects can easily be constructed through the use of alternative parametric forms for f(d). Also, cell-killing effects can be modelled by means of the inclusion of functions of dose in the exponential term.

In the work discussed here, parametric models for the background rates, $\rho(t;z)$, were fit to the data. Because of the nature of the methods used, this is essential for the generalized additive models. However, for the relative risk models, special algorithms have been developed which make it possible to use fully specified parametric models for the background or to consider non-parametric forms in which a large number of stratum-specific parameters are used to represent the background. In this latter case, the grouped data methods are closely related to stratified proportional hazards models as originally described by Cox (1972) and discussed further by Kalbfleisch and Prentice (1980). For the leukemia analysis, Pierce et al. assumed the function of dose f(d) to simply be proportional to dose and $\nu(e,t)$ to be linear in log(t), i.e.

$$\nu(e,t) = \alpha_i + \beta_i \log(t) \tag{2}$$

where i represents the age-at-exposure interval to which e belongs. Using this model with 5 age-at-exposure intervals, 8 dose intervals, and 8 time intervals, the acute leukemia incidence data were found to be adequately described.

Using the model developed by Pierce et al., one can calculate the lifetime probability of an individual's developing acute leukemia for a given radiation dose at a given age. Specifically, using life table methods and survival probabilities based on the 1970 U.S. Vital Statistics, the following quantity gives the probability of leukemia by age 80 for an individual in age-at-exposure category i

$$H(i,d) = \sum_{t=1}^{79-e} f(d)\exp(\alpha_i + \beta_i \log(t))p(t+e)/p(e) \tag{3}$$

where p(t) is the probability of being alive at age t and e is taken to be the average age for the corresponding age interval i. The following table gives the lifetime risk estimates for an exposure of 1 rad using the age-at-exposure categories in the Pierce et al. study.

Lifetime Probability of Radiation-Induced Acute Leukemia
Following Exposure of 1 rad

	Age-at-Exposure				
	0-9	10-19	20-34	35-49	50+
lifetime risk x 10^5 for t > 5	4.3	2.5	2.8	2.9	1.2

To obtain these values it was assumed that no radiation-induced cases occurred within the first five years after exposure.

A similar calculation made by the BEIR Report (p. 204) gave a lifetime risk for all leukemias and bone cancer to be 3.8 to 5.7 per 100,000 depending upon sex. Using weights based on U.S. population figures, the values in the above table give a weighted estimate of 2.7 per 100,000. This value should be increased by about one third to account for the chronic granulocytic leukemias and bone cancers included in the BEIR figure. Thus, we see a fair agreement between the two estimates.

Several major problems persist, however. The absence of incidence data for the first five years after exposure is a problem for the atomic bomb survivor analyses. In the ankylosing spondylitis data in Table 1, we observed that many excess leukemias occurred in the first 2 to 5 years after exposure. Therefore, in order to use the atomic bomb data for lifetime risk estimation, we are forced to speculate on the nature of the effects during what is possibly the most critical period after exposure. The individuals in the ankylosing spondylitis study were generally in the age group 25 to 50 years, with relatively few below the age of 25. The atomic bomb data (Figure 1) suggest that for the younger exposure groups, a greater proportion of the risk occurs soon after exposure. Thus, the acute leukemia risk for the 0-9 year cohort could be several times greater than what was estimated using the data from the atomic bomb survivors.

A second issue in the above risk estimates which was addressed by BEIR is the relationship between risk and dose. Specifically, whether one uses a linear, quadratic or linear-quadratic model can have a significant effect on risk estimates made at a low dose level, such as 1 rad. Further analyses on the acute leukemia incidence data involved extensions of the model used by Pierce et al. The model was expanded to include $\log(t)^2$, which potentially provided for a maximum excess risk at some time point. Also, a quadratic function of dose and a simple exponential cell-killing term were included. For the various age-at-exposure categories, there were generally no appreciable difference between the models.

For all age-at-exposure groups except the fourth (35-49 years), the linear model adequately fit the data. In three groups (0-9, 20-34, and 50+ years) the fit of the pure quadratic model was poorer, though not significantly so, than the pure linear model. In the 35-49 age-at-exposure category, the pure quadratic model fit significantly better than the pure linear model. For the 10-19 category the pure linear and pure quadratic models fit the data equally well. For all age-at-exposure groups, the addition of a simple exponential cell-killing term to the linear model did not improve the fit. In addition, it was observed that the coefficient of this term was negative. This indicates that deviations from the linear model are in the opposite direction from those predicted by cell-killing models. The addition of a cell-killing term to the quadratic models led to fits which were equal to or better than those of the pure linear model. For the 35-49 age category, however, the addition of a cell-killing term did not improve the fit. In these quadratic model cases, the sign of the cell-killing term was consistent with cell-killing, i.e. positive. This latter model is the one which has been proposed by Mole (1984) for leukemia in both animal studies and in the Japanese bomb survivors. The values of the cell-killing coefficient ranged from 0.003 to 0.005 which is somewhat smaller than the value 0.01 suggested by Mole for leukemia. However, the atomic bomb dose reassessment may change these estimates.

Models which included both a linear and a quadratic term for dose together with a possible additional cell-killing term were also considered. The results of fitting these models suggest that they are probably over-parameterized and do not lead to statistically significant improvements over the simpler models. Also, some problems arose because of negative estimates of coefficients which led to, in some instances, negative risk estimates at low dose levels.

The lifetime risk estimates, assuming no effect for the first five years after exposure, were fairly consistent across the age-at-exposure categories. The estimates for the linear model ranged between 1 and 4 per 100,000, whereas the quadratic model with and without cell-killing tended to give estimates two orders of magnitude smaller. All of this was assuming a single exposure of 1 rad. Table 2 provides some details on these risk estimates. Finally, since the dosimetry of the atomic bomb survivors is currently undergoing a reassessment, it is premature to make definitive statements concerning the linear versus quadratic issue.

EPITHELIAL CANCERS

The temporal patterns for radiation-induced non-leukemic cancers are quite different from the leukemias which exhibit a short latency followed by a peak in excess risk. The non-leukemia cancers are generally observed to have a latency period of ten years or more, with an approximately constant relative risk. Therefore, risk estimates have been based upon the observed relative risk for high doses and either linear or linear-quadratic extrapolation used to obtain low-dose estimates.

Models for describing the incidence rate of these non-leukemia cancers can also be developed as was described for acute leukemia in the previous section. To illustrate the models, we shall use the general category of epithelial cancer and base the data on death attributed to the cancer, as opposed to incidence data. We define the category of epithelial cancer as non-leukemias, not including multiple myeloma and those cancers which are hormone dependent, i.e. ICD 140-203 less 174, 180-183, 185, 203. The advantage of using such a large grouping of cancer types is, of course, the large numbers of cases which are available for modelling purposes. The drawback is that the temporal and dose-response patterns of the individual cancer types in the epithelial grouping may be quite different. It is, however, important to obtain some understanding of the radiation risk for total cancers. Generally, there is not sufficient data for risk modelling purposes if each cancer type is treated independently.

Table 2. Lifetime Risk for Acute Leukemia Effects
Estimated from 5 Years Post-Exposure of 1 rad
(incidence rate per 100,000)

Model	Age-at-Exposure				
	0-9	10-19	20-34	35-49	50+
Linear	3.7	2.3	3.6	**	1.3
Quadratic	*	0.09	*	0.01	*
Quadratic + Cell-Killing	0.03	0.00	0.05	0.01	0.03

* Poor fit to the data as compared with the other models

** Inadequate fit to the data

Working with the atomic bomb survivors, we have data available for over 5,000 cancer deaths in the epithelial category, with about 4,000 of them occuring in the last two age-at-exposure categories. As with leukemias, we shall use a very general additive risk model, which will depend upon the categories: city, sex, age-at-exposure, dose, and time since exposure. Specifically, using (1) we define

$$f(d) = \alpha_1 d + \alpha_2 d^2$$

$$\nu(e,t) = \beta_1 \log(a/50) + \beta_2 \log(t/20) + \beta_3 c + \beta_4 s + \sum_{i=1}^{4} \gamma_i I_i(e) \tag{4}$$

where $I_i(\cdot)$ is the indicator function for age-at-exposure group i

113

and c,s are zero-one variables with one indicating Nagasaki, female, respectively.

Using the same likelihood methods as with the leukemia data, a number of specific examples of the model were fit to the atomic bomb follow-up data. The parameter estimates are given in Table 3, along with some measures of the quality of the individual fits to the data.

There have been discussions concerning whether the excess risk is a simple addition to the background, or whether a relative risk model is more appropriate. For the epithelial cancers as a group, the purely additive model does not describe the data adequately, whereas a model which includes either a time or age dependency does provide an acceptable fit to the data. The one model which is purely age dependent, i.e. age-linear, has an estimated coefficient for age of 4.7, which is close to the coefficient found for the background, namely 4.5. This would suggest that a relative risk model may be a reasonable description of the epithelial data. In Table 3B, we see that the relative risk model is improved by including either a time or an age parameter. Therefore, the additive model, which includes time or possibly age and adjusts for age-at-exposure, appears to provide the best description of the

Table 3A. Epithelial Cancer Mortality Parameter
Values for Additive Model (age < 80)

	Constant	Age	Time	Time-Age	Quadratic
Dose x 10^6	6.15	1.69	30.5	346	S
Dose2 x 10^9	NS	NS	NS	NS	54.2
Age	S	4.74	NS	-4.56	NS
Time	S	S	2.51	5.17	2.33
City	-1.25	-0.66	-0.68	-0.63	-0.75
Sex	0.85	0.30	0.27	0.21	0.18
Age-at-Exposure					
0-9	-2.37	1.97	-3.66	-8.99	-2.78
10-19	-2.21	1.27	-3.11	-7.05	-2.47
20-34	-1.17	0.27	-2.94	-5.82	-2.77
35-49	-0.77	0.23	-1.75	-3.50	-1.29
Deviance	1081	1050	1043	1041	1055
Pearson χ^2	1385	1569	1314	1237	1345
D.F.	1135	1134	1134	1133	1134

S - statistically significant
NS - not statistically significant

Table 3B. Epithelial Cancer Mortality Parameter
Values for Relative Risk Model (age < 80)

	Constant	Time	Age	Time-Age
Dose x 10^3	0.99	1.39	0.89	362
Dose^2	NS	NS	NS	NS
Age	NS	S	0.31	-10.37
Time	NS	0.57	S	5.80
City	-0.69	-0.66	-0.68	-0.67
Sex	1.19	1.13	1.17	1.12
Sex x Age 0-9	-1.49	-1.38	-1.45	-1.76
Age-at-Exposure				
0-9	2.69	2.05	2.87	-9.45
10-19	1.27	0.78	1.43	-8.02
20-34	-0.01	-0.50	0.08	-6.81
35-49	-0.08	-0.46	-0.04	-4.23
Deviance	1050	1048	1050	1042
Pearson χ^2	1521	1638	1569	1250
D.F.	1134	1133	1133	1132

S - statistically significant
NS - not statistically significant

data. In both Table 3A and 3B, models are given which include both time and age. These two parameters are correlated and it may be the case that we are again over-parameterizing by including them both in the same model.

In comparing the age-linear model with a time-linear model, we find a preference for the latter. This suggests that the critical factor for the excess risk is "time since exposure", and not a simple multiplication of the existing background rate. This is consistent with a simple model of cell initiation.

Estimates of the coefficients for the sex and the city effects are given for both models. The city effect is significant in each instance and corresponds to about a doubling of the excess risk for a given dose in Hiroshima as compared to Nagasaki. This probably reflects problems with the dosimetry in the two cities since there is no difference in the cities with respect to background rates. The sex effect was not statistically significant in the additive model although it estimates an increased risk to females of about one-third. It is noted that the unrealistic constant additive risk model suggests factors of 3.5 and 2.3 for city and sex effects, respectively. The strong sex by dose interaction observed in the

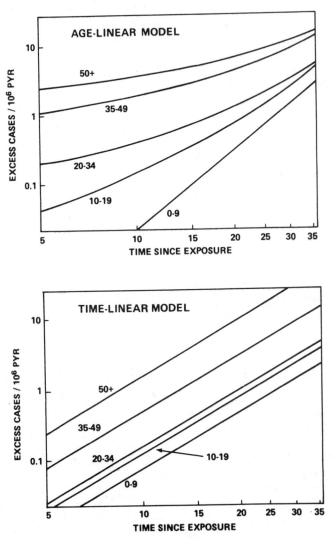

Figure 3. Plot of the age-linear model and the time-linear model found in Table 3A. Curves are given for each of the 5 ATB groups and calculated at an exposure of 1 rad.

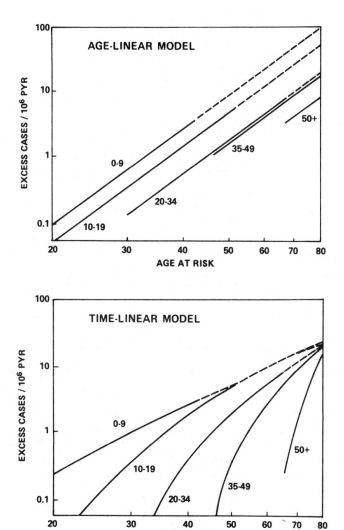

Figure 4. Same as Fig. 3 except the curves are for log-incidence versus log-age. The dashed lines are values given by the model but extrapolated beyond the observed data.

relative risk model results from the fact that the female background is about forty percent of the male rate. The estimates of excess risk for females are about the same as those obtained from the additive model, i.e. one-third higher than for males.

It is well known that the age-at-exposure is a critical component in risk estimation from ionizing radiation. Although not shown in Table 3, the models are significantly improved by incorporating age-at-exposure parameters for the excess risk. Looking at the age-linear model, one finds that the parameters for the age-at-exposure categories are decreasing. At the same time, one finds the opposite situation in the time-linear model. This is not the inconsistency it may seem since in the first model excess risk is described across age-at-exposure groups for a given age. The second model assumes a given time-since-exposure for the risk comparisons. Both models are illustrated in Figures 3 and 4.

Finally, we observe a definite preference for a linear model over a quadratic model. In fact, in all of the models considered, those with a purely linear term indicated that the addition of a quadratic term would not be of statistical significance. The quadratic models, on the other hand, indicated that the addition of a linear term would statistically improve the fit of the model to the data. When both a linear and a quadratic term are present, one would typically be negative. This may reflect possible cell killing at the higher doses. However, the addition of a dose term in the exponent of the model did not statistically improve the fit. If, however, a quadratic model with cell-killing is used then a fit equivalent to the linear model is observed. This is similar to the situation which was previously observed for acute leukemia incidence. The cell-killing coefficient is, in fact, essentially the same (0.004).

To compare risk estimates derived from the various models in Table 3, we use the same method for calculating a lifetime probability of a radiation-induced epithelial cancer, as was done for acute leukemia in the previous section. Specifically, the quantity

$$H(e,d) = \sum_{t=1}^{79-e} f(d)\exp(\nu(e,t))p(t+e)/p(e) \qquad (5)$$

gives the probability of an excess cancer occurring between the age-at-exposure and age 80 of the individual. These lifetime risk probabilities are given in Table 4 and correspond exactly with the models given in Table 3. The probabilities are obtained for each age-at-exposure category. Also, an average risk value is given, which is a weighted average of the age-at-exposure risks where the

118

weights are based on the population distribution in the U.S. for 1970.

Upon examining the values in Table 4, we observed first of all that, as one would expect, a purely quadratic model estimated practically no risk. This result is due to the absence of a linear term in the model. Simply adding a quadratic term to a linear model had little effect other than to possibly raise the risk somewhat due to the negative coefficient of the quadratic term. For the models which are either age-dependent or of a relative risk structure, we observed the highest lifetime risk estimates. This is especially true for the younger age-at-exposure individuals. The models which are additive and time-dependent have risk estimates which are less dependent on age-at-exposure. They tend to give lower values at the younger age-at-exposure groups than do the relative risk models. They all seem to coincide at the 35-49 age-at-exposure category. As mentioned previously, the estimated excess risk for females is about one-third larger than that for males, although the difference is not statistically significant. Finally, a time-linear model with a ten-year latency period was considered. The addition of a latency period has essentially no effect on either the model fit or the subsequent risk estimates.

To compare these values with those given in the BEIR Report (p. 207), we use the values for non-leukemia cancers which are reported to be 9.2 for males and 14.7 for females after an exposure of 1 rad. These values are lower than those average risk values we see in Table 4. This is due in part to the method which was used for calculating the BEIR estimates. In particular, they did not incorporate time into their model. The method used is to calculate relative risk over the various strata. The slope of the dose term does not vary with time or age. Using this slope, the expected number of excess tumors over the various strata is calculated and divided by the total person-year rads. (Pierce & Preston, 1984, provide a detailed discussion of this "average risk" approach.) This quantity will increase in time as more data becomes available from the follow-up of the cohort. Applying the technique to the Japanese epithelial cancers with city and sex combined, we estimated that the risk per person-year rad was 1.67, 1.87, 2.61, 2.93 per million for data collected through 1970, 1974, 1978, and 1982, respectively. These values led to lifetime average risk estimates of 6.4, 7.2, 10.1, 11.3 per 100,000. All of the foregoing is assuming 1 rad exposure and linear dose-response.

Table 4A. Lifetime Epithelial Cancer Risk Additive
Model (mortality rate per 100,000 for
Hiroshima males, age < 80, and 1 rad exposure)

Age-at-Exposure	Constant	Age	Time	Time-Age	Quadratic
0-9	3.6	92.6	30.8	12.8	0.11
10-19	3.6	46.2	31.0	25.0	0.09
20-34	4.8	17.2	17.1	17.3	0.03
35-49	7.9	16.4	16.1	15.9	0.04
50+	8.1	10.9	9.2	7.4	0.02
Average	5.6	35.4	20.4	15.5	0.06

Table 4B. Lifetime Epithelial Cancer Risk Relative
Risk Model (mortality rate per 100,000 for
Hiroshima males, age < 80, and 1 rad exposure)

Age-at-Exposure	Constant	Time	Age	Time-Age
0-9	85.8	112.8	99.3	11.7
10-19	41.1	56.4	46.5	20.6
20-34	16.1	19.1	17.1	15.3
35-49	16.1	16.4	16.3	15.0
50+	11.0	10.5	11.0	7.0
Average	32.9	41.5	36.7	13.7

CONCLUSIONS

All of the models and calculations which have been considered
indicate a number of points which are important for risk estimation
after low-level radiation exposure. First and foremost is the
issue of linear versus non-linear models. The purely quadratic
model clearly showed the reduced risk one estimates when compared
to a linear model or a linear-quadratic model. At a dose of 1 rad
we typically observed a factor of one to two orders of magnitude of
difference in the risk estimates. The second point for which we do
not really have the epidemiological data is the likelihood of a
reduced risk for protracted or low dose-rate exposures.
Information for risk assessment purposes must come from
experimental systems in order to properly account for dose-rate
effects. For the models we have presented, there are large

differences in the risk estimates, depending upon how time is treated. Also, there is the critical issue of possible increased effects for individuals exposed at younger ages. Here we observed differences of upwards of a factor of 20 in the risk estimates for epithelial tumors at the youngest category of 0-9 years.

Drawing any definite conclusions concerning the actual risk estimates is premature due to the reassessment of the dosimetry in the Japanese studies. Some comparisons can be made, however, with the BEIR estimates since any differences would be due primarily to differences in modelling approaches. For acute leukemia incidences, the estimates were similar, assuming linearity, except that for the lower age-at-exposure categories the ankylosing spondylitis data suggests that the risk may be underestimated. We observed some mix of linear or quadratic as the model choice. This could be due in part to the mixture of acute leukemia types, which have different age structures. Also, the data were consistent with a quadratic model which incorporated exponential cell-killing. The resolution of these leukemia model issues will no doubt depend upon further studies of the mechanisms of carcinogenesis and the influence of ionizing radiation.

For the epithelial cancers treated as a group, the temporal models suggest a somewhat higher risk than given in the BEIR study, assuming linearity. Our preference is for an additive model depending upon time since exposure. If, however, the relative risk model is the correct model, then the risks for the youngest age-at-exposure category would have been underestimated.

The epithelial cancers were adequately described by a linear dose-response function. The addition of a quadratic term did not improve the fit and had a negative coefficient. A quadratic model with a linear exponential cell-killing term was equivalent to the linear model although it produces much lower risk estimates. This should not be surprising since mathematically the quadratic model with an exponential cell-killing term can well approximate the linear model in the dose ranges which are observed in the Japanese data. Thus, as with leukemia, mechanism studies are needed to resolve this issue.

In conclusion, it is necessary to properly incorporate the effects of time into risk estimation models. The influence of the assumptions of time on risk estimates has been shown in this paper. While it is true that the linear-quadratic issue and the dose-rate issue are critical to risk assessment, the effects of time and age-at-exposure are also of crucial importance.

REFERENCES

Baker, R.J., and Nelder, J.A., 1978, The GLIM system. Release 3. Generalized linear interaction modelling. Numerical Algorithm Group, Oxford.

Cox, D.R., 1972, Regression models and life tables (with discussion). J. Royal Stat. Soc. (B), 34:187.

Holford, T., 1980, The analysis of rates and survivorship using log-linear models, Biometrics, 36:299.

Ichimaru, M., Ishimaru, T., Mikami, M., Yamada, Y., and Ohkita, Y., 1981, Incidence of leukemia in a fixed cohort of atomic bomb survivors and controls, Hiroshima and Nagasaki. October 1950 – December 1978, Radiation Effects Research Foundation Technical Report 13-81.

Kalbfleisch, J., and Prentice, R., 1980, "The Statistical Analysis of Failure Time Data," Wiley, New York.

Mole, R., "Dose-response relationships, radiation carcinogenesis: epidemiology and biological significance", Boyce, J. and Fraumeni, J., ed., Raven Press, New York.

National Research Council, 1980, Report of the committee on the biological effects of ionizing radiation: The effects on populations of exposure to low levels of ionizing radiation (BEIR Report), National Academy of Sciences, Washington, D.C.

Pierce, D., and Preston, D., 1984, Hazard function modelling for dose-response analysis of cancer incidence in the A-Bomb survivor data, in: "Atomic Bomb Survivor Data: Utilization and Analysis," SIAM, Philadelphia.

Pierce, D., Preston, D., and Ishimaru, T., 1983, A method for analysis of cancer incidence in Japanese A-bomb survivors, with application to acute leukemia, Radiation Effects Research Foundation Technical Report 15-83.

Smith, P., and Doll, R., 1982, Mortality among patients with ankylosing spondylitis after a single treatment course with x-rays, Clin. Res., 284:449.

FUNDAMENTALS OF DOSIMETRY AND MICRODOSIMETRY AND THE

RELATIVE BIOLOGICAL EFFECTIVENESS OF IONIZING RADIATIONS

Albrecht M. Kellerer
Institut für Medizinische Strahlenkunde
der Universität Würzburg
Versbacher Strasse 5
D-8700 Würzburg

INTRODUCTION

The effects of ionizing radiations have been explored in innumerable biological experiments, but they have also been inflicted - often with tragic negligence or irresponsibility - on human populations. The worldwide fascination with x-rays immediatedly after Röntgen's discovery was motivated by optimistic expectations and permitted little attention to biological damage seen immediately, such as skin-lesions, or to the later occurrence of leukemias in radiologists. Several decades after their discovery x-rays were still widely assumed to have general positive effects and nearly universal medical applicability. A painful process of learning then led to the stepwise development of adequate radiation-protection procedures and to a more realistic assessment of the beneficial and detrimental potential of ionizing radiations. As a reaction to past industrial misuses of radio-isotopes and errors in their medical application one has, today, in many ways gone to the other extreme. Beyond this, it has become difficult, after Hiroshima and Nagasaki, to draw a rational` balance between the uses and the misuses of nuclear energy.

The resulting attitude and public perception of ionizing radiations has made it difficult to discern similarities and dissimilarities between the actions of ionizing radiations and other agents, such as chemical carcinogens. In a discussion of fundamentals of dosimetry and microdosimetry one may, therefore, consider first presumed or real particularities of ionizing radiations and their biological effects. The subsequent short survey will deal with some of the essentials of radiation physics, with the attendant problems in dosimetry, particularly in epidemiological studies, with parameters that characterize radiation quality, and with some general implications for the action of radiations.

Absorbed dose is - in a simplified formulation - the energy transmitted from a radiation field to a small element of matter divided by its mass (1). The macroscopic distribution of absorbed dose in an irradiated body and the microscopic random fluctuations of energy deposition are the two essential factors that determine the effectiveness of different types and energies of ionizing radiations. The former are the objective of conventional dosimetry, the latter the objective of the more recent branch of radiation physics, microdosimetry. Before these two areas are considered it is helpful to illustrate the order of magnitude of the energy densities that cause observable biological effects.

It is sometimes thought that ionizing radiations produce specific deleterious effects, and that they produce them by extraordinarily small amounts of energy. Both assumptions are erroneous. There is no effect of ionizing radiations that can not also be produced by chemical compounds. The remarkable feature of ionizing radiations is merely the extremely broad spectrum of biological end points. The energies required to produce biological effects would seem to be minimal if compared to thermal energy. A lethal dose to man transfers an energy to the body that increases its temperature by less than 0.001 degree centigrade. However, the comparison to temperature - the most degraded form of energy - is misleading. It is somewhat more informative to consider the total energy corresponding to a lethal dose of 5 gray, which is 350 joule or 350 watt*seconds. An even better illustration is the comparison to mechanical energy. One gray corresponds to the energy required to lift the exposed object by 0.1 metre in the earth's gravitation; the lethal dose corresponds to an elevation by 0.5 metre, evidently sufficient energy to produce damage. Visualizations of the effects of ionizing radiations on the microscopic or the atomic level can be similarly disparate. At a dose of 1 gray, only one out of ten to hundred billion electrons in the exposed material is disturbed. On the other hand, there are, at this dose, roughly 100 000 electronic displacements in the nucleus of a mammalian cell.

CONVENTIONAL DOSIMETRY

The Macroscopic Distribution of Energy

All ionizing radiations work ultimately through the action of electrons. Electrons can be the primary radiation, or they can be produced as secondary radiation by x-rays or gamma-rays. The electrons can also be the secondary radiation produced along the tracks of heavy charged particles. Finally they can be the tertiary radiation occurring with high energy neutrons; they are then released by the heavy charged recoils of the neutrons. In radiation protection one deals mostly with uncharged primaries, i.e. with x-rays, gamma-rays, or neutrons, when the body is exposed to external sources. Charged primaries are of concern mostly in connection with internal emitters.

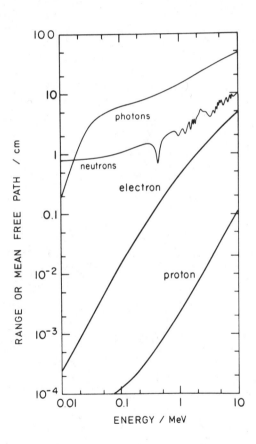

Fig. 1
Comparison of the mean free path of photons and neutrons in tissue, and of the ranges of their charged secondaries, electrons and protons.

The dosimetry of ionizing radiations is never trivial when one is concerned with large exposed objects, such as the human body. With energetic photons or neutrons beyond 20 MeV the total body irradiation may be nearly uniform. However, for these very energetic radiations cross-sections, and specifically the nuclear cross-sections, are still inadequately known. At the more common intermediate energies, in the range of 0.1 to 20 MeV, the cross-sections are adequately known, but the penetration of the radiation is then limited, and dose distributions in an exposed body are complex and depend on numerous parameters.

Fig.1 gives for uncharged and for charged particles their mean free path and their range for energies between 10 keV and 10 MeV. The essential observation is, that the mean free path of the uncharged particles is always considerably larger than the ranges of the charged secondaries. For many purposes one can, therefore, simplify dosimetric computations by neglecting energy transport by the charged secondaries. With this simplification one obtains the quantity kerma (Kinetic Energy Released in MAtter) instead of absorbed dose. It is evident that kerma and absorbed dose can be used interchangeably if, in a specified geometry, all dimensions of interest exceed the maximum ranges of charged particles. If this condition is not fulfilled, one must account for the different spatial distributions of the two quantities. Absorbed dose includes a further degradation process; the gradients of absorbed dose are therefore always less than those of kerma.

Beyond the facilitation of computations, the concept of kerma permits a further simplification. Kerma for any specified material is defined even in a receptor free geometry, e.g. in free space. A similar possibility does not exist for absorbed dose, which is always a complex result of attenuation and backscatter, and of the build-up of charged particle equilibrium in a specified geometry. These complexities of absorbed dose are sometimes disregarded with the silent assumption of a reference volume large enough to attain charged particle equilibrium but small enough that attenuation and backscatter can be disregarded. For crude estimates this may be an admissable procedure. In rigorous statements the reference to absorbed dose without specified geometry must be avoided. Fig.1 illustrates the difficulty by showing that the ranges of the released electrons can, at high energies, be equal to several percent of the mean free path of photons.

Although the use of exposure and its units röntgen or C/kg is now discouraged one may note that this quantity, too, is defined regardless of energy transport by charged particles, and that it is, therefore, defined even in receptor free conditions.

For dose planning and dose assessment in radiotherapy inaccuracies must not exceed a few percent. Precise measurements and accurate computations are thus required. Similar requirements for dose specification can be met in many radiobiological studies, either with cell cultures or with small laboratory animals. In epidemiological studies the inaccuracies are far greater and far more complex.

The difficulties and complexities of the dosimetric problems are exemplified by the studies on the atomic bomb survivers. The current reevaluation of the dosimetry has been necessitated by inaccuracies of the input data for the tentative Oak Ridge dosimetry of 1965 (TD 65). There were uncertainties concerning the yields and the energy spectra of the neutrons and the gamma-rays as well as the geometry of the bomb assemblies and the humidity of the atmosphere at the time of the bombings. Improvements in the transport codes, particularly for neutrons, are equally important. As a result the tissue-kerma values in air have been substantially changed. However, as a new consensus on the dosimetry appears to emerge there remain large areas of uncertainty. Perhaps most importantly, new individual shielding factors remain to be established. The free air kermas have to be reduced to kermas in the buildings where individuals were at the time of the bombing; the reduction can be appreciable and it depends strongly on energy. The further reduction from kerma within the building to organ doses is also substantial. For the deeper organs the reduction factors are 0.7 to 0.85 for gamma-rays, and 0.1 to 0.2 for neutrons (2,3). For the superficial organs, such as the breasts, there is the additional complexity of a dependence on the orientation of the person at the time of the explosion and during the subsequent seconds of delayed irradiation.

The relative contribution of the delayed radiation is still inadequately known. So are possible contributions from fall-out, including the possible role of the so-called black rain.

It is characteristic for radiation epidemiology that the dosimetric problems are further complicated by far less tangible uncertainties. Rules of compensation and medical care for the atomic bomb survivers were partly dependent on dose received; they may therefore have influenced the statements of individuals concerning their localization at the time of the blasts. There could also have been an opposite effect due to the desire to avoid any social stigma linked to heavy exposure. To name still another possible difficulty, there had been severe shortages of x-ray films in the period after the bombing, and this may have led to extensive use of fluoroscopy and thus to radiation doses in addition to those from the bomb.

The dosimetric studies for Hiroshima and Nagasaki have been referred to as examples of difficult and partly unresolved problems in radiation epidemiology. The same studies are, however, also exemplary and impressive efforts. Such efforts must continue, because the various collectives of substantially exposed persons are unique and will, hopefully, remain so.

The numerous investigations of the effects of internal emitters pose problems of comparable or even higher complexity (see for example (4)). Internal emitters produce - with few exceptions such as tritium - highly non-uniform exposures. For example in patients that have been exposed to the short lived radium-224 by far the largest doses were produced in narrow regions on the bone surfaces (5). Still further complexities occur with inhaled activity such as radon daughters. The study of the distribution of the radon daughters in different areas of the lung is, by itself, a specialized field of inquiery, as is the investigation of the dose dependence and the geometric and temporal distribution of lung tumors induced by the inhaled activity.

The microdistribution of absorbed dose in the vicinity of particulate alpha-emitters in the lung is an additional complexity of inhalation studies. This hot spot problem exemplifies further the wide range of dosimetric problems, and poses problems intermediate between conventional dosimetry and microdosimetry (6); it reaches beyond the scope of this survey.

MICRODOSIMETRY

The Microscopic Distribution of Energy

Absorbed dose is defined in terms of the expected value of the energy transferred by ionizing radiation to a mass element. It is, accordingly, a statistical concept that loses applicability when one deals with small doses, with small structures, and, especially, with densely ionizing radiations. The microscopic fluctuations of energy deposition can then be considerable. Fig.2 indicates, for sparsely and for densely ionizing radiations, the sizes of spherical regions in tissue and the doses where the standard deviations of energy deposition exceed 20%.

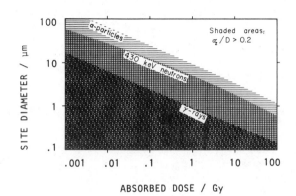

Fig.2. The shaded areas indicate those combinations of site sizes and absorbed doses where the standard deviations of energy imparted exceed 20%. Absorbed dose can then not be applied naively, and a treatment in terms of microdosimetry is required.

The figure is based on microdosimetric computations and measurements, but its meaning can be understood even before the principles of microdosimetry are formally introduced. At doses of several mGy, i.e. at the level of radiation protection, the absorbed dose is never meaningful, even if the entire nucleus of the cell or the cell itself is considered. Most cells receive, in this dose range, no energy deposition at all; those cells that are traversed by a charged particle receive energies that can be far in excess of the expectation value corresponding to absorbed dose. Although the affected cells are only a minor fraction of all cells, their total number is, of course, very large. The important consequence of this basic feature of ionizing radiations is that no threshold in absorbed dose can hold for cellular effects. For smaller cell structures, such as individual chromosomes, the dose concept remains inapplicable even at the highest doses of biological interest.

The discontinuous energy transfer by ionizing radiations has attracted attention early in the development of radiation biology. It has led to the hit and target theories (for surveys see (7-9)). Such theories, although they were valid as heuristic principles, have had only limited pragmatic success. They were based on the postulate of equal and statistically independent hit processes and of hypothetical cellular targets which have never been identified. A more successful approach requires realistic physical parameters of radiation quality. The most simplified, but still the most common, parameter is linear energy transfer (LET), also called collision stopping power, of charged particles. It characterizes the average local concentration of energy along the track of a charged particle, and it is still the parameter that determines the quality factor employed in radiation protection (10). However, LET itself is merely a statistical expectation value. Energy-loss straggling, the radial transport of energy away from the particle track by delta-rays, and the change of LET along the particle trajectory are factors that co-determine actual microscopic concentrations of energy. For heavy ions there are conditions where LET and its probability distributions permit adequate estimates of energy transfer by individual charged particles to the nucleus of the cell or comparable sites. For electrons the LET concept is never adequate (11).

The shortcomings of the LET concept have been responsible for the development of a new branch of radiation physics. When H.H.Rossi attempted to determine the LET distribution of the recoils produced by high energy neutrons he found that these distributions were not directly measurable. He then recognized that the seemingly inadequate response of the proportional counters was, in fact, more meaningful than the theoretical LET values. The spherical proportional counters - now known as Rossi counters - respond to energy actually imparted to their gas volume which simulates a microscopic tissue region. The basic principle of microdosimetry is that cellular effects are determined by actual energy concentrations, not by their expectation values. When this simple but fundamental principle was understood (12), the subsequent steps followed of necessity. A conceptional framework of microdosimetry was established and suitable experimental techniques were developed that could be applied to any radiation field to determine the probability distributions of energy concentrations on the microscopic scale (13-15).

There are a number of closely interrelated microdosimetric quantities:

The energy imparted, e, is the radiation energy transferred to a given reference volume of matter.

The specific energy, z, is the energy imparted, as defined above, divided by the mass, m, of the reference volume of matter:

$$z = e/m$$

The lineal energy, y, is the energy imparted, as defined above, divided by the mean chord length, l, resulting in straight random traversals of the reference volume *) :

$$y = e/l$$

The specific energy, z, is the random variable corresponding to the non-stochastic quantity absorbed dose, D. The linear energy, y, relates only to individual energy deposition events (i.e. individual charged particles), it is the stochastic counterpart of the non-stochastic quantity LET. In view of the simple relation between z and y, it is usually sufficient to use the specific energy, z, as will be done below.

----

*)
If the reference volume is a sphere of the diameter d, the mean chord length is l = 2d/3. For any convex volume the mean chord length is equal to four times the volume divided by the surface (16).

4000 simulations are performed per decade of dose for each graph. The decreasing number of points at low dose is due to the increasing number of events with zero specific energy.

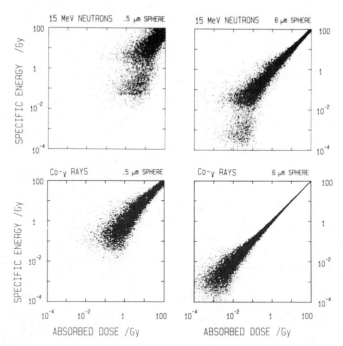

Fig.3. Scatter diagrams of the distribution of specific energy in small and large sites and for sparsely and densely ionizing radiation.

A definite value of the specific energy can not be predicted for a microscopic volume, even under fully defined irradiation conditions. Instead the possible values of the specific energy are described by a probability density, $f(z;D)$. The objective of microdosimetry is the calculation or the experimental determination of the probability densities of the specific energy for various types of radiation and specified reference volumes. The experimental determinations are carried out not directly in solid material, but in tissue equivalent gas volumes simulating microscopic regions in tissue. Without going into the technical details of the construction of the Rossi counters it is sufficient to note that the instruments can be used for measurements in a wide variety of radiation fields. It is possible to simulate tissue regions down to a diameter of about 0.3 micrometer. Microdosimetric data for much smaller regions are also of considerable interest, but they have to be obtained by computations. Experimental techniques to determine such data have not, as yet, been developed.

It is not necessary to measure the spectra of z for different values of the absorbed dose. Instead it is sufficient to determine the single-event spectra, $f(z)$, i.e. the densities of the increments of the specific energy due to single charged particles including their secondaries. If the single-event spectrum is known, it is possible to calculate the dose dependent spectra as solutions of a compound Poisson process (17). Fig.3 illustrates, in the form of scatter diagrams, the distributions of specific energy for a densely ionizing and a sparsely ionizing radiation and for sites of 0.5 and of 6 micrometer diameter. These diagrams illustrate the large fluctuations of specific energy; they also show, by the absence of points at small doses, the increasing probabilties for no energy deposition.

In most applications of microdosimetry to radiobiology and to radiation protection it is not actually required to utilize the dose dependent distributions of specific energy. Important conclusions can, instead, be based directly on the single-event spectra and their moments.

Typical examples of single-event distributions are shown in Fig.4. These spectra relate to spherical tissue regions of 1 micrometer diameter. The pronounced differences between sparsely ionizing and densely ionizing radiations are evident, but the very wide range of values of z for the different radiation types are equally notable. They extend over several orders of magnitude, i.e. a

densely ionizing radiation can always produce events with
relatively small energy deposition, and, vice versa,
moderate to high values of z occur even with sparsely
ionizing radiations. There is, accordingly, no sharp
dividing line between densely ionizing and sparsely
ionizing radiations.

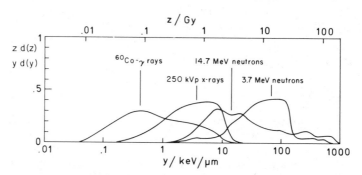

Fig.4. Single event distributions of specific energy and
lineal energy for a spherical tissue region of 1 micrometer diameter. Distributions of dose, rather than event
numbers, are given relative to the logarithmic scale
(18).

The larger the increments of specific energy per
event, the smaller is the mean number of events per unit of
absorbed dose. Table 1 shows event frequencies for various
types of radiation. Fig.5 indicates, largely in analogy to
Fig.2, those site sizes and doses where the mean event
frequency is less than 1. These data permit important
conclusions. In particular, dose-effect relations must
always be linear when the mean event number in the cell or
in the sensitive cell organelles is much smaller than 1.
With densely ionizing radiation this condition is met even
at doses of the order of several gray. However, the
argument applies only to dose-effect relations for
autonomous cells, i.e. to cells that are not influenced by
energy deposition in adjacent cells or by radiation induced
reactions of the tissue (22).

The postulate of radiation action on autonomous cells appears to apply to hereditary effects which are due to

Table 1: Event frequencies in spherical tissue regions of specified diameter.

SITE DIAMETER (μm)	^{60}Co-γ-Radiation ϕ (Gy^{-1})	NEUTRONS ϕ(Gy^{-1})		
		.43 MeV	5.7 MeV	15 MeV
12	2000	55	51	61
5	360	4.2	8.6	11
2	58	.39	1.2	1.6
1	12	.08	.32	.38
.5	1.7	.02	.07	.09

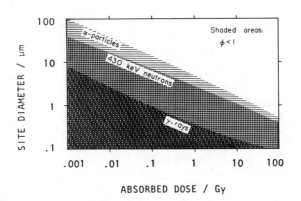

Fig.5. The shaded areas indicate combinations of site sizes and absorbed doses where the expected number of energy deposition events is less than 1, and dose dependences – for autonomous response – must accordingly by linear.

mutations or chromosome aberrations in individual cells. It is far less certain when applied to radiation carcinogenesis. In fact, non-linear dose-effect relations have been found at neutron doses far too small for an appreciable probability of multiple events in the cell (19-21). One must conclude that radiation tumorigenesis is co-determined by dose dependent tissue factors that are, as yet, unresolved. Linearity at low doses remains, therefore, a mere hypothesis for radiation carcinogenesis.

IMPLICATIONS FOR RADIATION PROTECTION

Dosimetry

Absorbed dose and the related quantity dose equivalent are utilized in the limitation principle of radiation protection. This principle is based on annual dose-equivalent limits which obviate the need to retain information on exposures of individuals in earlier calendar years. Another convenience has been - up to a recent change - that the maximum dose equivalent in any organ rather than a more complex quantity has been limited. A further feature of the limit system is the absence of any hypothesis concerning the form of the dose-effect relations.

However, there has been in past years a gradual change away from the limit to the assessment system. H.H.Rossi has recently analysed the change and its consequences in depth (22), and only some of the essentials will be considered here. For what has been called non-stochastic effects (10) -perhaps a somewhat artificial notion - the limit system has been retained. For the stochastic effects, i.e. hereditary effects and radiation carcinogenesis, which are of predominant concern in radiation protection, ICRP has shifted towards an assessment system that aims at an optimization of detriment and benefit. To be practicable such a system requires the assumption of linearity of the dose-effect relation at small doses, a postulate that is, at least for radiation carcinogenesis, entirely hypothetical.

The assessment system has also made it necessary to define and introduce into the practise of radiation protection a new quantity to replace the former dose equivalent. The new quantity, effective dose equivalent, is

a dose equivalent averaged with specified weight factors
over all organs of concern. The rules of radiation
protection for individuals retain numerically the earlier
annual limits. One may note that - except for uniform
exposures of the body - the limitation in terms of the new
quantity is less restrictive than the earlier limitation in
terms of the maximum dose equivalent in an organ. In fact,
it has been necessary to introduce additional limitations
on certain organ doses to ensure that non-stochastic
effects be avoided.

The new system and its implied assumption of linearity
have also been responsible for the increased use of
concepts such as collective dose (equivalent) or committed
collective dose (equivalent). It is not surprising that
these new, and somewhat contrived, notions lead to novel
conceptual difficulties when applied to specific situations. There have also been new problems in radiation-protection monitoring. It had been the practise to employ for
purposes of area monitoring, or for personal monitoring,
quantities that provide conservative rather than best
estimates. Within the new philosophy this is inadequate.
Accordingly the ICRU is about to present the definition of
operational quantities for radiation protection that can be
determined in area monitoring and personal monitoring.
These quantities, ambient dose equivalent and individual
dose equivalent, will serve as fair, if still somewhat
conservative estimates of effective dose equivalent. When
these quantities are introduced into the practise of
radiation protection a reasonable compromise between the
limit and the assessment system might be achieved. However,
it must be noted that any epidemiological investigation
will require information beyond the summary doses
determined for radiation protection monitoring. The rules
of radiation protection are aimed at keeping the risk
sufficiently low to be unobservable statistically. If
exposures beyond such safe levels occur, dosimetric
information is needed beyond routine requirements.
Effective dose equivalent, or its operational substitutes,
can not be suitable reference parameters for radiation
epidemiology.

Microdosimetry

The change from dose equivalent to effective dose
equivalent is to account for the macroscopic distribution

of absorbed dose. Another current development in radiation protection relates to the microscopic distribution of radiation energy. This is the possible revision of the quality factors.

Microdosimetric considerations (23) had first led to the recognition that the linear component of the dose-effect relation is related to the average energy concentration produced in subcellular regions by single events, while the quadratic component reflects a cumulative damage due to the interplay of several events. There is no certainty, as yet, on the critical distances for which the energy concentrations are relevant. However - largely independent of the distances - one has a ratio of average single event sizes for fast neutrons and for sparsely ionizing radiations of 30 to 60. At low doses where the linear component of the radiation action predominates one expects, therefore, RBE values of neutrons versus sparsely ionizing radiations of this magnitude. For neutrons of about 400keV the RBE was indeed found, in various experiments, to reach such values or still larger ones (23). Perhaps even more importantly, an inverse dependence of the neutron RBE on the squareroot of the neutron dose has been consistently found in these experiments, which corresponds to a linear-quadratic dose dependence of the underlying damage for both radiations. This has been so, even when the dose-effect relations were substantially different from the linear-quadratic relation. One concludes that the RBE-dose dependence is more fundamental and more closely indicative of the initial steps of radiation action than the dose-effect relation which may be co-determined by complex tissue factors.

On the basis of the T65 Oak Ridge dosimetry it appeared that the dose-effect relation for leukemia in Hiroshima compared to the one for Nagaski was in agreement with the high neutron RBE (24,25). The resultant high risk values for neutrons may have been an added motivation for the revision of the T65 dosimetry. As of now, the estimates of the neutron doses are so small, even for Hiroshima, that no conclusions on neutron RBEs can be expected from the Japanese data. This gives added importance to experimental data and to new evidence on high neutron RBE, such as the life shortening data from the Argonne experiments (26) and the transformation data obtained by Han et al.(27) with fractioned neutron exposures.

In view of these developments certain changes are envisaged. If, as it appears now, the RBE of densely ionizing radiations continues to rise at small doses below a few mGy, higher quality factors will have to be adopted for stochastic effects. The change will be unavoidable, because it is a basic tenet of the assessment system that risk estimates be realistic and that optimization be applicable even to doses substantially below annual limits. A substantial change of the quality factors will, on the other hand, make the new values inapplicable to non-stochastic effects. For these effects the limiting principle is still retained, with dose-equivalent limits in excess of 0.1 sievert. It is difficult to ignore the dualistic nature of the present system of radiation protection.

Acknowledgement

This work has been partly supported by EURATOM research contract BIO 286 D.

REFERENCES

1. ICRU Report 33, Radiation Quantities and Units, Int.Commission on Radiation Units and Measurements, Wash.D.C. (1980).
2. RERF, Reassessment of Atomic Bomb Radiation Dosimetry in Hiroshima and Nagasaki, 1st US-Japan Joint Workshop, D. J. Thompson, ed., RERF, Hiroshima, Japan, 1983.
3. RERF, Reassessment of Atomic Bomb Radiation Dosimetry in Hiroshima and Nagasaki, 2nd US-Japan Joint Workshop, RERF, Hiroshima, Japan, 1984.
4. Biological Effects of Radium-224 and Thorotrast, Proc. of an Int.Symp. at Alta, Utah, 1974, C. W. Mays, ed., Health Physics, Vol. 35, No. 1, Pergamon Press, New York, 1978.
5. W. A. Müller and H. G. Ebert, Biological Effects of Radium-224 - Benefit and Risk of Therapeutic Application -, Martinus Nijhoff Medical Division, The Hague/Boston, 1978.
6. NCRP Report 46, Alpha-Emitting Particles in Lungs, National Council on Radiation Protection and Measurements, Washington, D.C., 1975.
7. N. V. Timofeeff-Ressowsky and K. G. Zimmer, Das Trefferprinzip in der Biologie, Hirzel, Leipzig, 1947.
8. K. G. Zimmer, Studies on Quantitative Radiation Biology, Oliver and Boyd, London, 1961.
9. O. Hug and A. M. Kellerer, Stochastik der Strahlenwirkung, Springer-Verlag Berlin-Heidelberg-New York, 1966.
10. ICRP, Annals of the ICRP, Publication 26, Recommendations of the International Commission on Radiological Protection. Pergamon Press, Oxford-New York-Frankfurt, 1977.
11. A. M. Kellerer and D. Chmelevsky, Criteria for the Applicability of LET, Radiat. Res. 63:226 (1975).

12. H. H. Rossi, Specification of Radiation Quality, Radiat. Res. 10:522 (1959).

13. H. H. Rossi, Energy distribution in the absorption of radiation, in: "Advances in Biological and Medical Physics," J. H. Lawrence and J. W. Gofman, eds., Vol. 11:27, Academic Press, New York/London, 1967.

14. H. H. Rossi, Microscopic energy distribution in irradiated matter, F. H. Attix and W. C. Roesch, eds., Rad.Dosimetry, Vol.1, Fundamentals, 43-92, Academic Press, New York, 1968.

15. ICRU Report 36, Microdosimetry, Int.Commission on Radiation Units and Measurements, Wash.D.C. (1983).

16. M. G. Kendall and P. A. P. Moran, Geometrical Probability Griffin & Co., London, 1963.

17. A. M. Kellerer, Analysis of Patterns of Energy Deposition A Survey of Theoretical Relations in Microdosimetry, in: Proc. 2nd Symp.on Microdosimetry, H. G. Ebert, ed., 107-134, Euratom 4452 d-f-e, Brussels, 1970

18. A. M. Kellerer and H. H. Rossi, Biophysical Aspects of Radiation Carcinogenesis, in: "Cancer, A comprehensive treatise," F. F. Becker, ed., Vol.1, 2nd Edit., 569-616, Plenum Press, New York, 1982.

19. H. H.Rossi and A. M. Kellerer, Radiation Carcinogenesis at Low Doses, Science 175:200 (1972).

20. C. J. Shellabarger, D. Chmelevsky, and A. M. Kellerer, Induction of Mammary Neoplasms in the Sprague-Dawley Rat by 430-keV Neutrons and X-Rays, J.Natl.Cancer Inst. 64:821 (1980).

21. C. J. Shellabarger, D. Chmelevsky, A. M. Kellerer, J. P. Stone, and S. Holtzman, Induction of Mammary Neoplasms in the ACI Rat by 430 keV-Neutrons, X-Rays, and Diethylstilbestrol, J.Natl.Cancer Inst. 69:1135 (1982).

22. H. H. Rossi, Limitation and Assessment in Radiation Protection, Lauriston S.Taylor Lectures in Radiation Protection and Measurements, Lecture No.8, NCRP, Bethesda, 1984.

23. A. M. Kellerer and H. H. Rossi, The Theory of Dual Radiation Action, Curr.Top.Radiat.Res.Q. 8:85 (1972).

24. H. H. Rossi and A. M. Kellerer, The Validity of Risk Estimates of Leukemia Incidence Based on Japanese Data, Radiat.Res. 58:131 (1974).

25. H. H. Rossi and C. W. Mays, Leukemia risk from neutrons, Health Phys. 34:353 (1978).

26. J. F. Thomson, L.S. Lombard, D. Grahn, F. S. Williamson, and T. E. Fritz, RBE of Fission Neutrons for Life Shortening and Tumorigenesis, in: Proc."European Seminar on Neutron Carcinogenesis", J. J. Broerse and G. B. Gerber, eds., 75-93, EUR 8084 EN, Luxembourg, 1982.

27. A. Han and M. M. Elkind, Transformation of Mouse C3H/10T1/2 Cells by Single and Fractionated Doses of X-Rays and Fission-Spectrum Neutrons, Cancer Res. 39:123 (1979).

CRITICAL REVIEW OF CASE-CONTROL AND COHORT STUDY METHODOLOGIES

P. G. Smith

Department of Epidemiology
London School of Hygiene and Tropical Medicine
Keppel Street (Gower Street)
London WC1E 7HT

INTRODUCTION

Epidemiological studies are divided conventionally into those which are observational and those which are interventional. The latter are the easiest to interpret as they involve the application of some "exposure" in a carefully designed way to a defined group whilst, at the same time, maintaining an "unexposed" (control) group whose members are chosen to have the same characteristics as those in the exposed group except for the exposure under study. Both groups are followed over time in an identical fashion to ascertain disease events of interest. Any differences in disease rates between the two groups can be ascribed either to chance or to a consequence of the applied exposure, as the influence of other, potentially confounding, factors are eliminated through the study design. Randomized controlled trials of, for example, new drug therapies for specific diseases, are examples of such interventional studies. The circumstances in which such studies may be used to evaluate the effects of potentially hazardous exposures applied to ordinary (i.e. undiseased) members of the population are very limited because of the obvious ethical constraints and, in particular, very little of our knowledge of the long term carcinogenic effects of ionizing radiations on humans has been derived from such studies. Almost all estimates of the carcinogenic risks of radiation to humans are based on observational studies. In these studies the disease experience of individuals who have been irradiated for specific reasons (such as in warfare or in disease therapy or diagnosis) or accidentally (often as a consequence of their employment) has been contrasted with that of persons not so exposed in an attempt to measure the effects of the radiation exposure. Because individuals have not been allocated to the exposed or unexposed groups in a randomised or controlled fashion the groups may differ in their composition with respect to other risk factors for the diseases under study. Thus the question of whether disease differences are due to the radiation exposure or to other factors which differ between the compared groups is problematic. Careful statistical and epidemiological interpretation of such investigations may enable radiation effects to be segregated from the effects of confounding factors with a reasonable degree of confidence, but, because of their uncontrolled nature, individual studies rarely provide definitive conclusions. The strength of the evidence relating ionizing radiation to the induction of cancer derives from a variety of studies conducted in very different population groups that have yielded similar conclusions.

It is not the purpose of this paper to provide a comprehensive review of the major observational studies that have contributed to our knowledge of human radiation carcinogenesis. Nor is it the purpose to summarise those aspects of the results of observational studies that lead to the conclusion that a demonstrated association between radiation exposure and some disease is likely to represent a cause-effect relationship. What is attempted is a review, necessarily brief, of some critical issues in the design and interpretation of observational studies on radiation effects. Many of the issues discussed are relevant when investigating any exposure-disease association but the examples used have been selected because they have arisen, in general, in specific studies of radiation effects.

COHORT AND CASE CONTROL STUDIES

The principal types of observational study are "cohort" and "case-control". Various other names for these types of study have been used in the epidemiological literature but the two given are in most common use. In a cohort study the disease experience of some irradiated group is contrasted with that of either a non-irradiated group or a group whose members have received a lower radiation dose. Such studies may be retrospective, when the "exposed" and "unexposed" groups are defined on the basis of historical records and their disease experience is evaluated from the time of entry into the study up to the present, or recent, time, or prospective, when the compared groups are defined "now" and the disease experience of their members is followed into the future. Commonly, retrospective studies develop a prospective component as follow-up of the defined groups is continued once the initial retrospective evaluation has been conducted. Thus, cohort studies are exposure orientated in the sense that, in principle, any diseases that arise as a result of exposure may be studied.

In contrast, case-control studies are disease orientated. A group of persons with some specific disease (or group of diseases) is defined (the cases) and they are questioned, or documentary evidence is sought, regarding their exposure to radiation prior to the onset of disease (and regarding their exposure to any other factors which it is thought may also have caused the disease or may have interacted with radiation in causing the disease). A control group of individuals is chosen who do not have the disease(s) under study, but who, generally, are of similar age and sex as the cases, and their past exposure to radiation and other factors is determined in an identical manner as for the cases. Differences in the exposure histories between the cases and the controls may be used to identify potentially causative factors for the disease under study. Case-control studies are necessarily retrospective as information is sought after a case is diagnosed about past exposures.

Some of the critical issues in the design and interpretation of both cohort and case-control studies are discussed below.

CHOICE OF STUDY DESIGN

Cohort studies have been conducted more commonly than case-control studies in evaluating the late effects of radiation exposure. There are several factors that have militated against the choice of the latter study design. One of the possibly unique features of ionizing radiations is that they appear to cause cancers of nearly every body site to which exposure has occurred. As most radiation exposures involve irradiation of more than one organ, cohort studies are likely to give a better estimate of the overall effects of exposure as it is not necessary in such studies to select in advance the particular sites to be studied (as is so for case-control studies). There are exceptions, however. Stewart et al (1956) overcame this problem, when adopting the case-control approach to study the carcinogenic effects of in utero radiation, by including all childhood cancers in the study, but this is unlikely to be a profitable way of studying adult cancers. Firstly, it seems that the effect of radiation in utero may be greater than the corresponding doses given to adults - radiation exposure is likely to be responsible for only a small proportion of all tumours (see Smith in this volume). Secondly, large doses of radiation appear to be necessary to increase substantially the risk of most tumours, and only a small proportion of the population have been exposed to large radiation doses. In such circumstances the necessary study size to detect a hazardous effect through a case-control study is very large (see later section on Sample Size).

Neither case-control nor cohort approaches are likely to be of much value for quantitating directly the effects of radiation in populations exposed to low radiation doses. In general, groups with particularly high exposures have been studied and attempts made to extrapolate back from the results of these studies to estimate low dose effects. This procedure necessarily involves debatable assumptions about the shapes of dose-response relationships.

CHOICE OF COMPARISON GROUP

The choice of an appropriate "non-exposed" comparison group in cohort studies of an irradiated group is usually difficult. Ideally we want a group which is identical to the exposed group in all respects except for exposure (e.g. similar age, sex, smoking habits, diet etc). In practice, it is usually necessary to compromise on a group considerably short of this ideal. For the reasons discussed above, most cohort studies have focussed on individuals whose exposure to radiation has been considerably greater than "normal". In the earlier part of this century radiation was used to treat a variety of benign conditions (e.g. ringworm, enlarged thyroid, arthritis) and, because often large doses of radiation were used, a number of these groups have been the subject of (retrospective) cohort studies. Appropriate comparison groups would be patients with the same conditions but who were treated in other ways. Unfortunately, such groups are rarely available. Often it proved hard to find a source of such patients (radiotherapy records are often better maintained than other medical records). In some instances, even if such a group could be defined, problems of comparison would remain. Doll and Smith (1968) studied the mortality experience of women whose ovaries were irradiated to induce an artificial menopause. Alternative surgical methods of treatment would have removed some of the organs that were of special interest with respect to cancer induction by radiation and thus such women would have been an unsatisfactory control group. In many studies of patient groups the disease experience of the irradiated individuals has been compared with that of the general population. The principle concern with such comparisons is that the diseased group may differ from the general population with respect to their risk of other diseases independently of any effect of the radiation treatment. Perhaps, for example, women with benign menopausal bleeding (the symptom precipitating a radiation-induced menopause) are at increased risk of certain cancers, because of some hormonal disturbance of which the benign bleeding is a symptom. This might explain an excess of cancers of the uterus and ovary but can it also explain the excess of bladder cancer and leukaemia seen in these women? The answer must be possibly.

For all causes combined, the mortality rate of women given a radiation-induced menopause was very similar to that of the general population (Smith and Doll, 1976), but this was certainly not the case for the patients irradiated for ankylosing spondylitis (an

144

arthritic condition usually affecting the spine and sacro-iliac joint) studied by Court Brown and Doll (1965). They found that such patients had an overall mortality rate that was 60% higher than that of the general population of England and Wales. They ascribed the striking excess of leukaemia and the 60% excess of other cancers to the radiation treatment, but argued that the excess of deaths from non-malignant diseases was related to the presenting condition rather than the radiation treatment. Whilst this was plausible, others had argued that radiation might have a non-specific ageing effect, causing increased mortality rates from both malignant and non-malignant conditions. It would have been difficult to argue strongly against this on the basis of the findings of Court Brown and Doll (1965). Alternatively, it could be argued that patients with ankylosing spondylitis were at in-creased risk of many diseases, including leukaemia and other cancers, associated with their presenting condition and independent of the radiation exposure. Arguments were advanced against these inter-pretations (Court Brown and Doll 1965, Smith and Doll, 1982) but these depended, at least in part, on comparing the results in this study with those from other studies of different groups irradiated in quite different circumstances. Support for the original inter-pretation of Court Brown and Doll (1965) was provided by a study of a group of patients with ankylosing spondylitis who had not been treated with radiation. These patients showed no excess risk of cancer but an excess risk of non-malignant conditions similar to that of the irradiated group. This was a small study, however, and only 80% of the group were traced satisfactorily. Also it was impossible to be sure that the severity of their disease was the same as that of the irradiated patients.

Another illustration of the difficulty of finding a satisfact-ory comparison groups arose in the study of Court Brown and Doll (1958) of the mortality experience of British male radiologists. Three comparison groups were used: these were all men, all men in social class I, and all male doctors. Because the mortality rates for these groups were extracted from national statistics, the comparisons that could be made were limited. Of the three groups studied, male doctors would seem to be the most appropriate comp-arison group, but, for the whole study period, national death rates were only available for this group for a limited number of causes. Thus, many of the comparisons had to be limited to those with men in social class I (the class into which radiologists fall).

Seltzer and Sartwell (1965) overcame this problem by following-up, in their cohort study of American radiologists, not only radio-logists but also practitioners in other medical specialities (their study was consequently much larger because of the necessity of following-up the comparison groups). They were able, consequently, to make direct comparisons between radiologists and other doctors. Even so, it must be borne in mind that doctors are not allocated to specialities "at random" and differences in disease rates between specialities may not be ascribable to exposures related to those specialities. For example, Doll and Peto (1977) examined the variations in smoking related mortality rates between different British medical specialities and found a close correlation with the different smoking habits of the different groups.

Currently a number of studies are underway of workers in nuclear installations. The disease rates in such workers may be compared with national or regional disease rates, with disease rates of workers in a "similar" industry, of radiation exposed workers with non-exposed workers in the same plant, or of exposed workers who have received different radiation doses. Frequently there is a conflict between choosing the comparison group that provides greatest potential statistical power and that which is least likely to provide a biased comparison. Comparison of the irradiated spondylitics with the general population provides a study with the greatest power to detect an effect but comparison with the (small) non-irradiated group perhaps provides the least biased comparison.

Even in the studies of the atomic bomb survivors (in epidemiological terms, a reasonably unselected group) several different comparison groups have been used at various times, including the Japanese national population, those who moved into Hiroshima and Nagasaki after the explosions, and those in the cities who were estimated to have received a low radiation dose.

It would seem that, in most instances, there are no simple answers regarding the choice of an appropriate comparison group and, frequently, the design and interpretation of a study must take into account a number of different possibilities.

The problems with respect to the selection of appropriate comparison groups in case-control studies are, in general, no less. Indeed, the suitability of the control group chosen is, perhaps, the most common controversy in the interpretation of such studies. The problems are greatest when the cases included are a selected sample of all cases with the disease under study (for example, those attending a particular hospital) as, in such circumstances, the controls must be chosen in such a way so as to avoid confusing risk factors for the disease with risk factors for inclusion in the study. If the cases are all of those arising in a defined population, or a random sample of such cases, the issue of selecting controls is easier, at least in principle, as it is then appropriate to include as controls persons randomly selected from the population, usually matched to the cases with respect to factors such as age and sex. Stewart et al (1958) endeavoured to include all deaths from childhood cancers, nationwide, and selected controls from birth registers. While there were still potential

biases introduced by children in the control group who could not
be located or who had migrated away from their area of birth, the
method of control selection in this study seemed, on the whole, to
be satisfactory.

ASCERTAINING EXPOSURES

Quantification of the hazardous (and beneficial) effects of
exposure to radiation is essential for any rational evaluation of
the levels to which it is reasonable to expose members of the
general population and of specific groups. Thus it is highly
desirable that, in any epidemiological study of irradiated groups,
an attempt be made to relate any excess risk of cancer to the
radiation doses received. In some instances this has proved impossible because no adequate records of the exposures have been
maintained. The retrospective cohort studies of radiologists,
which extend back to the start of this century, suffer from this
defect (Matanoski et al, 1975; Smith and Doll, 1981). Fortunately,
however, radiation exposures have been documented more carefully
historically than exposures to most other carcinogens. As early
as the 1930's radiotherapists kept good records of the types and
doses of radiation given to their patients and, for several decades,
those at risk of radiation exposure as a consequence of their
employment have worn "film badges" from which exposures can be
assessed reliably.

Thus, for the studies of ankylosing spondylitics and women
given a radiation-induced menopause it was possible to go back to
the original radiotherapy records to extract details of the
radiation exposures and to use these to estimate the doses to
specific organs (Smith and Doll, 1976, 1982). Film badge assessments of dose have been used in studies of the mortality of workers
in nuclear plants (but the doses that such workers receive have
been too low, in general, to enable a precise quantification of
dose-effect relationships).

The studies of the survivors of the atomic bomb explosions
have contributed much to our knowledge of radiation effects but
the dosimetry has been particularly problematic. Great efforts
were made to estimate the doses that each individual included in
the study had received by questioning them regarding where they
were in the cities at the time of the explosion and by taking
account of the shielding effects of buildings between them and
the centre of the explosion. Such methods of evaluation, however,
are bound to be subject to quite considerable errors and, indeed,
recent evidence suggests that there were flaws in the methods
used to derive the dose estimates that have been used in the past
for quantifying the carcinogenic effects of exposure (Loewe and
Mendelsohn, 1981).

Cohort studies have focussed, usually, on groups for which the fact of exposure, or the amount of exposure, to radiation could be assessed with reasonable reliability. In case-control studies ascertainment of exposure is always retrospective and may be unreliable or biased if it is based on the recall of cases and controls. Of especial concern is that the reliability of the recall of cases may be different from that of controls because of the greater interest of the former group in the objectives of the study. This criticism has been levelled at the case-control study of childhood cancers and in utero radiation exposure of Stewart et al (1956). MacMahon (1962) overcame this potential bias, in his study of childhood cancers, by extracting the information on radiation exposures from the original maternity records, rather than relying on the recall of (the mothers) of cases and controls. This approach usually presents problems, however, in case-control studies as the records of exposure for different individuals may be scattered over a large number of different institutions, not all of which may have well maintained record systems. Though retrospective cohort studies are similarly dependent on the existence of exposure records, the source of the cohort may be confined to those places with record systems adequate for the purpose – as, for example, in the cohort study of in utero radiation of Court Brown et al (1960). The success of MacMahon's (1962) case-control approach was determined by his limitation of the cases (and controls) included to those born in institutions with reasonable maternity records. (He thus adopted a design now known as a case-control within a cohort study).

ASCERTAINING DISEASE EVENTS

Because the populations involved in cohort studies of the late effects of radiation are usually large, commonly involving several thousands of persons, it is not feasable to follow-up each individual for all disease events. This is especially the case for retrospective studies as in these it may be very difficult or impossible to collect the relevant data. This rules out the study of morbidity, as opposed to mortality, in most instances. In some countries it is possible to ascertain those in the study group developing non-fatal cancers through the records of cancer registries but, with a few exceptions, such registries have not operated on a national basis until relatively recently. National registries for other non-fatal diseases are rare. Thus retrospective cohort studies are based, generally, on mortality data. It might be argued, however, that this in itself has not posed too severe a limitation on the value of these studies. This is because the principal long term effect of exposure to radiation is the induction of cancer, and, with a few exceptions, cancers of most sites have a high associated mortality. (It is recognised that there is an element of circularity in this reasoning, in that there have been few studies of the long-term non-fatal consequences of radiation exposure!). It is relatively easy to follow-up individuals to determine if they are alive or dead and, if they are dead, it is possible in many countries to obtain a copy of the death certificate giving the certified cause of death. Mortality rates from specific diseases derived in this way may be compared with those from suitable "unirradiated" groups to assess the radiation risks. A problem is that the cause of death as written on a death certificate may not be an accurate record of the actual cause of death. This does not invalidate the comparison of mortality rates from specific causes in exposed and non-exposed groups, provided that the quality of the diagnoses are similar in both groups, but it does reduce the sensitivity of the comparisons and may lead to the under-estimation of radiation effects. Sometimes there are grounds for concern that the diagnostic accuracy may be different in the groups compared. For example, it is possible that doctors may be more careful in ascertaining the causes of death of their medical colleagues (e.g. radiologists) than they would be of other members of the population (which provides an additional reason for comparing the radiologists with other doctors rather than other members of the general population). Similarly, if an individual is known to be an atomic energy worker, it is conceivable that the death will be investigated more carefully than is usually the case for the possibility of an occupationally determined cancer. This argues in favour of comparing the mortality experience of such workers with that of fellow workers who have received different doses of radiation.

Determining the vital status of individuals in a cohort study is considerably easier than ascertaining their morbidity experience. Nonetheless even the former is not without difficulty in retrospective studies. Individuals migrate out of the country or are lost to follow-up for other reasons and this may bias the estimation of mortality rates. It is often assumed that the mortality rate of those lost to follow-up is similar to that of those successfully traced but this may not be so. If the proportion lost to follow-up is large there must be concerns about the representativeness of the mortality rates derived. This was the case, for example, in the study of the mortality of patients with ankylosing spondylitis who were not treated with radiation, in which only 80% were successfully traced (Smith et al, 1977) - whereas less than 2% of the irradiated patients were lost to follow-up (Smith and Doll, 1982).

Case-control studies have a potential advantage over cohort studies with respect to the ascertainment of disease status. Because in such investigations cases are included, usually, who have been diagnosed in the recent past, it may be possible to review the patient's case-notes, or examine pathological material, to obtain an accurate assessment of the disease classification.

In cohort studies the relevant deaths may be spread over a very long period and may have occurred over a wide geographical area, making uniform standards of diagnosis difficult to achieve.

CONFOUNDING FACTORS

As noted earlier, a fundamental problem with the interpretation of observational studies is that differences between the groups compared (with respect to disease experience in cohort studies, or radiation exposure history in case-control studies) may be explained completely or in part by factors unrelated to radiation. We have discussed earlier the problems inherent in comparing the mortality experience of patients irradiated for ankylosing spondylitis with that of members of the general population. It is possible that differences in mortality between these groups may be due to factors associated with the underlying condition rather than with the radiation treatment. A substantial part of the cancer excess in irradiated patients is due to cancers of the lung - an organ that was usually directly in the radiation treatment beams. We do not know, however, if the smoking habits of the patients differed from those of the general population as smoking habits were not recorded in the retrospective records. An explanation advanced for the association between in utero radiation and childhood cancers has been that it is due to those factors that precipitated the diagnostic x-rays rather than to the radiation exposure.

In a recent study Boice et al (1984) examined the incidence of second malignancies among women irradiated for treatment of cancer of the cervix. One of the striking findings of this large international study was a substantial deficit of cancers of the breast. It is possible that this was due, at least in part, to protection from this cancer being conferred by the artificial menopause that is likely to have been induced by the radiation treatment - a similar effect was postulated by Doll and Smith (1968) to explain the deficit of breast cancer in their study of women given a radiation-induced menopause. Some of the risk factors for cancer of the cervix, however, such as high parity and low socio-economic status, are also associated with a low risk of breast cancer. Thus some or all of the breast cancer deficit among patients irradiated for cervix cancer may be unrelated to the radiation treatment. One way in which these alternative possibilities may be evaluated is through the conduct of case-control studies within the defined cohorts in which it may be possible to obtain information about these other risk factors by direct questioning of individuals or their surviving relatives.

This illustrates one of the considerable design advantages of case-control over cohort studies. In the latter it is rarely possible to collect information on more than a few potentially confounding factors - either because the relevant records do not exist or because the task is too great for the thousands of persons under study. Case-control studies include, typically, only a few hundred individuals, and thus it may be feasable to collect information on many potentially confounding variables.

SAMPLE SIZE CONSIDERATION

One of the important determinants of the necessary size of a cohort study to detect an effect of a given magnitude, is the nature of the comparison group. Generally there are two broad options. Comparison may be made with the general population, or with some other large group, for which it is assumed that the sampling errors associated with the estimation of disease rates are negligibly small. Alternatively, the comparison may be with a specific "non-exposed" group who are followed-up in the same way as the exposed group. We have pointed out earlier that the latter comparison is likely to be less susceptible to bias. The consequence of adopting such a design, however, is to multiply the size of study needed to detect an effect of specified size by a factor of about four. Thus the statistical power associated with a study in which an exposed cohort, say of size N, is compared with the general population, is approximately the same as that of a study in which an exposed cohort of size 2N is compared with an unexposed cohort of the same size.

In some circumstances, only a subset of the "exposed" group may have a "high" exposure. If the exposure of the remaining members of the cohort is similar to that of the general population, or only slightly in excess, and the high exposure group is less than a quarter of the total exposed group, then the power of the comparison of the high exposure group with the general population is similar to that of the contrast of high and low exposure groups with each other. This situation might hold in some studies of occupational exposure to radiation.

Because radiation appears not to be a powerful carcinogen, very large studies are required to detect radiation effects even among populations exposed to quite large radiation doses. To illustrate this consider the design of a study to detect a leukaemia risk in a group whose members were each exposed to 5 rems (the present maximal permissible occupational exposure in a one year period). UNSCEAR (1977) have estimated that following exposure to one rem of radiation the leukaemia induction rate is of the order of one case per million per year for the 20 years following exposure. Among adults the "natural" rate of leukaemia varies from about 20 to 120 cases per million per year between the ages of 25 and 60 years (on average, say 70/million/year). To

have a reasonable chance of detecting the radiation effect on top
of this background risk would require a cohort study (with the
general population as the comparison group) in which the exposed
group accumulated approximately 25 million years-at-risk following exposure. Even if the radiation associated risk was 10 times
higher than the current estimate, a cohort study would need to
include about 400,000 person years-at-risk (e.g. 40,000 persons
followed for 10 years). It is for these reasons that most information on radiation effects has come from groups which, for various
reasons, have been exposed to unusually high radiation doses.

Most public health concern centres, however, on the much
larger groups whose members may be exposed to low radiation doses.
Current estimates of the health effects of such exposure are
derived by extrapolation back from effects seen in heavily exposed groups. It is clearly important to monitor the effects in
populations exposed to low doses in case the assumptions involved
in extrapolation are incorrect. It is an unfortunate fact,
however, that unless the estimates of low dose effects are out by
more than an order of magnitude there is little hope of this
being detected in studies of low-exposure groups. A more
extensive discussion of this issue is given by Land (1980).

The discouraging conclusions drawn above with respect to
cohort studies apply, with similar force, to case-control studies.
If only a small proportion of the population is exposed to
radiation, studies of prohibitive size are required to detect
radiation effects. For example, in the situation discussed above,
suppose 1% of the population have been exposed to 5 rems or
radiation, on top of background radiation (to which all are
exposed), and suppose further that the leukaemogenic effect is
10 times higher than is currently estimated. In these
circumstances we would need a study involving about 5000 cases
and a similar number of controls to have a reasonable chance of
detecting a statistically significant effect.

PROBLEMS IN EXTRAPOLATION

The effects of high radiation doses are of interest from a
scientific viewpoint, in that they offer clues to mechanisms of
carcinogenesis, but, short of a nuclear catastrophy, the major
public health interest is concentrated on the effects of low
doses - such as might be received through medical diagnostic
procedures, through employment in a nuclear industry, or through
environmental contamination from nuclear processes. We have seen
that the direct study of low dose effects may pose considerable
problems because of the large sample sizes required. Thus,
unless specific markers are found for radiation-induced cancers,
to distinguish them from cancers due to other causes, it seems

likely that estimates of low dose effects must continue to be based on backwards extrapolation from the effects seen in groups exposed to high doses.

The groups that have received high doses of radiation as a result of medical procedures are not ideal for this purpose for several reasons. Firstly the possibility must be considered that the members of such selected groups may be at an abnormal (high or low) risk of developing a malignant disease independently of any effect of radiation. Secondly, usually only part of the body or parts of organs were irradiated and it is likely that the effects of such exposure will be different from whole-body radiation - such as might be received by nuclear workers or from environmental contamination. Thirdly, the radiation exposure may be given at a relatively high dose rate and the total dose may have been delivered in a number of fractions separated in time by days or weeks. Both of these factors have been shown to modify the cell killing effect of radiation, and there are theoretical reasons, supported by some animal experimentation data, to suppose that both factors will also affect the rate of cancer induction, though it is not clear exactly what effect variations in these factors will have. The exposures in Hiroshima and Nagasaki are an extreme example of exposure at a very high dose rate.

A fundamental problem with extrapolation procedures is in the choice of the appropriate dose-response relationship. Until relatively recently the relationship between cancer induction and radiation dose was taken to be linear. There is now substantial evidence that this assumption is wrong, certainly at high doses, where the cell killing effects of radiation must also be taken into account. Possible forms of dose-response curve were discussed extensively in BEIR (1980), but they were unable to come to any final conclusion as to what was the most appropriate model.

CONCLUDING REMARKS

This review has been deliberately critical and has emphasised some of the problems in interpreting the available data on long-term radiation effects. It should be noted that ionising radiations have probably been studied more extensively than any other human carcinogen and, from the wealth of available data, it is possible to draw conclusions about their effects with some confidence, as will be discussed in other sections of this book. Nonetheless a number of outstanding problems remain, especially with respect to the estimation of low dose-effects, and it is likely that some, at least, will continue to be a source of controversy for the forseeable future.

REFERENCES

BEIR, 1980, The effects on populations of exposure to low levels
    of ionizing radiation: 1980. Committee on the Biological
    Effects of Ionizing Radiations. National Research Council.
    National Academy Press, Washington D.C.
Boice, J.D., Day, N.E., and 34 others, 1984, Cancer risk following
    radiotherapy of cervical cancer: a preliminary report, in:
    "Radiation Carcinogenesis: Epidemiology and Biological
    Significance", J.D. Boice, and J.F. Fraumeni, eds., Raven
    Press, New York.
Court Brown, W.M., Doll, R., 1958, Expectation of life and
    mortality from cancer among British radiologists, Brit.
    Med.J.,2:181-187.
Court Brown, W.M., Doll, R., and Hill, A.B., 1960, Incidence of
    leukaemia after exposure to diagnostic radiation in utero,
    Brit.Med.J., 4:1539-1545.
Court Brown, W.M., and Doll, R., 1965, Mortality from cancer and
    other causes after radiotherapy for ankylosing spondylitis,
    Brit.Med.J., 2:1327-1332.
Doll,R., and Peto,R., 1977, Mortality among doctors in different
    occupations, Brit.Med.J., 1:1433-1436.
Doll,R., and Smith, P.G., 1968, The long term effects of x-
    irradiation in patients treated for metropathia haemorrhagia,
    Brit.J.Radiol., 41: 362-368.
Land, C., 1980, Estimating cancer risks from low doses of ionizing
    radiation, Science, 209: 1197-1203.
Loewe, W.E., and Mendelsohn, E., 1981, Revised dose estimates at
    Hiroshima and Nagaski, Health Phys., 41: 663-666.
MacMahon, B., 1962, Prenatal x-ray exposure and childhood cancer,
    J.Natl.Cancer Inst., 5: 1173-1191.
Matanoski, G.M., Seltser, R., Sartwell, P.E., Diamond, E.L., and
    Elliott., E.E., 1975, The current mortality rates of
    radiologists and other physician specialists: specific cause
    of death, Am.J.Epidem., 101: 199-201.
Seltser, R., and Sartwell, P.E., 1965, The influence of occupational
    exposure to radiation on the mortality of American radiolo-
    gists and other medical specialists, Am.J.Epidem., 81:2-22.
Smith, P.G., and Doll, R., 1976, Late effects of x-irradiation in
    patients treated for metropathia haemorragica, Brit.J.Radiol.,
    49: 224-232.
Smith, P.G., Doll, R., and Radford, E.P., 1977, Cancer mortality
    among patients with ankylosing spondylitis not given x-ray
    therapy, Brit.J.Radiol., 50: 728-734.
Smith, P.G., and Doll, R., 1981, Mortality from cancer and all
    causes among British radiologists, Brit.J.Radiol., 54:
    187-194.

Smith, P.G., and Doll, R., 1982, Mortality among patients with
    ankylosing spondylitis after a single treatment course with
    x rays, <u>Brit.Med.J.</u>, 284:449-460.
Stewart, A., Webb, A., Giles, D., and Hewitt, D., 1956, Malignant
    disease in childhood and diagnostic irradiation in utero,
    <u>Lancet</u>, 2: 447.
UNSCEAR, 1977, Sources and effects of ionizing radiation. United
    Nations Scientific Committee on the Effects of Atomic
    Radiation, United, Nations, New York.

IN VITRO MALIGNANT TRANSFORMATION - A MULTI-STEPPED PROCESS

J. Justin McCormick   and Veronica M. Maher

Carcinogenesis Laboratory - Fee Hall
Department of Microbiology and Department of
Biochemistry
Michigan State University
East Lansing, MI   48824-1316

INTRODUCTION

In experimental studies with animals, cancer generally results only after multiple treatments with carcinogenic chemicals or radiation over an extended period of time. Analysis of such data has led to the conclusion that cancer results from a multi-stepped process (Peto, 1977). Similar conclusions have been arrived at in regard to human cancer, using epidemiological approaches (Peto, 1977). It should be noted, however, that there are a number of well-studied model tumor systems in which only a single high dose of the carcinogenic agent induces tumors in a majority of the animals. Examples of these include induction of rat mammary tumors by ethylnitrosourea (Stoica et al., 1984) and induction of rat brain tumors by this agent (Druckrey et al., 1966). Such experiments seem to indicate that carcinogenesis is not multi-stepped. However, they may actually represent a cryptic multi-stepped process in which the carcinogen causes the cells to advance only a single step through the transformation sequence and other steps occur spontaneously. Alternatively, they may represent cases in which two independent transforming events which are required for carcinogenesis are triggered simultaneously in some of the cells at risk because of the high dose of carcinogen used and the fact that the target population consists of a large number of rapidly proliferating cells at the time of carcinogen treatment. Rapid cell growth is known to enhance the risk of cells to carcinogenesis. In any case, these experiments using a single carcinogen treatment are the exception. The vast majority of the animal and human data indicate that carcinogenesis is a multi-stepped process, requiring repeated carcinogen treatment.

One of the major challenges of cancer research has been to identify the steps in this process. These steps can be of two types; 1) changes in the host which allow a tumor to grow, such as a depression in immunological function, and 2) changes in the cells which cause them to express the neoplastic phenotype. The development of techniques for growing mammalian cells in culture has provided excellent tools for arriving at an understanding of the cellular changes responsible for tumors, an area where animal experiments are weakest. This essay will concentrate on these latter phenomena. Cells in culture have served as target populations for investigating the process by which normal cells are transformed into tumor cells since the early 1960's. A variety of inducing agents have been used, including RNA tumor viruses, DNA tumor viruses, chemical carcinogens, and radiation, and cells from many vertebrate species have been the target cells. According to the definitions agreed to by the Tissue Culture Association (Schaeffer, 1983), when cells in culture acquire a heritable change(s) which confers a phenotype characteristic of tumor-derived cells, this is properly referred to as "in vitro transformation". Examples of such phenotypic changes are certain morphological changes, acquisition of anchorage independence, and focus formation. If cells acquire in vitro the ability to form benign or malignant neoplasms in appropriate animal hosts, the proper term is "in vitro neoplastic transformation". A more rarely used, but equally useful term is "in vitro malignant neoplastic transformation" which indicates that the cells have acquired in culture the ability to invade or metastasize when assayed in an appropriate animal host. Such definitions are the result of recent careful thinking about transformation. Because such careful distinctions were not made in some of the earlier studies, and even in some more recent studies, it is necessary to read the literature on transformation carefully, paying particular attention to the end points which are being considered.

As we examine the various cell systems, it is important to note that fibroblastic cells have been the target cells in the majority of the assays. This is because the techniques for cell culture were first developed with such cells and the methods and media used select for the growth of these cells. Even in assays in which one starts with primary or secondary embryo cultures which contain many different cell types (e.g., the Syrian hamster embryo system described below), the growth conditions are such that cells other than fibroblasts are lost from culture. Further evidence for this is the fact that in tumorigenicity assays carried out with the progeny of the mixture of embryonic cells transformed in vitro, one finds fibrosarcomas, i.e., malignant tumors of fibroblastic origin. The assumption in such studies with fibroblasts is that, despite the fact that fibrosarcomas are rare tumors in animals and in humans, the mechanisms by which fibroblasts become tumor cells are the same or similar to those for the more common tumors of humans which are epithelial or hematopoietic in origin.

STUDIES OF CARCINOGEN-INDUCED IN VITRO TRANSFORMATION

Assays with Primary or Early-Passage Cells with Finite Lifespans

Mammalian cells in culture were first used to propagate and titer various tumor viruses. Berwald and Sachs (1963) were the first to report the transformation of cultured cells with chemical carcinogens. In these studies, cells derived from primary or very early passage cultures of golden (Syrian) hamster embryos exhibited colonies with a transformed phenotype (cells were fusiform in shape and exhibited a random pattern of growth) after treatment with the carcinogen benzo(a)pyrene. A similar transformed phenotype had previously been noted in cells treated with polyoma, a DNA tumor virus (Sachs and Medina, 1961). The carcinogen-transformed cells were tested for their ability to form tumors, but no results were available at the time of publication of the paper by Berwald and Sachs (1963). A similar study using ionizing radiation as the transforming agent was carried out a few years later (Borek and Sachs, 1966). Similar morphologically-transformed colonies were seen among the radiation exposed cultures. These transformed colonies were isolated and grown continuously. When the cells were injected into 2-6 week-old hamsters at 2 and 8 months after irradiation they formed growths at the site of injection that reached a diameter of 7-10mm. These growths regressed 10-30 days after inoculation, but if excised before then and analyzed, they were identified as sarcomas.

These two pioneer studies are very important because they demonstrate in a simple, yet elegant manner the power of in vitro assays. This led to the use of the golden hamster transformation assay by many workers. In fact, this has remained the only commonly used transformation assay in which one begins with normal cells. However, several problems are raised by these assays which have only become clarified by recent studies. One important consideration is whether cells morphologically-transformed by chemicals or radiation (i.e., the cells in the original transformed colony) are tumorigenic per se, or only become so after further subculturing. Since one ordinarily injects $1-10 \times 10^6$ cells into animals for such tests, it is clear that one cannot assay the tumorigenicity of the $1 \times 10^3 - 5 \times 10^3$ cells in the original transformed colony, but rather must assay the progeny of such cells. For example, in the study of Borek and Sachs (1966), 6.5×10^6 cells were injected at 2 or 8 months after irradiation and, therefore, the cells necessarily underwent an extended period of proliferation before they were injected. Thus, it is not clear from this study in 1966 whether the morphologically-transformed colonies are tumorigenic or give rise to tumorigenic cells. Using the terminology discussed above, one properly speaks of the cells of the morphologically-altered colonies as "transformed", but not as "neoplastically transformed" as was originally done. Later elegant studies by Barrett and Ts'o (1978) and Newbold et al. (1982) have demonstrated that morphologically transformed hamster cells are not tumorigenic per se, but acquire this property after extended subculturing, i.e., when such cells acquire the anchorage independent phenotype.

A second finding in the studies of Borek and Sachs (1966) was that non-transformed hamster cells senesced after 40 to 60 days in culture, whereas the morphologically-transformed cells could be passaged indefinitely. Therefore, the effect of ionizing radiation or the carcinogen treatment might be understood as giving the cells an extended or indefinite lifespan. Interestingly, although this fact was noted in these and many other later studies, it was not usually considered an important point. However, recent studies by Newbold et al. (1982) have emphasized the point that carcinogen-treated populations of hamster cells give rise to cells that escape senescence, whereas control populations senesce. A study by Watanabe et al. (1984) has demonstrated that it is the progeny of the cells of the transformed foci that have escaped senescence. Whether morphogically-transformed cells have the property of indefinite lifespan or whether they acquire the property during subculturing is not yet clear. However, if it is the latter, it is clear that the ability to overcome senescence arises at a high frequency in such cells since in the study of Watanabe et al. (1984), 9 of 10 transformed colonies produced continuously proliferating tumorigenic cell lines.

Thirdly, the study of Borek and Sachs (1966) also found that even after a year in culture, the ionizing radiation-transformed cells still did not demonstrate anchorage independent growth, even though they had been able to form regressing tumors in animals. Later workers using a variety of inducing agents have found the opposite result, i.e., when cultures of carcinogen-treated Syrian hamster embryo cells have been propagated for a long time (have acquired an unlimited lifespan) and are able to form tumors in animals, they also exhibit anchorage independence (Barrett and Ts'o, 1978; Newbold et al., 1982).

A fourth important consideration is whether the observed morphological transformation could be the result of a somatic cell mutation. Borek and Sachs (1966) reported that the frequency of transformation induced by ionizing radiation was $5 - 8 \times 10^{-3}$

cells. Watanabe recently found that at a low dose of ionizing radiation (i.e. 200 rad), the frequency of morphological transformants was 2.3×10^{-3}, but the frequency of thioguanine resistant cells was only 1×10^{-5}. At a higher dose, i.e. 600 rad, the transformation frequency was 3×10^{-3} and the mutant frequency was 7×10^{-5} (M. Watanabe, unpublished studies). Barrett and Ts'o (1978) also reported that the frequency of morphological transformation, induced in these cells by benzo(a)pyrene was 25–125 fold higher than the frequency of ouabain resistant mutants. For this and other reasons it appears that morphological transformation does not arise mainly as a result of a classical mutation. Anchorage independence, on the other hand, may indeed arise as the result of a mutation. This is suggested by a variety of studies, including fluctuation test studies by Bellett and Younghusband (1979) in progeny of mouse embryo cultures and studies showing that the dose–dependent carcinogen induction of this phenotype in diploid human fibroblasts with finite lifespans occurs at frequencies much closer to those for induction of mutations to thioguanine resistance. (Sutherland et al., 1980, 1981; Silinskas et al., 1981; Maher et al., 1982).

Finally, the work of Borek and Sachs (1966) reported that only regressing tumors arose. Later work with this assay indicates that tumors created by anchorage–independent cells do not regress, but rather grow continuously (Newbold et al., 1982). Furthermore, in a minority of the animals in the latter study there was evidence for invasion and/or metastasis to various organs. It is possible that these differences in results are caused by differences in assay conditions or, perhaps, by the larger scale of the later experiments which allowed Newbold et al. (1982) to see less frequent events, or by a difference in inducing agents used. Additional light has been shed on this assay by studies that indicate that morphological transformation can be caused by agents such as diethylstilbestrol, which are unable to cause mutations in typical assays (Barrett et al., 1981). Workers have also shown that chromosomal aneuploidy correlates with morphological transformation (Tsutsui et al., 1983).

Taken together, the above results demonstrate that Syrian hamster embryo fibroblastic cells must undergo a series of independent changes to become tumorigenic. Some changes, such as loss of anchorage dependence, are probably mutational in origin. Some, such as morphological transformation, seem not to be. From these experiments, it seems clear that the changes take place within individual cells, and that these cells give rise to clonal populations which are capable of undergoing further changes. Because of various ambiguities in the work, one cannot yet be sure of how many steps are involved.

Assays with Continuous Cell Lines

Transformation assays have also been carried out using various continuous (indefinite lifespan) cell lines. Among the more commonly used cells are the mouse-derived Swiss-3T3, clone 4; C3H/10T½, clone 18; BALB/c 3T3, clone A-31 cells; and the Syrian hamster-derived BHK 21/clone 13 cells (see Mishra et al., 1980, for a more complete discussion of these assays). All of these cell lines are aneuploid. However, they lack the ability to grow in an anchorage independent manner and are not tumorigenic in suitable host animals under ordinary conditions. When treated with carcinogenic agents the three mouse cell lines form foci, i.e., clones of cells growing in a three dimensional array on a cell monolayer. Cells within such foci frequently exhibit a disordered growth pattern. Typically one exposes the cells to the carcinogen for a period of hours or days, removes the carcinogen-containing medium and then refeeds the cells with fresh medium. After a period of several weeks, foci appear as densely staining regions in the cell monolayer.

The BHK-21 cells are exposed to the carcinogenic agent in a similar manner. They are then grown for a few days, referred to as the expression period, and then assayed for their ability to express the anchorage-independent phenotype, i.e., suspended at clonal density in medium containing agar or methylcellulose so they cannot attach to the culture dish. Cells with the ability to grow in an anchorage independent manner form colonies which can be quantitated by scanning the dish with a microscope. When cells are isolated from the foci or the anchorage independent colonies and grown to large populations and injected into suitable animals, malignant tumors result. In the case of BALB/c 3T3 cells, angiosarcomas were reported (Boone et al., 1976), suggesting that this cell line is of endothelial origin (Porter et al., 1973). Fibroblasts and endothelial cells are closely related since both are mesodermal in origin. Therefore, this finding does not set the BALB/c 3T3 system apart from the others.

One can legitimately ask whether the cells from the foci or anchorage independent colonies are tumorigenic per se, or only become so as the populations are expanded to carry out the tumor assay. Most workers seem to assume that the cells of the foci or anchorage independent colonies are already tumorigenic, but it is difficult to find adequate evidence to support this conclusion. In addition, it should be noted that the tumorigenicity of transformed C3H/10T½ cells is usually demonstrated in athymic mice because these cells do not routinely give tumors in C3H mice. This problem has raised the question of whether the cells are actually from strain C3H.

Regardless of these problems, the value of these in vitro assays is their simplicity which allows one to determine whether specific agents are able to cause this type of cell transformation as well as to ask questions about mechanisms. What is often forgotten, however, is that by design, these assays can only measure the ultimate step in a carcinogenesis process, the step which makes these cells tumorigenic or the penultimate step, should the tumorigenic phenotype develop in the expansion of the transformed cell populations for tumor assays. It is only the fact that the progeny cells of the foci or the anchorage independent colony can form a tumor which allows one to conclude that these endpoints are relevant to carcinogenesis. However, since the target cells are not typical diploid cells of mouse or hamster, but are chromosomally abnormal, have an indefinite lifespan and may have other unknown changes, these cells cannot be used to identify the other critical cellular changes required for carcinogenesis. Yet if the primary or early passage hamster embryo cell system is a good model, such changes appear to be just as important as the "final step" studied with these continuous cell lines.

STUDIES ON THE SERIES OF CHANGES INVOLVED IN NEOPLASTIC TRANSFORMATION

Another type of analysis of the carcinogenic process has been carried out by workers who have begun with diploid or near diploid cells that have acquired an unlimited lifespan, but are apparently normal in other ways. These cells can be used to study what phenotypes a cell must acquire to become fully tumorigenic. The attribute of unlimited lifespan in cells allows one to carry out a series of sequential cloning assays in which one selects cells in a series for properties thought to be required for tumorigenicity. In a typical experiment, one selects for clones with property A, isolates and expands the cell population of one such clone, then selects for cells with property B and again isolates and expands the cell population of a clone. Obviously all cells with property B should also have property A. The experiment can be repeated until one has cells carrying several specific properties. (See Fig. 1.)

It should be clear why such studies cannot be carried out with normal diploid cells with their limited lifespan in culture, e.g., diploid human fibroblasts. Pouyssegur and his colleagues (Perez-Rodriguez et al., 1981; Perez-Rodriguez et al., 1982) have used a diploid Chinese hamster cell with an indefinite lifespan for their studies. They found that if these cells were to form progressively-growing tumors, visible 3 to 6 days following subcutaneous injection into a suitable animal host, it was necessary that the cells previously undergo three types of changes. (The short latent period of 3 to 6 days indicates that

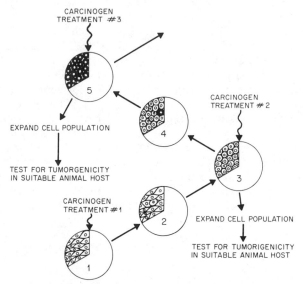

CARCINOGEN
TREATMENT #3

EXPAND CELL POPULATION

TEST FOR TUMORGENICITY
IN SUITABLE ANIMAL HOST

CARCINOGEN
TREATMENT #2

CARCINOGEN
TREATMENT #1

EXPAND CELL POPULATION

TEST FOR TUMORIGENICITY
IN SUITABLE ANIMAL HOST

SCHEMATIC VIEW OF CELL TRANSFORMATION

Fig. 1. Representation of an in vitro clonal selection assay for transformed cells. Petri Dish 1 represents a population of normal fibroblastic cells which are treated with a carcinogen; 2 shows the same dish in which a phenotypically-altered cell (round shape) arose as a result of the carcinogen treatment; 3 shows a pure population of round cells which arose by isolation of the round cell from Dish 2 and its subsequent propagation. This cell population can be expanded and tested for tumorigenicity. If the cells are not tumorigenic, one assumes that one or more changes are still required. The cells in Dish 3 are then treated with a carcinogen, and Dish 4 shows the same dish in which a cell having a new phenotypic alteration (black cell), induced by the carcinogen, has arisen. This cell is isolated and grown up as shown in Dish 5. The population of Dish 5 is expanded and tested for tumorigenicity. If the results are negative, the procedure is reiterated. Obviously the success of this procedure depends upon the investigator being able to make shrewd guesses as to which phenotypes are cancer-related. It does not, however, necessarily imply that each change induced is mutational in origin, only that the changes are stable and inherited.

essentially the entire cell population injected is tumorigenic, not some small fraction.) These required characteristics are: the ability to grow in an anchorage independent manner, a reduced requirement for the protein growth factors found in serum and some, as yet undefined, change that allows the cells to escape the residual immune function of athymic mice. Presumably these changes are required in addition to the indefinite lifespan which the cells already possess. Similar studies have also been carried out by Smith and Sager (1982), using another Chinese hamster cell line.

Thomassen and DeMars (1982) have carried out a similar study using a near-diploid mouse cell line which appears to be morphologically-transformed. These investigators demonstrated that to become fully transformed, the cells still need to acquire the anchorage independent phenotype and the ability to form a tumor. It is not clear from their results if these alterations represent two separate steps. If one assumes that morphological transformation occurs as a single step, these particular mouse cells need to go through a total of two, or perhaps three, steps for complete transformation.

STUDIES WITH DIPLOID HUMAN FIBROBLASTS

Obviously one would like to utilize human fibroblasts in such transformation studies since they would presumably allow one to determine the number and kind of steps required for malignant transformation in humans. In 1977, Freedman and Shin(1977) showed that human skin fibroblasts could be induced to form colonies in semi-solid medium. But cells from these colonies did not cause tumors in unirradiated athymic mice. Kakunaga (1978) was the first to demonstrate that after carcinogen treatment, normal diploid human cells can produce foci. The cells from these foci could be isolated and they sometimes produced tumors in athymic mice (Kakanaga, 1978). In Kakunaga's experiment, at least one cell line with an indefinite lifespan was obtained from a focus. This line, HUT 14, has been the subject of much additional work (Leavitt, et al., 1982) since it exhibits the malignant neoplastic phenotype producing progressively growing tumors which can kill athymic mice. Cells isolated from other foci had a finite lifespan (Kakunaga, personal communication). The cell populations derived from the foci of Kakunaga (1978) showed an increase in anchorage-independent growth and in saturation density at confluence. Because of the long expression period (>13 generations) required before the cells were placed in the focus assay, it is difficult to estimate the true frequency of transformation. This is because the replication rate of the cells that give rise to the foci may be faster or slower than that of the population as a whole. The formation of the HUT 14 line seems to represent a rare, chance event since human fibroblasts with an indefinite lifespan have never been reported to arise spontaneously. Namba et al. (1981), the only workers who have successfully generated such lines after carcinogen treatment, have found that repeated treatments were required and that even then, such lines appeared only rarely.

We have reproduced these focus assays with diploid human fibroblasts treated with carcinogens (McCormick et al., 1980; Silinskas et al., 1981) and find that the tumors formed after injecting progeny derived from the foci regress after reaching their maximal size. We also find that the foci formed are quite subtle so that they cannot readily be quantitated, which limits the usefulness of the assay. All the cells that we isolated from foci proved to have a finite lifespan.

Milo and his collaborators have published studies in which chemical carcinogen or UV radiation treatment of human fibroblasts induced anchorage independent growth (Milo and DiPaolo, 1978; Milo and DiPaolo, 1980; Milo et al., 1981a,b). When cells from colonies growing in semi-solid medium were isolated and grown to large populations, Milo found they produced nodular growths in irradiated athymic mice. These growths were variously described as myxofibromas (Milo et al., 1981b), fibrosarcomas (Tejwani et al., 1981) or undifferentiated mesenchymal tumors (Milo and DiPaolo, 1978). Milo and his co-workers have not indicated in their studies whether or not the tumors regress. They also have not shown evidence for invasion of the tumor into mouse tissue or for metastasis, although they have shown that the anchorage independent cells can invade embryonic chicken skin. (Milo et al., 1981a).

We have reproduced these kinds of experiments, i.e., induced anchorage independence in diploid human fibroblasts by exposure to carcinogens, and find the induction occurs in a dose-dependent manner (McCormick et al., 1980; Silinskas et al., 1981; Maher et al., 1982). When the cells from the colonies are isolated and grown to large populations, they sometimes produce tumors in irradiated athymic mice. We find that these tumors reach a maximum size of 7-10mm in diameter, stop growing, and then, if not removed, regress completely. Pathology studies of such regressing tumors showed infiltration of lymphocytes. Regression of such tumors also has been noted by Newbold et al. (1982). In our studies, cells derived from these anchorage independent colonies do not have an unlimited lifespan, but appear to have a lifespan which is slightly longer or shorter than the age-matched control cells of clonal origin. Our interpretation of these experiments is that, in terms of the definitions given above, the anchorage independent cells are transformed since they show this tumor-cell-like phenotype. However, since the cells form tumors in only a percentage of the animals, eventually regress, and characteristically do not invade, it is not clear whether the term "neoplastic transformation" is proper.

Examples of other studies on carcinogen-induced transformation of diploid human fibroblasts include Borek (1980), Joseph et al. (1983), Miyaki et al. (1980, 1982), Newbold et al. (1982), Shimada et al. (1976), Sutherland et al. (1980, 1981), and Zimmerman and Little (1981, 1983a,b). Further studies are needed if one is to induce human cells to progress through the several steps to neoplastic transformation.

STUDIES WITH TRANSFORMING VIRUSES

Use of RNA Tumor Viruses

The most efficient transforming agents are the acute transforming RNA tumor viruses. They have a small simple genome and carry only a single gene for cell transformation (or two, for example, in the case of avian erythroblastosis virus). The prototype acute transforming RNA tumor virus, Rous sarcoma virus (RSV), was discovered by Peyton Rous in 1911 (Rous and Murphy, 1911). This virus, which is of chicken origin, readily transforms chicken fibroblasts in culture as well as the cells from many other species. Various studies have clearly demonstrated that the transforming activity resides in the src sequence. Chicken fibroblasts treated with RSV form foci similar to those described above for mouse cells. When the cells of the foci are isolated and assayed they are also found to exhibit anchorage independent growth and cytoskeletal anomalies. A further proof that these phenotypes are the result of the src gene is that cells transformed with a RSV carrying a temperature sensitve src exhibit the morphological change typical of the cells in the focus, i.e., anchorage independent growth and cytoskeletal anomalies, only when grown at the permissive temperature (Weiss et al., 1982).

RSV-transformed chicken cells have a finite, although slightly extended, life span in culture and form regressing tumors in chickens. This is in contrast to the effect of infecting susceptible chickens with the RSV virus itself. RSV forms progressively growing fibrosarcomas in such birds. However, these tumors are believed to result form viral spread (sequential viral infection and transformation of additional cells) in the bird. Further evidence for this interpretation is the fact when DNA carrying the isolated src gene is injected into chickens, the subsequent tumors regress. Since no virus is produced in this case, the tumors are self-limiting, presumably because of the limited lifespan of the transfected cells. In contrast, the injection of DNA from the entire RSV virus into susceptible chickens results in tumors similar to those found when the birds are infected with intact RSV virus (Fung et al., 1983).

Traditionally, RNA tumor virus workers have not placed as much stress on tumorigenicity of the transformed cells as the ultimate criterion for transformation as have workers with other kinds of transforming agents. This may be because the typical virus infected cells are highly antigenic because they produce virus and this antigenicity often limits the growth of such cells as a tumor. Because of this and because of the problem of viral spread in animals in which cells infected with whole virus are assayed for tumorigenicity, it is difficult to analyze with precision the steps involved in transformation by many different acute transforming RNA tumor viruses. However, it is now commonly believed that such viruses will effect only a partial transformation of cells since they carry only one transforming gene.

Use of DNA Tumor Viruses

DNA tumor viruses are quite different from the acute transforming RNA tumor viruses since they have long been understood to have the ability to make the infected cells fully tumorigenic, i.e., to act as if carcinogenesis were a single-stepped process. However, the results of recent studies at the molecular level indicate that the process is, indeed, multi-stepped. For example, in polyoma virus, it has now been demonstrated that there are three oncogenes, and these must act in a coordinated manner to cause the virus-induced malignant transformation of rat embryo cells (Cuzin et al., 1984). Three overlapping genes, located in a single region of the viral genome but with alternate translational reading frames, direct the synthesis of distinct proteins via the production of distinct mRNA's by means of different splicing processes operating on a common primary transcript (Kamen et al., 1980). The adenoviruses are also known to carry multiple oncogenes (van der Eb, et al., 1980).

FURTHER EVIDENCE OF THE MULTI-STEPPED NATURE OF NEOPLASTIC TRANSFORMATION

A recent study by Land et al. (1983a) is perhaps the most dramatic demonstration of the multi-stepped nature of neoplastic transformation. Transfection of secondary rat embryo fibroblasts (finite lifespan) with the Ha-ras oncogene isolated from the EJ human bladder carcinoma cell line gave no foci or morphological transformation, nor did the cells have an indefinite lifespan or form tumors. However, when assayed in soft agar, the cells exhibited anchorage independent growth, and if individual cells which had taken up DNA were isolated from those that had not, they appeared morphologically-transformed. These cells produced only small, subcutaneous, cartilaginous nodules when injected into animals and thus were non-tumorigenic. The above results suggest that the presence of normal cells prevented the expression of the anchorage independent growth and of morphological transformation. In contrast, a continuous rat cell line did form foci when transfected with this same oncogene and when injected into suitable animals, the progeny cells from the foci produced progressively-growing tumors. However, when the secondary culture of rat embryo fibroblasts carrying the ras oncogene was transfected with a second oncogene (myc), the cells produced foci, and, when the cells of the foci were expanded to large populations,, and injected into suitable animals, tumors grew to a size of about 2 cm and remained stationary thereafter. When the myc gene was transfected into the secondary rat cells in which the ras gene had not been transfected, there was no apparent change in the cells.

Other studies (reviewed by Land et al., 1983b) have shown that the Ha-ras oncogene can be substituted by N-ras or by polyoma middle T gene. Similarly, the myc oncogene can be replaced by polyoma large T or by the Ela gene of adenovirus. There are minor variations in the phenotype of the cells transfected with genes from a single complementation group (reviewed in Land et al., 1983b). Since the tumors created by the progeny of the doubly-transfected rat fibroblasts of Land et al., (1983a) remained static in size, it is obvious that these experiments have not fully recapitulated the process of malignant transformation. Perhaps, as they suggest, a third gene may need to be transfected into these cells. One recent study by Spandidos and Wilkie (1984) is of special importance because they found that when vectors containing transcriptional enhancers were linked to the Ha-ras oncogene, it was capable of transmitting the full malignant phenotype to normal rat or Chinese hamster cells. The transformed cells showed an expression of Ha-ras-1 which was more than 20 to 60 times that found in cells transfected with Ha-ras-1 not linked to these transcriptional enhancer sequences. Although these cells show full transormation after a single event (transfection), they clearly demand an expression of the oncogene to levels not found when such genes are linked to their normal promoters and enhancers. Thus, they seem to represent a special case not found in nature.

As noted earlier, most transformation studies have made use of fibroblasts. It seems unlikely that all the transforming genes for diverse cell types including epithelial cells and the hematopoietic system will be identical to those identified for fibroblasts. Nevertheless, of all the studies cited in this essay, these transfection studies perhaps most clearly indicate the multi-stepped nature of transformation.

CONCLUSION

It is obvious from this wide-ranging survey of cell transformation that the bulk of the evidence indicates that multiple changes are required for a normal cell to become a true cancer cell. The data clearly suggest that this can result from a number of different types of processes. Careful analysis of various cell systems should allow us to come to an understanding of the cellular and underlying molecular changes which take place during this process. It seems likely that the sequence of changes one observes in cultured cells as they become fully tumorigenic is arbitrary and follows a pattern most convenient to the investigator. However, in vivo there may be a predetermined sequence in which the changes usually, or indeed must, take place. As in vitro assays become fully developed, it will be interesting to compare the in vitro and in vivo processes. It will also be of interest to see whether cells in vitro can be blocked at specific steps in the transformation process, and if such treatments can be used to prevent transformation in vivo in individuals at high risk for cancer.

ACKNOWLEDGEMENT

The research from our laboratory reported in this essay was supported by D.O.E. Contract 04659 and D.H.H.S. Grant CA21289 from the National Cancer Institute.

REFERENCES

Barrett, J. C., and Ts'o, P. O. P., 1978, Evidence for the progressive nature of neoplastic transformation in vitro, Proc. Natl. Acad. Sci. (U.S.A.), 75:3761.

Barrett, J. C., Wong, A., and McLachlan, J. A., 1981, Diethylstilbestrol induces neoplastic transformation without measurable gene mutation at two loci, Science, 212:1402.

Bellett, A. J. D., and Younghusband, H. B., 1979, Spontaneous, mutagen-induced and adenovirus-induced anchorage independent tumorigenic variants of mouse cells, J. Cell Physiol., 101:33.

Berwald, Y., and Sachs, L., 1963, In vitro cell transformation with chemical carcinogens, Nature, 200:1182.

Boone, C. W., Takeichi, N., Paranjpe, M., and Gilden, R., 1976, Vasoformative sarcomas arising from BALB/3T3 cells attached to solid substrates, Cancer Res., 36:1626.

Borek, C., 1980, X-ray-induced in vitro neoplastic transformation of human diploid cells, Nature, 283:776.

Borek, C., and Sachs, L., 1966, In vitro cell transformation by x-irradiation, Nature 210:276.

Cuzin, F., Rassoulzadegan, M., and Lemieux, L., 1984, Multigenic control of tumorigenesis: three distinct oncogenes are required for transformation of rat embryo fibroblasts by polyoma virus, in: "Cancer Cells: Oncogenes and Viral Genes," Cold Spring Harbor Laboratory, Cold Spring Harbor, New York.

Druckrey, H., Ivankovic, S., and Preussman, R., 1966, Teratogenic and carcinogenic effects in the offspring after single injection of ethylnitrosourea to pregnant rats, Nature, 210:1378.

Freedman, V., and Shin, S., 1977, Isolation of human diploid cell variants with enhanced colony-forming efficiency in semi-solid medium after a single step chemical mutagenesis: Brief Communication, J. Natl. Cancer Inst., 6:1873.

Fung, Y., Crittenden, L., Fadly, A., and Kung, H., 1983, Tumor induction by direct injection of cloned v-src DNA into chickens, Proc. Natl. Acad. Sci. (U.S.A.), 80:353.

Joseph, L. B., Stephens, R. E., Ottolenghi, A. C., Lipetz, P. D., and Newman, H. A.I., 1983, Morphological transformation of in vitro of normal human fibroblasts of chrysotile, Environ. Hlth. Perspect., 51:17.

Kakunaga, T., 1978, Neoplastic transformation of human diploid fibroblast cells by chemical carcinogens, Proc. Natl. Acad. Sci. (U.S.A.), 75:1334.

Kamen, R., Favaloro, J., Parker, J., Triesman, R., Lania, L., Fried, M., and Mellor, A., 1980, Comparison of polyoma virus transcription in productively infected mouse cells and transformed rodent cell lines, Cold Spring Harbor Symposium Quant. Biol., 44:63.

Land, H., Parada, L. F., Weinberg, R. A., 1983a, Tumorigenic conversion of primary embryo fibroblasts requires at least two cooperating oncogenes, Nature, 304:596.

Land, H. Parada. L. F., and Weinberg, R. A., 1983b, Cellular oncongenes and multistep carcinogenesis, Science, 222:771.

Leavitt, J., Goldman, D., Merril, C., and Kakunaga, T., 1982, Actin mutations in a human fibroblast model for carcinogenesis, Clin. Chem, 28:850.

Maher, V. M., Rowan, L. A., Silinskas, K. C., Kateley, S. A., and McCormick, J. J., 1982, Frequency of UV-induced neoplastic transformation of diploid human fibroblasts is higher in xeroderma pigmentosum cells than in normal cells. Proc. Natl. Acad. Sci. (U.S.A.), 79:2613.

McCormick, J. J., Silinskas, K. C., and Maher, V. M., 1980, Transformation of diploid human fibroblasts by chemical carcinogens. in: "Carcinogenesis: Fundamental Mechanisms and Environmental Effects," 13th Jerusalem Symposium on Quantum Chemistry and Biochemistry, D. Reidel Publ. Co., Dordrecht.

Milo, G. E., and DiPaolo, J. A., 1978, Neoplastic transformation of human diploid cells in vitro after chemical carcinogen treatment, Nature, 175:130.

Milo, G. E., and DiPaolo, J. A., 1980, Presensitization of human cells with extrinsic signals to induced chemical carcinogenesis, Int. J. Cancer, 26:805.

Milo, G. E., Oldham, J. W., Zimmerman, R. Hatch, G. G., and Weisbrode, S. 1981a, Characterization of human cells transformed by chemical and physical carcinogens in vitro, In vitro, 17:719.

Milo, G. E., Weisbrode, S. A., Zimmerman, R., and McCloskey, J. A., 1981b, Ultraviolet radiation-induced neoplastic transformation of normal human cells, in vitro, Chem. Biol. Interactions, 36:45.

Mishra, N., Dunkel, V., and Mehlman, M. (eds.), 1980, "Mammalian Cell Transformation by Chemical Carcinogens," Senate Press, New York.

Miyaki, M., Akamatsu, N. Hirono, U. Ono, T., Tonomura, A., and Utsunomiya, J., 1980, Transformation of fibroblasts from a patient with adenomatosis coli by treatment with a chemical carcinogen, Gann, 71:741.

Miyaki, M. Akamatsu, N. Ono, T., Tonomura, A., and Utsunomiya, J., 1982, Morphological transformation and chromosomal changes induced by chemical carcinogens in skin fibroblasts from patients with familial adenomatosis coli, J. Natl. Cancer Inst., 63:563.

Namba, M. Nishitani, K. Fukishima, F., Kimoto, T., Utsunomiya, J., and Hayflick, L., 1981, Neoplastic transformation of human diploid fibroblasts treated with chemical carcinogens and Co-60 -rays, Gann, 27:221.

Newbold, R. F., Overell, R. W., and Connell, J. R., 1982, Induction of immortality is an early event in malignant transformation of mamalian cells by carcinogens, Nature, 299:633.

Perez-Rodriguez, R., Chambard, J. C., Van Obberghen-Schilling, E., Franchi, A., and Pouyssegur, J., 1981, Emergence of hamster fibroblast tumors in nude mice - evidence for in vitro selection leading to loss of growth factor requirement, J. of Cellul. Phys., 109:387.

Perez-Rodriguez, R., Franchi, A., Deys, B. F., and Pouyssegur, J., 1982, Evidence that hamster fibroblast tumors emerge in nude mice through the process of two in vivo selections leading to growth factor "relaxation" and to immune resistance, Int. J. Cancer, 29:309.

Peto, R. 1977, Epidemiology, multistage models, and short-term mutagenicity tests, in: "Origins of Human Cancer," Cold Spring Harbor Laboratory, Cold Spring Harbor, New York, 1403.

Porter, K. R., Todaro, G. J., and Fonte, V., 1973, A scanning electron microscope study of surface features of viral and spontaneous transformants of mouse BALB/3T3 cells, J. Cell. Biol., 59:633.

Rous, P, and Murphy, J. B., 1911, Tumor implantations in the developing embryo, J. Am. Med. Assoc., 56:741.

Sachs, L. and Medina, D., 1961, In vitro transformation of normal cells by polyoma virus, Nature, 189:457.

Schaeffer, W., 1983, Usage of vertebrate, invertebrate, and plant cell, tissue and organ culture terminology, Tissue Culture Report, 17:19.

Shimada, H., Shibuta, H. and Yoshikawa, M., 1976, Transformation of tissue-cultured xeroderma pigmentosum fibroblasts by treatment with N-methyl-N'-nitro-N-nitrosoguanidine, Nature, 264:547.

Silinskas, K. C., Kateley, S. A., Tower, J. E., Maher, V. M., and McCormick, J. J., 1981, Induction of anchorage-independent growth in human fibroblasts by propane sultone, Cancer Res., 41:1620.

Smith, B. L., and Sager, R., 1982, Multistep origin of tumor-forming ability in Chinese hamster embryo fibroblast cells, Cancer Res., 42:389.

Spandidos, D. A., and Wilkie, N. M., 1984, Malignant transformation of early passage rodent cells by a single mutated human oncogene, Nature, 310:469.

Stoica, G., Koestner, A., and Capen, C., 1984, Neoplasms induced with high single doses of N-ethyl-N-Nitrosourea in 30-day-old Sprague Dawley rats, with special emphasis on mammary neoplasia, Anticancer Research, 4:5.

Sutherland, B. M., Cimino, J. S., Delihas, N. Shih, A. G., and Oliver, R. P., 1980, Ultraviolet light-induced transformation of human cells to anchorage-independent growth, Cancer Res., 40:1934.

Sutherland, B. M., Delihas, N. C., Oliver, R. O., and Sutherland, J. C., 1981, Action spectra for ultra-violet light-induced transformation of humna cells to anchorage-independent growth, Cancer Res,, 41:2211.

Tejwani, R. Witiak, D. T., Inbasekaran, M. N., Cazer, F. D., and Milo, G. E., 1981, Characteristics of benzo(a)pyrene and A-ring reduced 7,12-dimethylbenzo(a)anthracene induced neoplastic transformation of human cells in vitro, Cancer Letters, 13:119.

Thomassen, D. G., and DeMars, R., 1982, Clonal analysis of the stepwise appearance of anchorage independence and tumorigenicity in CAK, a permanent line of mouse cells, Cancer Res., 42:4054.

Tsutsui, T., Maizumi, H., McLachlan, J. A., and Barrett, J. C., 1983, Aneuploidy induction and cell transformation by diethylstilbestrol: a possible choromosomal mechanism in carcinogenesis, Cancer Res., 43:3814.

van der Eb, A. J., van Ormondt, H. Schrier, P. I., Lupker, J. H., Jochemsen, H., van den Elsen, P. J., DeLeys, R. J., Maat, J., van Beveren, C. P., Dijkema, R., and de Waard, A., 1980, Structure and function of the transforming genes of human adenoviruses and SV40, Cold Spring Harbor Symposium Quant. Biol., 44:383.

Watanabe, M., Horikawa, M., and Nikaido, O., 1984, Induction of oncogenic transformation by low doses of x-rays and dose-rate effect, Radiation Res., 98:274.

Weiss, R., Teich, N., Varmus, H., and Coffin, J. (eds.), 1982, "RNA Tumor Viruses," Cold Spring Harbor, New York.

Zimmerman, R. J. and Little J. B., 1981, Starvation for arg and glu sensitizes human diploid cells to the transforming effects of N-acetoxy-2-acetylaminofluorene, Carcinogenesis, 2:1303.

Zimmerman, R. J. and Little J. B., 1983, Characterization of a quantitative assay for in vitro transformation of normal human diploid fibroblasts to anchorage independence by chemical carcinogens, Cancer Res., 43:2176.

Zimmerman, R. J. and Little J. B., 1983, Characteristics of human diploid fibroblasts transformed in vitro by chemical carcinogens, Cancer Res., 43:2182.

PROBLEMS IN DOSE RESPONSE AND RISK ASSESSMENT : THE EXAMPLE OF

ASBESTOS*

Julian Peto

Section of Epidemiology
Institute of Cancer Research
Sutton, Surrey, SM2 5PX
England

The selection of an inappropriate model of carcinogenesis
can lead to gross errors in the predicted effects of exposure to
a carcinogen. For example, the increase in lung cancer incidence
caused by cigarette smoking is approximately proportional to the
product of the dose (number of cigarettes smoked per day) and the
fourth or fifth power of duration of smoking (Doll, 1978; Doll
and Peto, 1978; in fact, the dose-dependence may include linear
and quadratic terms). It is therefore impossible to base useful
predictions on the cumulative dose (total number of cigarettes
smoked), as the eventual risk caused by smoking 10 cigarettes/day
for 40 years may be 50 times greater than that caused by smoking
40 cigarettes/day for 10 years. The term "dose" should therefore
be used only to describe the dose-rate of exposure to a carcinogen
(cigarettes per day, or fibres/ml of asbestos), and the effects
of temporal variables (age, time since first exposure, duration
of exposure) should be examined separately. There is no useful
general formula that describes the effects of all carcinogens.
Asbestos appears to act as an initiator (early stage carcinogen)
in mesothelioma induction but as a promoter (late stage carcinogen)
for lung cancer (Peto et al., 1982); cigarette smoking seems
to both initiate and promote lung cancer induction: and ionising
radiation probably acts primarily at one or more intermediate or
late stages in the induction of most or all carcinomas (Doll, 1978).
These different effects may lead to very different predictions of
lifelong risk, although they can all be explained within the

---

* Originally presented at a meeting at the Banbury Center, Cold
Spring Harbor Laboratory, New York, 11714, 13-16 May 1984.

framework of a simple multi-stage model of carcinogenesis (Day and Brown, 1980).

CANCER INCIDENCE IN ASBESTOS WORKERS

Assumption of Linear Dose-response, Fibre Type Differences and Measures of Exposure

The dependence of lung cancer and mesothelioma incidence rates on age, duration of asbestos exposure and smoking are reasonably well established. Four further assumptions are required for low-dose extrapolation from observations on heavily exposed industrial cohorts, however, and all are open to serious doubt.

1. Linear dose-response is assumed in the following models, but existing exposure data, although consistent with this assumption, are not accurate enough to exclude other models, particularly at low doses.

2. Conditions in most sectors of the asbestos industry have greatly improved, and the working conditions 30 or more years ago that caused very high cancer rates among asbestos workers were measured, if at all, with various instruments that counted particles rather than pathogenic fibres. There is no satisfactory uniform conversion factor from particle to fibre counts, and any estimate of dose-specific risk under current working conditions is therefore extremely unreliable.

3. The observed increase in lung cancer risk at the same nominal level of exposure varies more than 50-fold between different cohorts, such as chrysotile (white asbestos) miners and U.S. chrysotile textile workers (McDonald et al., 1983) and it is not clear which provides the best estimate for other conditions of industrial or environmental exposure. Dose-specific lung cancer rates are given below to illustrate the qualitative implications of the assumed models, but these figures, although compatible with certain published studies, are not intended as "best estimates" that can be applied generally.

4. Crocidolite (blue asbestos) appears to be particularly liable to cause mesothelioma, and it is suspected that at least some mesothelioma among workers exposed principally to chrysotile with occasional exposure to crocidolite are due to the effects of crocidolite. Few formal estimates of the dose-specific mesothelioma risk have been published, however, and the mesothelioma rates assumed below have been chosen to make the predicted mesothelioma risk among men first exposed to asbestos at age 20 approximately half the predicted lung cancer excess,

which is similar to the ratio observed among insulation workers
exposed to a mixture of fibre types. They may therefore be too
high for chrysotile but too low for crocidolite.

Age and Time Dependence

Mesothelioma incidence rises sharply with time since first
exposure to asbestos but is unrelated to age at first exposure or
smoking, while lung cancer incidence is strongly related to both
smoking and age, as well as to time since first exposure. The
differential effects of these relationships in North American
insulation workers are shown in Table 1. The rate of mesothelioma
to excess lung cancer (observed minus expected) was more than 4:1
in non-smokers, about 1:2 in smokers first exposed to asbestos below
age 25, and about 1:4 in smokers first exposed at age 25 or over
(Peto et al., 1982). The relative risk for lung cancer (observed/
expected) was however virtually the same irrespective of age or
cigarette smoking, which suggests that asbestos simply multiplies
the lung cancer risk caused by natural or other processes. (Note that
the expected numbers in Table 1 are smoking-specific; a relative risk
of 2 would thus mean that asbestos exposure increases the risk of
developing lung cancer from about 1 in 200 to about 1 in 100 in
non-smokers, and from about 1 in 10 to about 1 in 5 in smokers.)

Table 1. Observed and expected deaths due to lung cancer and
deaths due to mesothelioma among North American
insulation workers (Peto et al., 1982).

	Lung Cancer				Mesoth-elioma	Ratio of mesothelioma to excess lung cancer
	Obs	Exp*	Obs/Exp*	Obs-Exp*	Obs	
Smokers aged under 25 at first exposure	211	32.67	6.5	178.33	99	0.56
Smokers aged 25 or over at first exposure	237	48.05	4.9	188.95	48	0.25
Non-smokers (all ages)	5	1.04	4.8	3.96	18	4.55

* Expected numbers are smoking-specific

A Model for Lung Cancer

The relative risk for lung cancer increases with both dose and
duration of asbestos exposure, and a simple model that is now widely
accepted, at least as a useful approximation, for the resulting
incidence I_A in asbestos workers of a given age, history of smoking
and asbestos exposure is

$$I_A = I_U [k_L (f.d)+1],$$

where f is the average exposure level in fibre/ml, d is duration of
exposure, k_L is a constant that probably depends on fibre dimension
and type, and I_U is the 'normal' lung cancer incidence among
unexposed individuals of the same age and smoking history (Peto, 1978).
This model can be modified in various ways to accommodate the delay
of about 10 years before the maximum relative risk caused by brief
intense exposure is reached (Seidman et al., 1979) and the
observation in several cohorts that the relative risk eventually
falls (Walker, 1984). The effects of such adjustments are however
likely to be smaller than the uncertainty in the appropriate value
of k_L.

As the majority of lung cancers in both smokers and non-smokers
occur in old age, this model implies that the lifelong risk caused
by asbestos exposure will be virtually independent of age at exposure
and will be almost proportional to eventual cumulative dose. It
should perhaps be emphasised that the average age at which asbestos-
induced lung cancers occur will under this model be virtually the
same as that of lung cancers in unexposed individuals, even if
asbestos exposure occurs only in childhood or throughout life due
to ambient exposure.

To illustrate the calculation, suppose that the risk of dying
of lung cancer is 0.5% among non-smokers and 10% among moderate
smokers, and that the relative risk for lung cancer is increased by
2.0 (i.e. from 1.0 to about 3.0) by a cumulative exposure of 200
fibre/ml years. (This would correspond to 20 years at an average
level of 10 fibre/ml, which is typical of the exposure conditions
in certain factories 30 or 40 years ago.) Twenty years' exposure
to a level of 0.001 fibre/ml (about 10,000 times lower than
industrial conditions in the past) throughout the working day would
therefore produce an increase in relative risk of 2.0/10,000, or
0.0002, and the increase in life-long lung cancer risk would be
about 2 in 10^5 in smokers and about 1 in 10^6 in non-smokers. For
ambient exposure at this level 7 days a week throughout the day
and night for 20 years these estimates would be increased by a
factor of about 5, and for lifelong ambient exposure by a further
factor of about 3 or 4. The lifelong risks for various durations
of exposure corresponding to these assumptions are shown in
Table 2.

Table 2. Predicted excess numbers of deaths before age 80 among 1,000 men due to lung cancer (LC) or mesothelioma (M) caused by asbestos exposure during working hours at 1.0 fibres/ml. (Calculated from the models described in the text, using current England and Wales male death-rates for lung cancer and all causes)

Age at first exposure (years)		Duration of exposure (years)			
		5	10	20	40
0	LC:	3.7	7.3	14.4	28.4
	M:	7.5	13.1	20.1	24.7
20	LC:	3.7	7.4	14.7	27.4
	M:	2.1	3.5	5.0	5.6
40	LC:	3.7	7.3	13.2	16.8
	M:	0.3	0.5	0.6	0.7

A Model for Mesothelioma

For both pleural and peritoneal mesothelioma the incidence appears to be proportional to the third or fourth power of time since first exposure irrespective of duration of exposure, age or cigarette smoking (Peto et al., 1982), although the magnitude of the risk is of course related both to level and to duration of exposure. A simple model that predicts this sort of pattern is that the risk is increased by each day of exposure by an amount proportional to the level of exposure on that day and to the cube of time since that day. For an exposure of duration T_0 years at a constant level of f fibre/ml, the incidence T years after first exposure will then be given by the formula

$$I = f.k_M [T^4 - (T-T_0)^4],$$

where k_M is a constant that depends on fibre dimension and type. It is not clear to what extent the incidence of pleural mesothelioma differs between fibre types for a given fibre concentration and size distribution, although peritoneal mesothelioma is almost never caused by exposure to pure chrysotile.

Predicted lifelong risks for different durations of exposure and ages at first exposure are shown in Table 2. These suggest that the mesothelioma risk increases in approximate proportion to duration for exposures of up to about 10 years, but then rises more

179

slowly, and is not greatly increased by continuing exposure beyond about 20 years. The model also implies that the lifelong risk for mesothelioma will be very much greater if exposure occurs early in life. Ambient exposure in childhood may cause similar risks for lung cancer and mesothelioma among smokers, and in non-smokers, as Table 1 suggests, the mesothelioma risk will probably exceed the lung cancer risk irrespective of age at first exposure.

NICKEL REFINING

The very high lung and nasal sinus cancer rates suffered in the past by nickel refinery workers provide a further example of site-specific differences in incidence patterns (Table 3; Peto et al., 1984). Working conditions in this factory had greatly improved by 1930, and high cancer risks occurred only in men first exposed before about 1925. Follow-up began in 1934 and was thus restricted to men whose exposure had virtually ceased. The subsequent absolute excess risk for lung cancer was approximately constant beyond 30 years after first exposure and was unrelated to age at first exposure. In contrast, for nasal sinus cancer the risk was very much higher in those first exposed at older ages, and continued to rise sharply for at least 50 years.

Table 3. Estimated lung (LC) and nasal sinus (NS) cancer death rates in pre-1925 Welsh nickel refinery workers (relative rates adjusted for period and intensity of exposure; see Peto et al., 1984).

Age at first exposure (years)		Years since first exposure				
		Under 20	20–	30–	40–	50 or over
Under 25	LC:	1.0	2.9	5.5	6.0	4.8
	NS:	1.0	4.7	6.2	12.5	16.7
25 – 34	LC:	1.3	3.7	7.0	7.6	6.0
	NS:	3.0	13.8	18.3	37.0	49.3
35 or over	LC:	1.3	3.7	6.9	7.5	6.0
	NS:	10.0	46.8	61.9	125.4	167.2

MODELS OF CARCINOGENESIS

The multi-stage model of carcinogenesis, according to which a normal cell must undergo an ordered sequence of heritable changes to become a cancer cell, predicts that agents acting at the first stage will cause a cancer incidence roughly proportional to a power of time since first exposure independent of age at exposure, while the cancer risk caused by agents acting at a later stage will appear more quickly and will be greater when exposure occurs at older ages (Day and Brown, 1980). The pattern of mesothelioma incidence therefore suggests that asbestos acts at the first stage in carcinogenesis, while the lung cancer pattern suggests that it acts at a later stage. It is thus impossible to classify carcinogens as early or late acting, except in relation to particular types of tumour. This is a further limitation on any extrapolation from animal data to predict human cancer risks, particularly when the route of administration or tumour type are not the same. Carcinogenicity experiments are rarely conducted on large enough numbers of animals of various ages for such differences to be studied at all, but even if they were it is not at all certain that the cancer incidence patterns in man would be similar to those observed in the laboratory. Moreover, the striking differences in both age and time dependence between lung cancers and mesotheliomas in asbestos workers and between lung and nasal sinus cancers in nickel refiners, together with laboratory evidence that various carcinogens act at more than one stage in carcinogenesis, suggest that such heterogeneity of effect is probably the rule rather than the exception (Peto, 1985).

Initiation and Promotion

The current fashion for classifying agents as initiators or promoters on the basis of experimental studies and inferring that a certain pattern of dose or time dependence will necessarily be observed in man, and in particular the suggestion that promoters are likely to exhibit a dose threshold, are of dubious relevance to risk assessment. The terms "initiation" and "promotion" were coined to describe the effect whereby exposure to one agent followed later by exposure to another causes a very much greater tumour incidence in experimental animals than the same agents applied in the opposite order. It was therefore natural that the same terms should be adopted to describe epidemiological observations suggesting early or late effects in a multi-stage process, but it cannot be assumed that this speculative analogy implies any particular mode of action.

Duration of Exposure

The "natural" incidence of many cancers increases in proportion to the fifth or higher power of age, and the conventional explanation

of this phenomenon is that the background rates at which the
different cellular accidents postulated by the multi-stage model
occur remain roughly constant throughout life. The implications
of this effect in relation to duration of exposure to a carcinogen
are however uncertain. An agent that acts only at the first stage
would be expected to produce a cancer rate similar to that of
mesothelioma, rising very sharply with time since first exposure but
increasing sub-linearly with increasing duration of exposure. For
agents that act at several stages, however, the risk will be very
much greater when exposure is prolonged, as the lung cancer risk is
among continuing smokers. Ionising radiation provides a nice example
of this problem. Conventional calculations of the cancer risk at a
given total dose have been based almost entirely on the effects of
brief exposure from nuclear weapons or therapeutic irradiation. If
the biological effects of radiation were analogous to those of smoking,
however, prolonged exposure to the same total dose might cause a
very much higher cancer risk than these brief intense exposures. The
limited data on humans and animals who have suffered prolonged low-
level irradiation do not in fact indicate that the risk at a given
total dose is increased enormously; but it is remarkable that this
major weakness in the assumptions implicit in the conventional risk
calculation should have received so little attention, and further
studies of the effects of chronic irradiation would certainly be
worthwhile.

PERCEPTION AND ACCEPTANCE OF RISK

     A curious aspect of risk assessment is that the actual value
of the calculated risk is almost universally ignored. In view of
the dubious nature of such calculations it could be argued that this
is just as well; but until the meaning of a risk of 10^{-1}, 10^{-3} or
10^{-6} is better understood, slogans such as 'one asbestos fibre can
kill' will continue to dominate the public debate. The history
of asbestos control provides one example of the irrational way in
which risks may be ignored or exaggerated, but there are many others.

Environmental and Industrial Asbestos Exposure

     In the case of asbestos, direct observation showed that about
20 years' exposure at an average level of the order of 10 fibres/ml
had caused substantial risks, and the resulting prediction that a
working lifetime at 2 fibres/ml (the asbestos standard in force in
Britain until 2 years ago) might cause a risk of the order of 1 in 10
therefore seemed unlikely to be wrong in either direction by a large
factor (Peto, 1978). This dose-specific risk estimate was however
based on a study in an asbestos textile factory, and subsequent
studies in other working environments suggested lower dose-specific
risks. Using one of the higher risk estimates and assuming linear

dose-response leads to the prediction that the average asbestos levels usually encountered in schools and other buildings containing asbestos will cause a risk of the order of 10^{-5}. (Ontario Royal Commission, 1984. The level in such buildings is usually less than 0.001 fibres/ml, counting fibres longer than 5μm and having an aspect ratio exceeding 3 to 1 with an electron microscope. The same criterion based on optical microscopy is used for industrial measurements, but as very fine fibres cannot be seen with an optical microscope the "optical equivalent" count in buildings would be even lower.) I do not know what proportion of the British or U.S. population live or work in buildings containing substantial amounts of asbestos, but if it is about one in five a risk of the order of 10^{-5} would correspond to about one excess death per year in Britain, and about four in the U.S. The dust levels and extent of exposure assumed in this calculation need to be properly estimated by further surveys, but unless they can be shown to be much too low my personal view is that the wholesale removal of asbestos now occurring in Britain and the U.S. is in most buildings an unjustified waste of money. I would not object to myself or my own family being exposed to a risk of this order, and nor, I suspect, would most people if they understood what it means. A smoker probably reduces his life-long risk by about 10^{-5} by smoking one less cigarette a year.

This is an interesting example, as the conclusions are of immediate practical importance. It is my personal judgment that the predicted risk is unlikely to be much too low, and thus provides a sensible basis for policy decisions; but I reached this conclusion by offsetting the conservative aspects of the calculation (ignoring the progressive reduction in the relative risk for lung cancer observed after exposure ceases, and using one of the highest reasonable dose-specific risk estimates) against its obvious uncertainties (the dubious quality and comparability of the exposure estimates, and linear extrapolation over four orders of magnitude), and such a process cannot be justified formally.

The sequel to the asbestos story is also instructive. The industrial risk, which in my opinion was unacceptably high, was not adequately controlled in Britain until several years after it was recognised, and then only in response to a media scare, while the minute environmental risk generated an hysterical over-reaction which still continues. Informed public debate would probably have led to the opposite response in both cases, with much quicker industrial action and a more balanced environmental response. Few people have any clear idea of the meaning or magnitude of everyday risks. A substantial proportion of Americans have now rejected smoking, but as saccharin was rejected with almost equal fervour this can hardly be attributed to a cool appraisal of the evidence, and most smokers are still not aware that about one in four of them will be killed by the habit.

DISCUSSION

Predicted risks due to agents such as cigarette smoke or asbestos for which there are extensive epidemiological data should certainly be calculated from an appropriate model. For carcinogens for which such data are not available, however, the examples discussed above merely indicate that model-dependent error must be added to the many other uncertainties that such extrapolation entails. It would evidently be prudent to assume a "most pessimistic" model, and the assumption that the increase in relative risk will remain after exposure ceases may for most carcinogens provide a useful upper limit, but this is of little practical value in relation to agents for which there are no epidemiological data, as relative risks in animals and humans are unlikely to be similar. There are, however, several known carcinogens for which better information on the dependence on age and duration of exposure and the evolution of risk after exposure ceases could be obtained, either by re-examining existing data or by further studies. The collation of such results, together with similar data on the effects of the same agents in animals, would be a useful exercise.

It is very much easier to dismiss risk assessment out of hand than to criticise it constructively, as the mode of carcinogenic action, the measures of dose, and above all the validity of extrapolation from mouse or salmonella to man are for many agents so uncertain that it can be equally plausibly argued either that the risk is unacceptable or that it is negligible. The problem is real, however, and independent scientists can and must be influential in the debate between a conservative industry, erratic regulatory policy and campaigning zealots, although most of this audience must know from personal experience that it is extremely difficult to be objective when the choice between plausible assumptions is so arbitrary. For the next decade or two we can only refine the rules of risk assessment, ensure that they are observed and await the day when the molecular basis of carcinogenesis is finally understood. The risk assessment game will then no longer be played, and its passing will be mourned only by those who weren't fit to play it anyway.

REFERENCES

Day, N.E., and Brown, C.C.,1980, Multistage models and primary prevention of cancer, J. Natl. Cancer Inst., 64 No.4: 977.
Doll, R., 1978, An epidemiological perspective of the biology of cancer, Cancer Res., 38:3573.
Doll, R., and Peto, R., 1978, Cigarette smoking and bronchial carcinoma: dose and time relationship among regular smokers and lifelong non-smokers, J. Epidemiol. Community Health, 32:303.

McDonald, A.D., Fry, J.S., Wooley, A.J., and McDonald, J.C., 1983, Dust exposures and mortality in an American chrysotile textile plant, Brit. J. Industr. Med., 40:361.

Ontario Royal Commission, 1984, Report of the Royal Commission on matters of health and safety arising from the use of asbestos in Ontario (3 vols.), Ontario Ministry of the Attorney General.

Peto, J., 1978, The hygiene standard for chrysotile asbestos, Lancet, i:484.

Peto, J., Seidman, H., and Selikoff, I.J., 1982, Mesothelioma mortality in asbestos workers: implications for models of carcinogenesis and risk assessment, Br. J. Cancer, 45:124.

Peto, J., Cuckle, H., Doll, R., Hermon, C., and Morgan, L.G., 1984, Respiratory cancer mortality of Welsh nickel refinery workers, in:"Nickel in the Human Environment,"F.W. Sunderman, ed., I.A.R.C. Scientific Publications No.53, p37, International Agency for Research on Cancer, Lyon.

Peto, J., 1985, Early and late stage carcinogenesis in mouse skin and in man, in:"Models, Mechanisms and Aetiology of Tumour Promotion,"M. Börzsönyi, N.E. Day, K. Lapis, and H. Yamasaki, eds., I.A.R.C. Scientific Publications No. 56, p359. International Agency for Research on Cancer, Lyon.

Seidman, H., Selikoff, I.J., and Hammond, E.C., 1979, Short-term asbestos work and long-term observation, Ann. N.Y. Acad. Sci., 339:61.

Walker, A.M., 1984, Declining relative risks for lung cancer after cessation of asbestos exposure, J. Occup. Med., 26:422.

ROLE OF DNA DAMAGE AND REPAIR IN THE MUTAGENESIS OF HUMAN CELLS

BY CARCINOGENS

Veronica M. Maher and J. Justin McCormick

Carcinogenesis Laboratory - Fee Hall
Department of Microbiology and Department of
Biochemistry
Michigan State University
East Lansing, MI   48824-1316

INTRODUCTION

It is clear from numerous studies on the induction of cancer in animals and from epidemiologic studies, as well as from recent studies with cells in culture, that carcinogenesis is a multi-stepped process. Although studies with animals are indispensable in analyzing many aspects of carcinogenesis, the use of cells in culture permits a more direct experimental manipulation and quantitation of the individual steps involved and can yield information on the nature of these steps (cf. McCormick and Maher, this volume). Another reason for using cells in culture is that this permits experimental studies with <u>human</u> cells which would otherwise be impossible for obvious ethical reasons.

As part of our on-going studies of the mechanisms of carcinogenesis, we and our co-workers have examined the effects of DNA damage and DNA repair-processes on the induction of mutations and transformation in diploid human fibroblasts by chemical carcinogens and radiation. The results of a series of investigations comparing cells with normal rates of DNA repair and repair-deficient cells indicate that cell killing, mutations, and transformation to anchorage independence are directly related to the number of DNA lesions remaining unrepaired in the cell at critical times posttreatment. DNA repair in human fibroblasts acts to eliminate potentially cytotoxic, mutagenic, and transforming damage from DNA before these can be transformed into permanent cellular effects.

COMPARING CELLS THAT DIFFER IN RATE OF DNA NUCLEOTIDE EXCISION REPAIR

The source of diploid human fibroblasts with a normal capacity for excision repair was skin biopsies from normal persons or circumcision material from newborn males. Skin fibroblasts from patients with xeroderma pigmentosum (XP) disease provided the DNA repair-deficient cells. These XP patients are characterized by an inherited pre-disposition to sunlight-induced skin cancer. Their cells are deficient in ability to carry out nucleotide excision repair of ultraviolet light-induced DNA damage and have been classified into complementation groups which differ in their rates of excision (Cleaver and Bootsma, 1975). In our studies the cytotoxic effect of various agents was determined from loss of ability to form a colony. The genetic marker used was resistance to 8-azaguanine (AG) or 6-thioguanine (TG), the result of any kind of mutation that causes inactivation of the gene coding for hypoxanthine(guanine)phosphoribosyltransfer-ase (HPRT) (see McCormick and Maher, 1981 for experimental details).

To investigate the effect of DNA excision repair on the cytotoxicity and mutagenicity of ultraviolet (UV) radiation, we irradiated a strain of XP cells that are virtually incapable of excision repair (XP12BE cells, from complementation group A); a strain of XP cells with an excision rate approximately 20% that of normal (XP2BE, from complementation group C) and cells with a normal rate of excision (derived from the foreskin of a normal neonate). The results (Figure 1) indicated a dose-dependent increase in cell killing and mutations in all three strains, but the normally-excising cells were far more resistant than the repair-deficient XP cells. At low doses, e.g., 0.5 J/m^2, the strain that cannot remove UV-induced pyrimidine dimers (XP12BE) showed a survival of 6%; the cells with some residual repair capacity (XP2BE) showed a survival of 30%; whereas the normal cells with rapid excision repair had 100% survival. A similar effect was seen for mutation induction. At low doses mutations were induced in the XP cells at high frequencies, but the normal cells did not exhibit any measureable increase in mutations to AG resistance. Only when exposed to much higher doses of UV did the normal cells show a response. This is the result expected if there is a certain amount of time available for excision repair between the UV irradiation and the critical cellular events responsible for cell killing and mutation induction. The faster a cell can remove the potentially lethal and/or mutagenic damage from DNA, the lower the degree of cell killing and mutations. Thus, excision repair acts not to introduce mutations, but to prevent them.

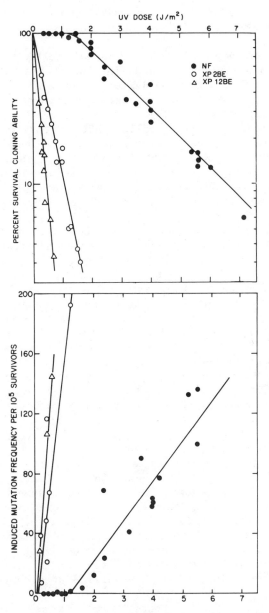

Fig. 1. Comparison of the cytotoxic and mutagenic effect of increasing doses of UV radiation in normal human skin fibroblasts (NF) and in XP cells with an excision rate ~20% that of normal (XP2BE) or with little or no detectable excision-repair capacity (XP12BE). Cells were plated into culture dishes at appropriate densities, allowed ~12 hr to attach, irradiated, and allowed to develop into colonies. Selection in situ with 20uM 8-azaguanine was begun after 5-8 days of expression. (Taken from Maher, et al., 1979, with permission).

EFFECT OF LENGTHENING THE TIME BETWEEN EXPOSURE TO THE DNA DAMAGING AGENT AND THE ONSET OF DNA SYNTHESIS

XP cells do not differ from normal cells in the initial number of photolesions induced in their DNA by particular doses of UV radiation, but do differ in rate of excision repair of such damage. Therefore, the data in Figure 1 suggest that the loss of ability to form a clone and the frequency of mutations induced in these cells reflect the average number of lesions remaining unexcised in the DNA at the time of some "critical event". We hypothesized that this event was semi-conservative DNA synthesis (S-phase). This hypothesis predicts that if UV-irradiated cells are prevented from replicating for various lengths of time post-irradiation, normal cells with their rapid rate of repair and even those XP cells with residual repair capacity (slower than normal rate) would exhibit a higher survival and lower frequency of mutants than if the radiation were given to the cells in exponential growth. No such difference should be seen with the XP12BE cells which are essentially incapable of repair. To test this, a series of cultures were grown to confluence and starved for mitogens until they ceased replicating (G_0 state) (Maher et al., 1979). They were irradiated with a dose that had been shown to reduce their survival to $\sim 25\%$ of the unirradiated control. One set was immediately released from confluence and allowed to cycle and assayed for cell killing and for mutations. The other sets were maintained in the non-replicating state and released after various hours in confluence.

The results showed a gradual increase in the percent survival of the normal cells and the XP cells with a slow rate of repair. The cells held in confluence and allowed to repair for 24 hr showed 100% survival upon release from G_0. But there was no change in the percent survival of the XP12BE cells (Maher et al., 1979). Similarly, the frequency of mutants induced in the XP12BE cells did not decrease with time held in confluence post-irradiation. But the frequency of mutants gradually decreased in the normal cells until by 24 hr, it was equal to that of the unirradiated control.

In a separate study, Konze-Thomas et al. (1979) in our laboratory showed that UV-irradiated normal human cells, maintained in this non-replicating state, were capable of excision of pyrimidine dimers and of incorporating thymidine into parental strands of DNA (repair replication). However, it was not possible to measure the rate of excision of these DNA lesions at very low doses of UV light, i.e., the doses used for the biological studies. Therefore, we carried out similar investigations with normal and XP12BE cells using chemical carcinogens that cause lesions in DNA that resemble in some fashion the kinds of damage induced in DNA by pyrimidine dimers. We showed that XP cells from various complementation groups are much more sensitive than normal cells to the cytotoxic and mutagenic effect of these agents. Examples are reactive derivatives of aromatic amides (Maher et al., 1975, Heflich et al., 1980, Maher et al., 1981); polycyclic aromatic hydrocarbons (Maher et al., 1977; Heflich et al., 1977, Yang et al., 1980); and aflatoxin (Mahoney et al., 1984).

Using radioactive labeled 7,8-diol-9,10-epoxide of benzo(a)pyrene (BPDE) of high specific activity, it was possible determine that the kinetics of recovery of human cells from the potentially lethal and potentially mutagenic lesions induced by BPDE was highly correlated with the kinetics of removal of the covalently-bound residues (adducts) from DNA (see Figure 2). For this study, normal and excision repair-minus XP12BE cells were grown to confluence, starved for mitogens for 72 hr and treated with radioactive BPDE. A concentration of 0.2uM and 0.3uM was used for the normal cells in order that the survival of the cells assayed immediately would be 27% and 12%, respectively. The XP12BE cells were treated with a much lower concentration (0.025uM) so that their survival would also be 27%. One set of each treated series was harvested immediately after the 2 hr exposure to BPDE and analyzed for the number of BPDE residues bound per 10^6 DNA nucleotides (middle panel of Fig. 2) and for percent survival (upper panel) and mutant frequency (lower panel). The rest were similarly assayed after 2, 4, or 8 days in confluence posttreatment.

The results showed that BPDE adducts were gradually removed from the DNA of the normal cells over a period of 4 days, but then excision slowed. Similarly, the extent of cell killing and the mutant frequency in cells released from confluence on Day 2 or 4 were decreased compared to those assayed on Day 0, but this decrease slowed considerably after Day 4. There was no loss of adducts from the DNA of the XP12BE cells with time held in the resting (G_0) state and no change in survival or mutant frequency. Thus, excision repair protects the normal cells by reducing the number of potentially cytotoxic and mutagenic lesions (adducts) remaining in the cells' DNA.

EFFECT OF SHORTENING THE TIME AVAILABLE FOR EXCISION REPAIR BEFORE THE ONSET OF DNA SYNTHESIS

These results supported the hypothesis that the cells' rate of excision repair and the time available for repair

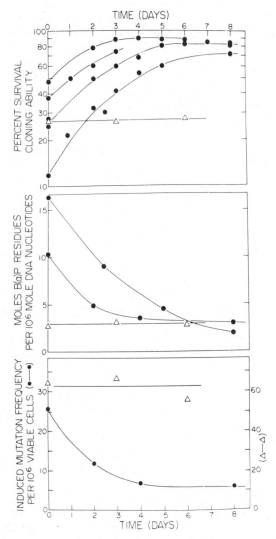

Fig. 2. Kinetics of removal of covalently bound adducts (middle panel) and recovery of normal (circles) or XP12BE cells (triangles) from the potentially cytotoxic (upper panel) or mutagenic (lower panel) effects of BPDE. The cells were treated in the G_0 state, released on the designated days, and assayed for survival of colony-forming ability, for the number of residues bound to DNA, and after a suitable expression period, for the frequency of induced mutations to TG resistance. (Taken from Yang, et al., 1980, with permission).

before some critical cellular event, such as DNA synthesis on a template containing DNA lesions (photoproducts or adducts), was responsible for determining the ultimate biological consequences of exposure to DNA damaging agents. However, it was clear that the frequency of mutants induced in cells treated in confluence and released immediately was much lower than what was found for cells treated in exponential growth (data not shown). Investigation (Watanabe et al., 1984) showed that confluent cells released from the resting G_0 state by being plated at lower cell density, e.g., 10^4 cells/cm^2, are synchronized and proceed as a cohort through G_1 phase and enter S-phase synchronously about 16 hr later. (If cells are plated at still lower densities, S-phase does not begin until~22 hr after release (Konze-Thomas et al., 1982, Yang, et al., 1982).

We hypothesized that the low frequency of mutants observed in cells treated in confluence and immediately released reflected the degree of excision repair that took place during G_1 phase before the potentially mutagenic DNA adducts could be converted into a mutation during S-phase. If so, it should be possible to synchronize cells in this way and vary the time available for excision repair by treating the cells just prior to the onset of S-phase or 16, 18, or 24 hr earlier. If DNA synthesis were the critical cellular event, normal cells treated just before the gene for HPRT was to be replicated during S-phase might be much more sensitive to mutation induction than cells treated in early G_1.

Figure 3 (lower panel) shows the result of such a study using UV radiation as the DNA damaging agent (Konze-Thomas et al., 1982). A similar result was found by Yang et al. (1982) and by Watanabe et al. (1984) with BPDE. The slope of the curve for induced mutant frequency in cells treated at the beginning of S-phase was 8-fold higher than that of cells treated 18 hr earlier in the cell cycle. Cells treated in confluence and released to proceed through the cycle to begin S-phase after ~ 24 hr showed still lower frequencies. No such difference in induced mutant frequencies was found for the XP12BE cells.

As can be seen in the upper panel of Figure 3, although the cytotoxic effect of UV in the normal cells was much less than in the excision repair-minus XP cells, there was no significant cell cycle dependence. Cells irradiated at the onset of S-phase or 18 hr prior to the onset of S-phase showed the same survival. Cells irradiated in the confluent state and released by plating at cloning density appeared to be somewhat less sensitive, but studies indicated that part of

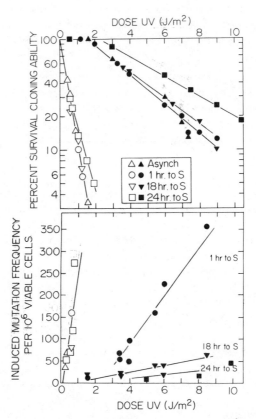

Fig. 3. Cytotoxicity and mutagenicity of UV in normal (closed symbols) or XP12BE cells (open symbols) irradiated under conditions designed to allow various lengths of time for excision repair to take place prior to the onset of S-phase. Cells irradiated in confluence (G_0) and immediately plated at lower densities to begin S-phase after 24 hr ($\square$, $\blacksquare$); cells released from G_0 and irradiated 6 hr later (18 hr to S-phase) ($\triangledown$, $\blacktriangledown$); cells released and irradiated 24 hr later just at the beginning of S-phase ($\bigcirc$, $\bullet$); cells replated from asynchronously growing cultures, and irradiated 16 hr later ($\triangle$, $\blacktriangle$). (Taken from Konze-Thomas et al., 1982, with permission.)

this resistance results from the shielding effect of cells in the confluent cultures. These results suggest that S-phase is responsible for the induction of the mutations and that the frequency of mutants is directly related to the number of unexcised lesions remaining at the time the cell begins to replicate its DNA. However, something other than DNA replication is responsible for the cell killing by these agents.

We interpreted these results as follows: After DNA is damaged by these agents, the time available for repair of potentially lethal lesions is determined by the cell's need for critical cellular proteins and their respective mRNA's. If the DNA template for transcription of these mRNA's by RNA polymerase is still blocked by lesions at the time the cell has need of them, reproductive death (i.e., inability to form a colony) is the result. This would explain why holding cells for a few days in a resting state following exposure to DNA damaging agents before releasing them into the cycling state results in a higher survival than does immediate release. Cells held in confluence have a lower metabolic state than do cells in exponential growth and, therefore, following treatment fewer critical proteins are needed before the cell has time to remove the blocking DNA damage. We suggest that reproductive death from exposure to UV-radiation or these chemical agents results indirectly from faulty or blocked transcription from DNA containing photoproducts or adducts because of the resulting lack of required protein synthesis. This conclusion is consistent with the fact that the XP12BE cells which do not remove such lesions from their DNA show no dose modifying effect on being held in the G_0 state (Maher et al., 1979, Yang et al., 1980).

EFFECT OF EXCISION REPAIR ON THE FREQUENCY OF TRANSFORMATION OF HUMAN CELLS

We have recently succeeded in inducing loss of anchorage dependence in normal diploid human fibroblasts following exposure to chemical carcinogens (Silinskas et al., 1981, Maher et al., 1982). Cells capable of forming colonies in semi-solid medium (soft agar) were produced with high frequency and in a dose dependent manner. The cells derived from such colonies were isolated, propagated and assayed for ability to form tumors upon injection subcutaneously into sublethally X-irradiated athymic mice. In many instances tumors arose at the site of injection within a few weeks. These attained a maximum size of 7 to 10mm in diameter and then stopped growing and eventually regressed. We suggest that acquisition of anchorage independence is a preliminary or initial step in

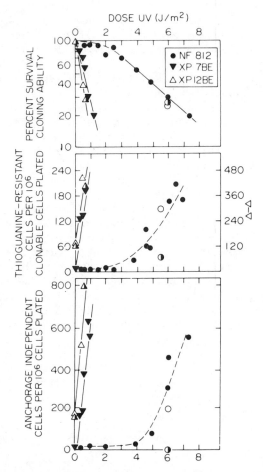

Fig. 4. Cytotoxicity, mutagenicity, and transforming activity of UV radiation in normal (circles) and XP cells (XP12BE, triangles; XP7BE, inverted triangles). The frequency of TG resistant cells was assayed after 6 doublings; that of anchorage independent cells after 9 doublings. Solid symbols, populations irradiated in exponential growth; open symbols, cells synchronized by release after confluence and irradiated shortly before onset of S-phase; half-solid symbols, cells irradiated 18-20 hrs prior to S-phase. (Figure taken from McCormick and Maher, 1983, with permission.)

the transformation of normal human fibroblasts and that cells with this property are partially transformed (see McCormick and Maher, this volume). We suggest, further, that acquisition of this particular phenotype occurs as the result of a mutagenic event (see below).

The role of excision repair in preventing induction of anchorage independence was investigated by exposing normal human cells and XP cells from complementation groups A and D to UV radiation (Figure 4). The XP cells irradiated with 8- to 10-fold lower doses of UV than the normal cells exhibited approximately the same degree of cell killing, the same frequency of mutations to TG resistance, and, more importantly, the same frequency of UV-induced anchorage independent cells in the population as did the normal cells. As discussed above, this is the result expected if induction of anchorage independence as well as thioguanine resistance results ultimately from DNA damage remaining unexcised in the cell at some critical time after irradiation and if, because of the difference in their respective rates of excision repair, the average number of lesions remaining at this critical time is approximately equal in the three populations.

If, like TG resistance, anchorage independence results from an event "fixed" during semi-conservative DNA synthesis on a template which still contains unexcised lesions, the frequency of such cells should be much higher in populations of normal human cells UV-irradiated just before the onset of S-phase than in cells irradiated 18 to 20 hr prior to S-phase. XP12BE cells should not show such a cell-cycle dependence. We tested this prediction and found it to be correct. The results are included in Figure 4 as open and half-solid symbols. The transformation frequencies of the normal cells irradiated with 6 J/m^2 ~3 hr prior to onset of S-phase yielded 200 anchorage independent cells per 10^6 cells plated; the cells irradiated 18 hr prior to onset of S-phase showed no colonies per 10^6 cells plated; the control cells in this experiment also gave no colonies out of 2 x 10^6. In contrast, the frequency of anchorage independent cells in the XP12BE population irradiated in early G_1 did not decrease; in fact it was somewhat higher. In the corresponding mutation experiment, the frequencies of thioguanine resistant XP12BE cells irradiated at the two times were equal. In the mutagenesis experiments with normal cells from which the data in the middle panel were taken, the frequency of mutant cells did not decrease completely to the background level. However, in this particular mutagenesis experiment, the cells irradiated in G_1 had somewhat less time for excision repair before onset of S than was available in the transformation experiments.

The fact that allowing substantial time for excision before DNA synthesis eliminated the potentially mutagenic and transforming effect of UV radiation in normal cells, but not in XP12BE cells, suggests that DNA synthesis on a template still containing unexcised lesions is the cellular event responsible for "fixing" the mutations and transformation.

EFFECT OF REPAIR OF O^6 METHYL GUANINE IN HUMAN CELLS TREATED WITH METHYLATING AGENTS

Recently, Domoradzki et al. (1984) investigated the biological significance of another type of DNA repair system, i.e., O^6-methylguanine DNA methyltransferase (MT), an acceptor protein that specifically removes methyl groups from the O^6 position of guanine in alkylated DNA. Three human cell lines were identified as being extremely deficient in this methyltransferase activity. One is an XP cell line (XP12RO) transformed to a infinite life span by Simian virus 40 (SV40); one, GM3314 from the Institute of Medical Research (Camden, NJ), is a fibroblast cell line from a skin biopsy of a patient with an inherited predisposition to colon cancer (Gardner's syndrome) and one, GM0011 from Camden, is a skin fibroblast cell line from an apparently normal fetus. A fourth cell line obtained by SV40 virus transformation of normal fibroblasts (GM637), exhibited an intermediate level of methyltransferase activity. The level of MT activity was measured using high pressure liquid chromatography to determine the number of methylated bases remaining in a DNA substrate after exposure to cell extracts as described by Pegg et al. (1983). Accompanying studies using a methylated poly(dT) · poly(dA) substrate (Dolan et al., 1984) indicated that cell extracts from human fibroblasts with active MT do not remove methyl from the O^4 position of thymine (Domoradzki et al., 1984).

These repair-deficient cells and a series of cell lines with normal levels of MT were compared for sensitivity to the killing and mutagenic effect of N-methyl-N'-nitro-N-nitroso-guanidine (MNNG). Figure 5 (upper panel) shows that three repair-deficient cell lines were extremely sensitive to the cytotoxic action of MNNG compared to cells with a normal ability to remove this lesion and that the response of the GM637 cells was intermediate. These data suggest that O^6-methylguanine is a potentially cytotoxic lesion in human fibroblasts and that this repair system protects the cells. The data in the lower panel of Figure 5 show that mutations were induced by low doses of MNNG in the three cell lines that lack the ability to remove methyl groups from the O^6-position of guanine, but in the methyl repair-proficient cells there was no significant

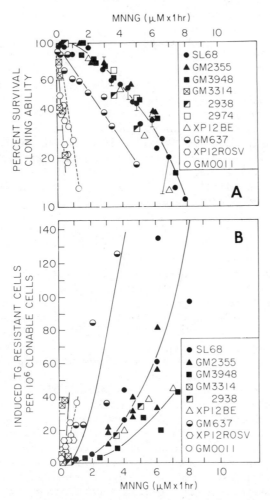

Fig. 5. Comparison of cytotoxicity (A) and mutagenicity (B) induced by MNNG in human fibroblasts. Cells in exponential growth were treated with MNNG for 1 hr at a density of not more than 8 x 10^5 cells per 150mm diameter dish for mutagenicity determination. Symbols without error bars represent individual determinations of survival or determinations for which the symbol drawn is greater than the error bar. The mutant frequencies have been corrected for cloning efficiency. (Adapted from a figure in Domoradzki et al., 1984.)

increase in the frequency of mutants at these low doses. Only at much higher concentrations did induction of mutations occur. The GM637 cells gave an intermediate response to mutation induction (Domoradzki et al., 1984).

Taken together, the biochemical and the biological data indicate that O^6-methylguanine, or any other lesion that the MT can remove from methylated DNA, but not O^4-methylthymine, is the lesion responsible for mutation induction by MNNG in human cells. They also indicate that lack of MT activity is not necessarily a characteristic of skin fibroblasts of persons with a predisposition to colon cancer. This is because included in the series of normal cells shown in Figure 5 are cell lines derived from several patients with Gardner's syndrome (GM3948, 2938, 2974) and one with familial polyposis coli (GM2355). Unlike GM3314, these cell lines had a normal level of MT activity and a normal response to MNNG.

CONCLUSION

In summary, these series of comparative studies with various repair-deficient or normal cells indicate that excision repair in diploid human fibroblasts is essentially an error-free process and that the ability to carry out excision repair of potentially cytotoxic and potentially mutagenic or transforming lesions induced in DNA by UV radiation or by various classes of chemical carcinogens determines their ultimate biological consequences. The data suggest that there is a certain amount of time available between the initial exposure and the onset of the cellular events responsible for mutation induction, for cell transformation, and for cell killing. They suggest that the critical event for the induction of mutations and transformation to anchorage independence is DNA replication on a template that still contains unexcised lesions. In contrast, the cell cycle studies indicate that although a population's survival is determined by the extent of excision repair of potentially lethal damage from DNA before some critical cellular event takes place, the critical event is not DNA synthesis on a damaged template, but rather involves failure to produce needed mRNA's and proteins.

ACKNOWLEDGEMENTS

We thank our colleagues J. C. Ball, M. E. Dolan, J. Domoradzki, P. L. Grover, R. H. Heflich, J. W. Levinson, B. Konze-Thomas, E. M. Mahoney, A. E. Pegg, K. C. Silinskas, D. H. Swenson, M. Watanabe, and L. L. Yang for their invaluable contributions to the research summarized here. The excellent technical assistance of N. Birch, R. Corner, D. J. Dorney, R. M. Hazard, S. A. Kateley, L. Lommel, A. Mendrala, J. R. Otto, D. Richmond, L. Rowan, and J. E. Tower is gratefully acknowledged. The research summarized in this report was supported in part by Contract EV-78-4659 from the Department of Energy and by Grants CA21253 and CA21289 from the Department of Health and Human Services, National Cancer Institute, N.I.H.

REFERENCES

Cleaver, J. E., and Bootsma, B, 1975, Xeroderma pigmentosum: Biochemical and genetic characteristics, Annu. Rev. Genet., 9:19.

Dolan, M. E., Scicchitano, D., Singer, B., and Pegg, A. E., 1984, Comparison of repair of methylated pyrimidines in poly (dT) by extracts from rat liver and Escherichia coli, Biochem. Biophys. Res. Commun., 123:324.

Domoradzki, J., Pegg, A. E., Dolan, M. E., Maher, V. M., and McCormick, J. J., 1984, Correlation between 0^6-methylguanine-DNA methyltransferase activity and resistance of human cells to the cytotoxic and mutagenic effect of N-methyl-N'-nitro-N-nitrosoguanidine, Carcinogenesis, in press.

Heflich, R. H., Dorney, D. J., Maher, V. M., and McCormick, J. J., 1977, Reactive derivatives of benzo(a)pyrene and 7,12-dimethylbenz(a)anthracene cause S_1 nuclease sensitive sites in DNA and "UV-like" repair, Biochem. Biophys. Res. Commun., 77:634.

Heflich, R. H., Hazard, R. M., Lommel, L., Scribner, J. D., Maher, V. M., and McCormick, J. J., 1980, A comparison of the DNA binding, cytotoxicity and repair synthesis induced in human fibroblasts by reactive deriatives of aromatic amide carcinogens, Chem. Biol. Interact., 29:43.

Konze-Thomas, B., Levinson, J. W., Maher, V. M., and McCormick, J. J., 1979, Correlation among the rates of dimer excision, DNA repair replication, and recovery of human cells from potentially lethal damage induced by ultraviolet radiation, Biophys. J., 28:315.

Konze-Thomas, B., Hazard, R. M., Maher, V. M., and McCormick, J. J., 1982, Extent of excision repair before DNA synthesis determines the mutagenic but not the lethal effect of UV radiation, Mutat. Res., 94:421.

Maher, V. M., Birch, N., Otto, J. R., and McCormick, J. J., 1975, Cytotoxicity of carcinogenic aromatic amides in normal and xeroderma pigmentosum fibroblasts with different DNA repair capabilities, J. Natl. Cancer Inst., 54:1287.

Maher, V. M., McCormick, J. J., Grover, P. L., and Sims, P. 1977, Effect of DNA repair on the cytotoxicity and mutagenicity of polycyclic hydrocarbon derivatives in normal and xeroderma pigmentosum human fibroblasts, Mutat. Res., 43:117.

Maher, V. M., Dorney, D. J., Mendrala, A. L., Konze-Thomas, B., and McCormick, J. J. 1979, DNA excision repair processes in human cells can eliminate the cytotoxic and mutagenic consequences of ultraviolet irradiation, Mutat. Res., 62:311.

Maher, V. M., Heflich, R. H., and McCormick, J. J., 1981, Repair of DNA damage induced in human fibroblasts by N-substituted aryl compounds, in: "Carcinogenic and Mutagenic N-Substituted Aryl Compounds," National Cancer Institute, Bethesda.

Maher, V. M., Rowan, L. A., Silinskas, K. C., Kateley, S. A., and McCormick, J. J., 1982, Frequency of UV-induced neoplastic transformation of diploid human fibroblasts is higher in xeroderma pigmentosum cells than in normal cells, Proc. Natl. Acad. Sci. (U.S.A.), 79:2613.

Mahoney, E. M., Ball, J. C., Swenson, D. H., Richmond, D., Maher, V. M., and McCormick, J. J., 1984, Cytoxocity and mutagenicity of aflatoxin dichloride in normal and repair deficient diploid human fibroblasts, Chem.-Biol. Interact., 50:59.

McCormick, J. J., and Maher, V. M., 1981, Measurement of colony-forming ability and mutagenesis in diploid human cells, in: "DNA Repair: A Laboratory Manual of Research Procedures," Vol. 1, Part B, Marcel Dekker, New York.

McCormick, J. J., and Maher, V. M., 1983, Role of DNA lesions and DNA repair in mutagenesis and transformation of human cells, in: "Human Carcinogenesis," Academic Press, New York.

McCormick, J. J., and Maher, V. M., 1985, In vitro malignant transformation - a multi-stepped process, in: "Epidemiology and Quantitation of Environmental Risk in Humans: Potential and Limitations," Plenum Press, New York.

Pegg, A. E., Wiest, L., Foote, R. S., Mitra, S., and Perry, W., 1983, Purification and properties of 0^6-methylguanine-DNA transmethylase from rat liver, J. Biol. Chem., 258:2327.

Silinskas, K. C., Kateley, S. A., Tower, J. E., Maher, V. M., and McCormick, J. J., 1981, Induction of anchorage independent growth in human fibroblasts by propane sultone, Cancer Res., 41:1620.

Watanabe, M., Maher, V. M., and McCormick, J. J., 1985, Excision repair of UV- or benzo(a)pyrene diol epoxide-induced lesions in xeroderma pigmentosum variant cells is "error-free", Mutat. Res., in press.

Yang, L. L., Maher, V. M., and McCormick, J. J., 1980,
  Error-free excision of the cytotoxic, mutagenic
  N^2-deoxyguanosine DNA adduct formed in human fibroblasts
  by (±)-7β,8α-dihydroxy-9α,10α-epoxy-7,8,9,10-tetrahydro-
  benzo(a)pyrene, Proc. Natl. Acad. Sci. (U.S.A.), 77:5933.
Yang, L. L., Maher, V. M., McCormick, J. J., 1982, Relationship
  between excision repair and the cytotoxic and mutagenic
  effect of the "anti" 7,9-diol-9,10-epoxide of benzo(a)pyrene
  in human cells, Mutat. Res., 94:435.

VARIATIONS IN DNA REPAIR AMONG PEOPLE

R.B. Setlow

Biology Department
Brookhaven National Laboratory
Upton, New York 11973

INTRODUCTION

A number of inherited, cancer-prone diseases are associated with severe defects in the abilities of cells to repair damaged DNA (Setlow, 1978; Friedberg, 1985; Maher, this volume; Paterson, this volume). The diseases with the largest defects in repair are xeroderma pigmentosum (XP) and ataxia telangiectasia (AT), the former showing high levels of skin cancer as a result of sunlight irradiation and the latter, high levels of lymphoreticular cancer whose etiologic origins are unknown. The cytotoxic effects of ultraviolet radiation (UV) are much greater on XP cells than on normal cells, whereas the cytotoxic effects of X-rays are much greater on AT cells than on normal ones. It is known that XP cells are defective in one or more DNA repair pathways, but the molecular nature of the defect(s) in AT cells is not known. In XP, the skin cancer susceptibility to sunlight and the cytotoxic effects of UV on their cells in vitro show good correlations with the ability to repair UV-damaged DNA by the process of nucleotide excision. The repair defects range from approximately 20 to 95 percent. It is important to recognize that the repair defects are not 100 percent and actually average somewhere in the neighborhood of 80 percent. This 80 percent average repair defect is associated with an approximately 10^4-fold increase in skin cancer prevalence (Setlow, 1980; Kraemer et al., 1984) and an approximately 12-fold increase in internal cancers at sites not exposed to sunlight (Kraemer et al., 1984).

One reason for the large increase in skin cancer with decreases in DNA repair is related to the apparent exponential increase of skin cancer with UV flux (Scotto et al., 1983). A small increase in effective dose results in a large effect. This exponential model has been used to estimate that DNA repair in normal cells reduces the effective UV dose to the cells by approximately 95 percent (Setlow, 1980). Thus it seems as if UV is possibly a special case, because the doses to which people are exposed make tremendous numbers of damages per cell compared to those made by exogenous or endogenous chemicals in the environment (Setlow, 1985). UV-damaged DNA represented by the well-described bulky lesions, pyrimidine dimers, is repaired by a complex set of enzymic steps not fully elucidated. These enzymic reactions also work on other bulky damages; hence, it is not surprising that the level of internal cancers (obviously not arising from UV exposure) is higher in XP than in unaffected individuals. Since the etiologic agents producing the putative damages to DNA are not known, it is not possible to assess quantitatively the role of DNA repair in these internal cancers.

In XP, an 80-percent defect in DNA repair results, on the average, in a 10^4-fold increase in cancer susceptibility. Such a large change in susceptibility, with a less than complete defect in DNA repair, leads one to hypothesize that the variation in repair in an apparently normal population could result in large changes in susceptibility to cancer-initiating agents (Fig. 1) It is conceivable that small variations in DNA repair--variations that one would not describe as abnormal--could result in large variations in susceptibility which would only show up if an individual were exposed to a carcinogenic agent. Such variations in susceptibility could account for the fact that usually only a small fraction of exposed individuals develops cancer. If the idea represented in Fig. 1 is correct, it implies that there are nonstochastic processes involved in cancer induction in a population uniformly exposed to a carcinogenic agent. It is not known whether the small deviations from the average amount of DNA repair shown in Fig. 1 are inherited, are the result of lifestyle, or both.

DNA REPAIR

There are five reasonably well understood DNA repair processes: (1) photoreactivation, (2) nucleotide excision, (3) base excision, (4) alkyl transfer, and (5) X-ray damage repair consisting of many component parts, all poorly understood. Photoreactivation is important not only for its repair characteristics but because it is a repair process specific for one particular type of damage--UV-induced pyrimidine dimers. It works by the direct monomerization of the dimers catalyzed by visible light absorbed by an enzyme bound to the dimer. It is highly efficient and carries no risk. It is difficult to study in human cells in culture because the level of enzyme activity depends, in as yet unknown ways, on the composition of the medium (Sutherland and Oliver, 1976). Nevertheless, it is clear that the enzyme exists in human cells and can reverse the dimers made in skin by ultraviolet radiation (Sutherland et al., 1980; D'Ambrosio et al., 1981).

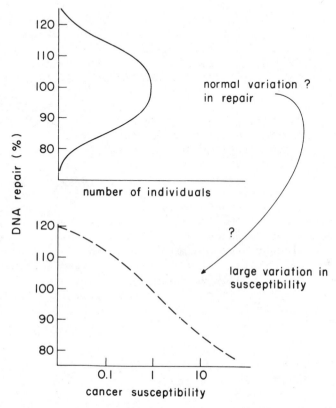

Fig. 1. The upper part shows the hypothetical variation in repair for an apparently normal population. The lower part indicates a hypothetical variation in cancer susceptibility. A high susceptibility is associated with a less-than-average amount of DNA repair capability.

Reasonable amounts of data exist on the variations in the levels of nucleotide excision and alkyl transferase repair among people. Nucleotide excision represents the removal of a bulky lesion from DNA by an endonucleolytic attack on the polynucleotide chain so as to remove the adduct plus an oligonucleotide surround-

207

ing it. It is characterized by the introduction of single-strand breaks into DNA and their closure as repair replication and ligation take place. An often-used technique to measure nucleotide excision repair is the measurement of the incorporation of ^{3}H-thymidine into the DNA of cells during non-S periods of the cell cycle. This incorporation, called unscheduled DNA synthesis (UDS), represents the incorporation during the repolymerization step of nucleotide excision. It is a relatively simple measurement to make, but it is difficult to put it on an absolute basis since the magnitude of UDS per cell depends upon the number of lesions repaired, the size of the gap repolymerized, and the specific activity of the DNA precursor within the cell. Nevertheless, it is a good comparative measure in most systems.

Alkyl transfer, on the other hand, cannot be measured by UDS. In this repair system, an alkyl group on DNA, in particular O^6-alkylguanine (Lindahl, 1982; Pegg, 1984) is transferred to an acceptor protein by a methyl transferase reaction. The transferase and the receptor are presumably the same protein. The transfer does not result in any attack on the polynucleotide chain. The alkyl group is transferred to a cysteine residue on the acceptor protein and uses up that acceptor site. Hence, this repair system is stoichiometric; the number of alkyl groups that can be repaired equal the number of acceptor groups--a result quite different from the repair of other types of damages in which repair enzymes are used over and over again. Alkyl transfer in vivo is rapid (15 to 30 minutes). It is usually detected by the disappearance of O^6-alkylguanine either in vivo or in vitro using cell extracts and radioactive substrate DNAs, or by the transfer of radioactive alkyl groups to protein.

VARIATIONS IN DNA REPAIR

UV-Radiation

Wide variations have been observed in the abilities of apparently normal fibroblasts or leukocytes to repair UV damage (Setlow, 1983). The measurements that have been made all utilize UDS or a similar method. The standard deviations from the mean range from approximately 20 to 50 percent in three extensive studies. Such a variation also is found for epidermal cells (Fig. 2). The range of UDS is almost sixfold in the population studied in Fig. 2. That particular population included a wide range in ages, and some of the variation can be ascribed to an age dependence of UDS, but even when the age dependence is removed, large deviations from the mean are still observed.

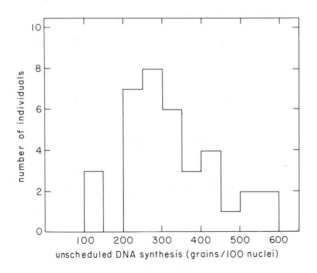

Fig. 2. The distribution of UV-induced UDS among epidermal cells of a number of individuals (Nette et al., 1984).

Alkyl Transfer

A number of measurements have been made on the abilities of cell and tissue extracts to repair O^6-methylguanine. The latter is a presumptive mutagenic and carcinogenic lesion (Pegg, 1984). Large variations are shown not only for lymphocytes but also for normal human tissues (Waldstein et al., 1982; Myrnes et al., 1983; Grafstrom et al., 1984). The range of activity per mg of protein is extensive and, depending on the tissue, ranges from approximately 2- to 42-fold, with an average in the neighborhood of 5-fold. The distribution curve, shown in Fig. 3 for human lymphocytes, indicates the wide variation among normal cells and the fact that cells from individuals with chronic lymphocytic leukemia have much greater activity than the normal. A similar wide range of activity is shown for human liver samples (Fig. 4). The range of acceptor activity is similar to that of lymphocytes.

CONCLUSIONS

There are large variations in DNA repair among the cells of apparently normal individuals. The range of values is in the neighborhood of 5-fold and is appreciable compared to those for the inherited repair-deficient diseases that have been well studied. Such large variations raise the possibility that cancer, or other indications of ill health, may have a strong deterministic component that outweighs the stochastic ones of exposure to exogenous or endogenous environmental chemicals.

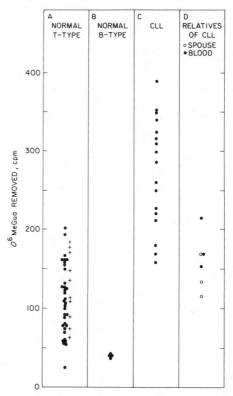

Fig. 3. The amount of acceptor activity measured as O^6-methylguanine removed from an exogenous substrate per 100 μg of protein (one count per minute is approximately one fmol). Data are for normal lymphocytes, chronic lymphocytic leukemia lymphocytes (CLL) and relatives of CLL (Waldstein et al., 1982).

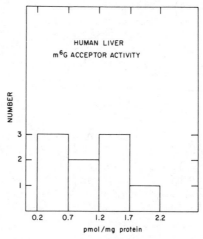

Fig. 4. The distribution of O^6-methylguanine acceptor activity among human liver samples (Grafstrom et al., 1984).

The variations observed are real and not just experimental error. However, it is not clear whether these variations are genetic, whether they are stable (What is the result of repeated measurements on the same individual over several years?), or whether they are influenced strongly by the various parameters that go under the heading of lifestyle. A typical lifestyle effect is observed in the cells washed out of the lungs of smokers or non-smokers. The lung lavage cells from nonsmokers have normal levels of alkyl acceptors (Setlow, 1985). Those from smokers, on the other hand, have much lower levels (Cao, Setlow, and Janoff, unpublished), indicating that smokers have a double risk. They are exposed to alkylating agents--nitrosamines in smoke--and at the same time have a low level of alkyl repair. At present, DNA repair measurements have no prognostic value. Only a long-term study will indicate whether the observed wide variations in DNA repair among the normal population are associated with a greater prevalence of disease.

ACKNOWLEDGEMENT

This work was supported by the U.S. Department of Energy.

REFERENCES

D'Ambrosio, S.M., Whetstone, J.W., Slazinski, L., and Lowney, E., 1981, Photorepair of pyrimidine dimers in human skin in vivo, Photochem. Photobiol., 34:461.

Friedberg, E.C., 1985, "DNA Repair," W.H. Freeman, New York.

Grafstrom, R.C., Pegg, A.E., Trump, B.F., and Harris, C.C., 1984, O^6-alkylguanine-DNA alkyltransferase activity in normal human tissues and cells, Cancer Res., 44:2855.

Kraemer, K.H., Lee, M.Y., and Scotto, J., 1984, DNA repair protects against cutaneous and internal neoplasia: evidence from xeroderma pigmentosum, Carcinogenesis, 5:511.

Lindahl, T., 1982, DNA repair enzymes, Annu. Rev. Biochem., 51:61.

Myrnes, B., Giercksky, K.E., and Krokan, H., 1983, Interindividual variation in the activity of O^6-methylguanine-DNA methyl-transferase and uracil-DNA glycosylase in human organs, Carcinogenesis, 4:1565.

Nette, E.G., Xi, Y.-P., Sun, Y.-K., Andrews, A.D. and King, D.W., 1984, A correlation between aging and DNA repair in human epidermal cells, Mech. Ageing Dev., 24:283.

Pegg, A.E., 1984, Repair of O^6-methylguanine in DNA by mammalian tissues, in: "Biochemical Basis of Chemical Carcinogenesis," pp. 265-274, H. Greim, R. Jung, M. Kramer, M. Marquardt, and F. Oesch, eds., Raven Press, New York.

Scotto, J., Fears, T.R., and Fraumeni, J.F., Jr., 1983, "Incidence of Nonmelanoma Skin Cancer in the United States," DHHS Pub. No. (NIH) 76-1029, Bethesda, MD.

Setlow, R.B., 1978, Repair deficient human disorders and cancer, Nature (London), 271:713.

Setlow, R.B., 1980, Different basic mechanisms in DNA repair, Arch. Toxicol. Suppl. 3:217.

Setlow, R.B., 1983, Variations in DNA repair among humans, in: "Human Carcinogenesis," pp. 231-254, C.C. Harris and H.N. Autrup, eds., Academic Press, New York.

Setlow, R.B., 1985, Saturation of Repair, in: "Assessment of Risks from Low-Level Exposure to Radiation and Chemicals," in press, A.D. Woodhead, C.J. Shellabarger and V. Pond, eds., Plenum Press, New York.

Sutherland, B.M, Kochevar, I., and Harber, L., 1980, Pyrimidine dimer formation and repair in human skin, Cancer Res., 40:3181.

Sutherland, B.M., and Oliver, R., 1976, Culture conditions affect photoreactivating enzyme levels in human fibroblasts, Biochim. Biophys. Acta, 442:358.

Waldstein, E.A., Cao, E.-H., Miller, M.E., Cronkite, E.P., and Setlow, R.B., 1982, Extracts of chronic lymphocytic leukemia lymphocytes have a high level of DNA repair activity for O^6-methylguanine, Proc. Natl. Acad. Sci. USA, 79:4786.

CANCER-PRONE FAMILIES: A RESOURCE FOR ETIOLOGIC STUDIES

Mark H. Greene

Environmental Epidemiology Branch
National Cancer Institute
Bethesda, Maryland   20205

INTRODUCTION

Familial aggregations of malignancy have suggested that host
susceptibility factors play an important role in the pathogenesis
of many human cancers. Although many such familial aggregations
are quite striking, single gene (Mendelian) inheritance is not
readily demonstrable in the majority of cases (1). It is often
difficult to know how much importance to attach to such familial
clusters, since many of the cancers implicated are among the most
common in the general population; as a consequence, such
occurrences are to be expected on the basis of chance alone. In
addition, the presence of multiple cancers of the same type in a
given family does not necessarily implicate a genetic mechanism.
Families share many other potential risk factors including similar
diet, similar occupation or common environmental exposures.
Nonetheless, the importance of genetic factors as determinants of
cancer in humans has been clearly established; Mulvihill has
listed in excess of 200 single gene disorders, each of which is
associated with an increased risk of malignancy (2). In view of
the wide international variations in cancer incidence rates (3),
many investigators have suggested that up to 90% of all human
malignancies can be attributed to environmental exposures. While
this may be true in a general sense, the role of host
susceptibility to potentially carcinogenic environmental exposures
is also clearly important (4). Since the broad concepts of
genetic and familial risk factors in cancer susceptibility have
been extensively reviewed (1, 2, 4-6), this presentation will
focus upon a research strategy designed to investigate newly-
identified constellations of familial cancer, with the goal of

elucidating mechanisms of cancer pathogenesis. This inter-disciplinary approach to the study of cancer-prone families has been described previously (7); in this presentation, our experience in investigating familial cutaneous malignant melanoma (CMM) will be used to illustrate this approach. First, I will present a brief summary of those syndromes which are associated with an increased risk of neoplastic disease, in order to place the discussion which follows in its proper context.

MEDICAL CONDITIONS ASSOCIATED WITH INCREASED CANCER RISK

In spite of the rare occurrence of various cancer-prone disorders, they have been intensively investigated because they may serve as illustrative models which permit insight into broader mechanisms of cancer susceptibility. Conditions predisposing to malignancy can be separated into several broad categories. The HAMARTOMATOUS DISORDERS include conditions such as neurofibromatosis (Autosomal Dominant) – prone to neural sarcomas and leukemia; tuberous sclerosis (AD) – astrocytoma; Von-Hippel Lindau (AD) - kidney, pheochromocytoma, brain tumors; multiple exostosis (AD) - chondrosarcoma; Peutz Jeghers syndrome (AD) – ovarian tumors; and Cowden's Disease (AD) – breast, thyroid, and brain cancer. These conditions are characterized by faulty embryonic development which results in a localized proliferation of tissues which are embryologically diverse (8). This disordered pattern of tissue development appears to be an indicator of a growth defect which in some situations gives rise to an increased risk of cancer. The precise mechanism for the cancer susceptibility in the aforementioned diseases is not well understood. A second category of cancer susceptibility states are the GENODERMATOSES. Examples of this class of conditions include xeroderma pigmentosum (Autosomal Recessive) - skin cancers of all types, oral cancers; albinism (AR) - skin cancers of all kinds; and adult progeria (AR) - sarcomas. Xeroderma pigmentosum has been an invaluable model of genetically determined carcinogenesis in man. It represents the first and best characterized disorder of DNA repair identified in humans (9). Patients with this disorder are unusually susceptible to the development of cutaneous neoplasms including both ordinary skin cancer and malignant melanoma. This susceptibility appears to be a consequence of an inherited enzyme deficiency which prevents effective cellular repair of ultraviolet light induced DNA damage. A third category of predisposing conditions can be classified as CHROMOSOME BREAKAGE DISORDERS. These include such conditions as Down's syndrome, Bloom's syndrome, and Fanconi's syndrome. All three conditions appear to be associated with an increased risk of acute leukemia. Finally, a series of IMMUNE DEFICIENCY STATES have also been described in which cancer susceptibility appears to be heightened. Disorders in this group include ataxia telangiectasia (AR) - leukemia, lymphoma, gastric, and brain cancer; the Wiskott-

214

Aldrich Syndrome (X-linked Recessive) - lymphoreticular cancers;
X-linked agammaglobulinemia (XR) - lymphocytic leukemia; and the
X-linked lymphoproliferative disease described by Purtilo and
colleagues (XR) - various lymphoproliferative cancers. More
specific information on these predisposing conditions has been
reviewed by Fraumeni (1). Familial and hereditary cancers per se
have also been described in some detail. HEREDITARY CANCERS
include those conditions in which a single gene (Mendelian) mode
of inheritance has been documented. Included in this category are
retinoblastoma, the nevoid basal cell carcinoma syndrome, multiple
endocrine neoplasia types I, II and III, chemodectomas, familial
polyposis coli, Gardner's syndrome, tylosis and the dysplastic
nevus syndrome. I will return to a discussion of this latter
condition as a model of how cancer-prone families can be
investigated. A variety of FAMILIAL CANCER SYNDROMES have also
been reported (6), in which either site-specific aggregations of
specific tumors (breast, endometrium, ovary, prostate, Hodgkin's
disease, non-Hodgkin's lymphoma, gastric cancer, chronic
lymphocytic leukemia, colon cancer without polyposis, lung cancer,
bladder cancer, kidney cancer, and testicular cancer) or non-site
specific aggregations (the familial adenocarcinoma syndrome,
Turcot's Syndrome, Li-Fraumeni Syndrome, Torre's Syndrome) are
observed. Familial aggregations of such cancers, be they clearly
hereditary or not, frequently offer a unique opportunity to
conduct etiologic studies which may help clarify mechanisms of
cancer susceptibility and pathogenesis. Close collaboration
between etiologically oriented clinicians and laboratory
investigators has proven particularly fruitful in this approach,
as the following example illustrates.

HEREDITARY CUTANEOUS MELANOMA AND THE DYSPLASTIC NEVUS SYNDROME

   The notion that nevi (common moles) might be precursors to
cutaneous malignant melanoma dates back to the early part of the
nineteeth century. The French investigator Recamier described a
patient with a long-standing pigmented lesion which began to
change, ulcerate and bleed. Histologically, this lesion was found
to be a malignant tumor. In fact, the first report of malignant
melanoma in the English language literature described malignant
transformation of a pigmented nevus in a patient with multiple
large moles (10). This report is further of interest in that
Norris noted that his patient's father, who also had multiple
nevi, died of metastatic malignant melanoma as well. Thus, he
described the first melanoma-prone family, and suggested that the
cancers which developed in that context arose from pre-existing
pigmented nevi. Cawley's seminal report of familial melanoma in
1952 (11) opened the modern era of investigation into the causes
of familial melanoma. Since that time, multiple melanoma-prone
kindreds have been described (for review, see Reference 12) but by
the time we initiated our initial investigations into the

pathogenesis of familial melanoma, an explanation for the cancer susceptibility in these kindreds was not apparent. With the recognition that familial melanoma occurred with surprising frequency, we planned an interdisciplinary research investigation of such high-risk kindreds. On a rainy afternoon in April 1976, we examined 25 members of a family in which four individuals were known to have had malignant melanoma. During the course of that afternoon, we noted two critical findings. The first was the presence "funny-looking" moles or nevi on the skin of the three surviving melanoma patients and a number of their close relatives. Larger and more numerous the ordinary moles, these skin lesions were haphazardly colored, had irregular borders and sometimes occurred in areas where moles usually do not develop, such as the scalp and buttocks. The second finding was that one family member with the unusual mole pattern also had a previously-undiagnosed melanoma, which upon surgical excision was found to be an early (surgically curable) invasive melanoma. Six additional families were investigated and all seven kindreds were found to exhibit this unusual mole pattern, which we designated the B-K mole syndrome (13). These initials were derived from the surnames of the first two families studied and were chosen to reflect our lack of understanding of the nature of these pigmented lesions during the initial phases of our investigation. Subsequently, we introduced the more precise and descriptive term, dysplastic nevus syndrome (DNS) (14), when it became apparent that nuclear atypia and disorderly growth patterns, i.e., dysplasia of melanocytes were the histologic hallmarks of these nevi (15, 16).

The early clinicaly studies of these melanoma-prone families were conducted by a team of investigators including dermatologists, pathologists, and epidemiologically-oriented clinicians. These studies clarified the natural history of ordinary, common acquired nevi, an understanding of which proved to be necessary for a clearer conceptualization of the nature of dysplastic nevi. In brief, the typical Caucasian adult has 25 to 40 acquired common nevi on his or her skin. These lesions begin as pinpoint macules that expand circumferentially, evolve into pigmented papules which eventually lose their pigmentation (17). Such lesions may disappear completely in the latter years of life. In general, common acquired nevi are small, round, uniformly pigmented (tan or brown), have a smooth border and predominate on sun-exposed skin above the waist. This evolution (from a pigmented pinpoint macule to a larger one, to a pigmented, and then a non-pigmented papule, and finally to clinically normal skin) takes many decades and may stop at any point along this developmental pathway. Proliferation of common acquired nevi seems to peak in early middle age, with relatively few additional lesions occurring later in life. In contrast, dysplastic nevi are often more numerous and larger than ordinary moles, have irregular borders and varigated pigmentation. Although lesional size does

tend to exceed 5mm in diameter (sometimes reaching 10 to 15mm) and
although lesional number can be 200 or more in an individual with
the syndrome, enough exceptions in both respects have been
observed to indicate that neither is as important as the other
morphologic and histologic features that are diagnostic of the
syndrome. Our cross-sectional observations suggest that the
earliest clinically detectable abnormality signalling the
expression of the DNS is an increase in the number of
morphologically normal nevi. This occurs in children of 5 to 6
years of age and typically involves the development of 20 to 40
small, uniform and deeply pigmented lesions. As the affected
individual enters adolescence, a second proliferation occurs and
some of the nevi acquire the morphologic features of dysplastic
nevi. By the late teens and early twenties, the DNS is usually
manifest in those individuals who are destined to be affected
(18). It it important to note that dysplastic nevi continue to
develop and affect individuals throughout their life, in contrast
with the behavior of common acquired nevi. Generally, family
members who have clinically normal skin in their mid-twenties
remain normal. The early clinical studies of melanoma-prone
families also serve to clarify the histologic characteristics of
dysplastic nevi. As mentioned earlier, the sine qua non is
cytologic nuclear atypia of melanocytes. Specifically, melanocytes in these lesions show nuclear hyperchromatism and pleo-
morphism which may involve many or only a few cells, usually most
notably those at the dermal-epidermal junction. These nuclear
abnormalities are invariably accompanied by a lymphocytic
infiltrate and series of mesenchymal changes that have been
designated "lamellar fibroplasia" (stacks of alternating layers of
attenuated fibroblast-like cells and collagen at the tips of rete
ridges) and "concentric eosinophilic fibroplasia" (a broad band of
acellular collagen that is parallel to the dermal-epidermal
interface and involves up to four rete and intervening dermal
papillae) (15, 16). In other tissues, such distorted architecture
and cytologic changes have commonly been termed dysplasia.
Although sometimes misunderstood or misused, dysplasia here simply
implies the presence of a disordered pattern of growth which is
associated with an increased risk of progression to overt
neoplasia.

Our clinical studies have documented that, like other familial
cancers, hereditary CMM is characterized by a younger than usual
age at onset and predisposition to multiple independent primary
tumors. Thus, of the 69 hereditary CMM patients in the fourteen
high-risk families which comprise our formal study cohort, the
median age at first melanoma diagnosis was 32 years (in contrast
to the median age in the general population of 52 years.)
Altogether, 21 patients (30%) developed more than one primary
malignant melanoma. The back was the most common site of origin
in men, while the calf and back predominated in women.

Superficial spreading melanoma accounted for 102 (88%) of 116 histologically-reviewed cases of primary melanoma, with nodular melanoma a distant second (7%). The majority of melanomas were thin, that is Clark Level II or less (63%) or less than .76 mm in thickness (61%). Over 90% of the familial CMM patients examined to date have also had the DNS. Detailed histologic evaluation of these familial neoplasms revealed a dysplastic melanocytic precursor at the tumor margin in 69% of cases, compared to one-third of unselected melanomas.

In an attempt to quantify the risk of CMM in members of these high-risk families, person-years of observation for family members with and without DNS were accumulated. After excluding the first two melanoma patients from each of the fourteen families (to minimize ascertainment bias), we divided the observations made on these families into three periods: the retrospective interval (that period of time prior to the onset of our survey), the prevalence period (information collected at the time of first study exam), and the prospective interval (information acquired during prospective follow-up of the members of these families). The risk quantification is purest if one considers the prospective interval and excludes from observation all patients known to have had a prior melanoma. Thus, among 77 members with DNS, 4 persons developed their first melanoma during follow-up, compared with 0.027 cases expected (O/E = 148; 95% CI = 40-379). The age-adjusted melanoma incidence rate was 14.3 cases per 1,000 DNS patients per year and the cumulative risk of first melanoma 7.2% ($\pm$3.6 at 8 years). The cancer risk was similar in males and females. When considering the 40 family members with DNS in whom melanoma had occurred prior to the prospective interval, the melanoma rates were approximately five times greater than those observed in the group just described. In contrast, 122 family members without DNS accrued 564 person-years of observation; no melanomas developed in this group (0.04 cases expected). Thus, dysplastic nevi are clearly markers which identify the specific individuals at high risk of melanoma in melanoma-prone families and they comprise the actual precursors of these melanomas (19). Family members with dypslastic nevi experience a dramatic excess risk of melanoma, several hundred times that of the general population, with a melanoma incidence rate of 1.4% to 5.4% per year, depending upon the presence or absence of prior melanoma.

The magnitude of melanoma risk in this setting becomes more understandable when one realizes that familial melanoma represents a single gene autosomal dominant disorder (20). The fourteen families comprising the core study cohort were subjected to standard segregation analysis. When the analysis was performed considering as affected only those family members with melanoma, an autosomal dominant mode of inheritance was found to be the hypothesis most consistent with the data. In a second analysis, however, we considered individuals with melanoma or DNS as affected; no genetic model fit these data. In view of the evidence that most familial melanomas occur in the context of DNS and that such tumors evolve directly from dysplastic nevi, the latter finding was surprising. Our inability to corroborate an autosomal dominant mode of inheritance when DNS was considered was a consequence of there being too many affected individuals in the families studied. It is well recognized that segregation analysis is most useful in detecting the affect of a major locus when the trait in question is rare in genotypically normal individuals. If phenocopies of the trait are relatively common and if the phenocopies cannot be distinguished from the genetically determined phenotype, the affect of a major gene may be masked. Thus, one possible explanation for our findings is the possibility that DNS is not rare in the general population and that sporadic phenocopies of the trait were included among subjects in our study who were classified as genetically affected. This is a plausible explanation, as data presented below indicate. The likelihood of an autosomal dominant mechanism being the correct model for familial CMM was provided additional support in the results of the linkage analysis that we conducted on the same patients. We measured 24 common genetic markers in blood samples from members of these fourteen families and tested for linkage of these markers to the DNS/melanoma trait. The finding of greatest interest was suggestive evidence for linkage between the DNS/melanoma trait and the Rh locus, which is located on the short arm of chromosome 1. The lod score reached its maximum value of 2.00 at a recombination fraction of 30%. This finding provided additional support for an autosomal dominant mode of inheritance for the melanoma/DNS trait and also suggested that if a susceptibility gene for this disorder exists, it may be loosely linked with the Rh locus. This is a possibility that is currently being explored in greater detail using genetic markers at the DNA level (i.e., restriction fragment length polymorphisms).

Thus, our clinical investigations of melanoma-prone families resulted in the identification of a new preneoplastic syndrome (i.e., DNS) and permitted us to characterize these precursor lesions both clinically and histologically. Furthermore, we were able to derive quantitative estimates of the risk of melanoma in individuals with familial DNS and document that these lesions provide a clinical marker which permits specific identification of high-risk family members. Prospective medical surveillance of family members with the DNS has resulted in the diagnosis of a substantial number of surgically-curable malignant melanomas. Formal genetic analysis of these families documented an autosomal dominant mode of inheritance for this disorder and suggested that the melanoma susceptibility gene might be located on the short-arm of chromosome 1. This latter observation has provided an important lead for subsequent molecular studies.

The broader relevance of these studies also deserves emphasis. These observations are not simply of passing interest, based as they are on a small subgroup of patients drawn from a pool of individuals with a relatively rare cancer. Having identified the DNS in the setting of hereditary melanoma, we subsequently evaluated a series of unrelated CMM patients, all of whom had a negative family history for CMM, and found that a fraction of them had on their skin nevi that were clinically and histologically indistinguishable from those observed in high-risk family members (21). This observation has been confirmed by multiple investigators, leading us to designate this disorder as the non-familial (sporadic) variant of the dysplastic nevus syndrome. Current evidence suggests that somewhere between 30% and 50% of all primary melanomas arise in histologic contiguity with a dysplastic melanocytic precursor (16). This observation has recently been confirmed in a case-control study of malignant melanoma in which the presence of dysplastic nevi was evaluated in 131 melanoma cases and 108 controls. Twenty-one cases and zero controls had multiple dysplastic nevi (22). This study also revealed a strong dose-response relationship between counts of nevi and risk of melanoma; melanoma patients were twenty-five times more likely to have more than 25 nevi and fifteen times more likely to have more than 5 "large" nevi than were controls. Furthermore, nevus surveys in various cohorts of non-cancer patients have suggested that from 2% to 5% of such persons have dysplastic nevi. The most impressive report in this regard describes the presence of histologically-confirmed dysplastic nevi in 43 (4.9%) of 881 consecutive patients examined in a community dermatology practice (23). Thus, the study of high-risk families has led to the recognition of what now appears to be the most common and best characterized precursor to malignant melanoma, be it familial or sporadic (24).

Members of cancer-prone families represent a source of biologic materials which can be utilized in laboratory studies designed to unravel mechanisms of cancer susceptibility. For example, it is well known that there is an increased risk of malignant melanoma in various immunosuppressed populations (25). Immunologic studies conducted on members of melanoma-prone families have suggested the presence of impaired immune function in members of these high-risk kindreds (26-28), although a specific, reproducible abnormality has yet to be pinpointed. Similarly, solar (ultraviolet) radiation has clearly been linked with the development of non-melanoma skin cancers and has also been implicated as a major risk factor in sporadic melanoma. We undertook laboratory investigations designed to evaluate the possibility that cells derived from members of melanoma-prone families might be unusually sensitive to injury by ultraviolet radiation. In the first set of experiments, six fibroblast strains from melanoma/DNS patients showed modest but significantly enhanced cell killing compared with controls, after exposure to 254 nm ultraviolet irradiation (29). The magnitude of ultraviolet radiation sensitivity was similar to that observed in the variant form of xeroderma pigmentosum. Biochemical studies revealed that repair of UV-induced thymine dimers was normal in the melanoma/DNS strains, indicating that this UV sensitivity has a different basis than that documented in patients with XP. Australian investigators have subsequently replicated these observations (30), and further indicated that this UV sensitivity appears to be distributed in melanoma-prone families in a pattern suggestive of autosomal dominant inheritance. A second set of experiments employed the chemical carcinogen, 4-nitroquinoline 1-oxide (4-NQO). This agent was selected because it is believed to be a UV-like chemical carcinogen. Three of the six melanoma/DNS fibroblast strains were sensitive to killing by 4-NQO (31). The magnitude of sensitivity observed was considerably greater than that for UV radiation. However, neither study was able to define a specific DNA repair defect as the cause for the cellular sensitivities observed.

How then can one explain this enhanced cellular sensitivity to environmental carcinogens? Furthermore, what relevance do such observations have to the etiology of hereditary melanoma? In our most recent studies, we have considered the possibility that the in vitro sensitivity to various carcinogens may reflect an abnormality in the mutation rate of these cells. Preliminary results with hereditary melanoma/DNS lymphoblastoid cell lines (32) and fibroblast strains (33), indicate that these cells are indeed hypermutable after exposure to ultraviolet radiation and 4-NQO respectively. Since the cancer-prone condition XP is currently the only known hypermutability state in man, this evidence of enhanced mutation following exposure to environmental carcinogens in hereditary melanoma/DNS suggests that an interaction between host susceptibility factors (genetic) and environmental exposures are important in the pathogenesis of familial CMM. Thus, carefully designed laboratory studies utilizing the unique biological materials available from members of melanoma-prone families have permitted a series of more basic observations which have provided clues into the etiology of malignant melanoma. Furthermore, these observations provide a basis for planning subsequent studies which may produce still further important information.

SUMMARY

Thus, it can be seen that the interdisciplinary research strategy for studying cancer-prone families can provide a broad spectrum of both clinical and laboratory insights into mechanisms of cancer pathogenesis. In brief, one identifies a familial cancer constellation of interest, develops an appropriate interdisciplinary research protocol, assembles a series of appropriately-selected families for study, examines study participants, collects the required biospecimens, and analyzes the data in search of an explanation for the cancer susceptibility observed in the families under study. In the case of familial melanoma/DNS, presented as a model for this type of investigation, an observation made in the course of studying cancer-prone families resulted in the characterization of what now seems to be the most important precursor of melanoma in general, with significant implications for both clinician and researcher. For the investigator, the recognition of DNS makes cutaneous melanoma a useful model for studying neoplastic diseases in man. It has the considerable advantages of involving an accessible, directly observable tissue and both hereditary and non-familial types of preneoplastic and neoplastic disease. For the clinician, recognition and proper management of patients with DNS promises to facilitate prevention, diagnosis, and cure of melanoma (24, 34-36).

REFERENCES

1. Fraumeni JF, Jr: in Cancer Medicine (Holland & Frei, eds.), pp 5-12, Lea & Febiger, Philadelphia, 1982.
2. Mulvihill JJ: in Genetics of Human Cancer (Mulvihill, Miller & Fraumeni, eds.), pp 137-143, Raven Press, New York, 1977.
3. Higginson J: Am J Med 69: 811-813, 1980.
4. Strong LC: in Cancer Epidemiology & Prevention (Schottenfeld & Fraumeni, eds.), pp 506-516, WB Saunders, Philadelphia, 1982.
5. Swift M: op. cit., pp 475-482.
6. Anderson DE: op. cit., pp 483-493.
7. Blattner WA, et al: in Human Carcinogenesis (Harris & Autrup, eds.), pp 913-939, Academic Press, New York, 1983.
8. Warkany J: in Genetics of Human Cancer (Mulvihill, Miller & Fraumeni, eds.), pp 199-204, Raven Press, New York, 1977.
9. Cleaver JE: Nature (London) 218: 652-656, 1968.
10. Norris W: Edinburgh Med Surg J 16: 562-565, 1820.
11. Cawley EP: AMA Arch Dermatol 65: 440-450, 1952
12. Greene MH, et al: in Human Malignant Melanoma (Clark, Goldman & Mastrangelo, eds.), pp 136-166, Greene & Stratton, Philadelphia, 1979.
13. Reimer RR, et al: JAMA 239: 744-746, 1978.
14. Greene MH, et al: Lancet 2: 1024, 1980.
15. Clark WH Jr, et al: Arch Dermatol 114: 732-738, 1978.
16. Clark WH Jr, et al: Human Pathology, in press, 1984.
17. Greene MH, et al: N Engl J Med, in press, 1984.
18. Tucker MA, et al: J Pediatrics 103: 65-69, 1983
19. Greene MH, et al: Proc ASCO 3: 262 (Abstr #1027), 1984.
20. Greene MH, et al: Proc Natl Acad Sci USA 80: 6071-6075, 1983.

21. Elder DE, et al: Cancer 46: 1787-1794, 1980.
22. Swerdlow AJ, et al: Lancet 2: 168, 1984.
23. Crutcher WA, et al: Lancet 1: 729, 1984.
24. National Institutes of Health Consensus Development Conference Statement: Precursors to Malignant Melanoma. JAMA 251: 1864-1866, 1984.
25. Greene MH, et al: Lancet 1: 1196-1198, 1981.
26. Dean J, et al: J Natl Cancer Inst 63: 1139-1145, 1979.
27. Vandenbark A, et al: J Natl Cancer Inst 63: 1146-1151, 1979.
28. Hersey P, et al: Brit J Cancer 40: 113-122, 1981.
29. Smith PJ, et al: Int J Cancer 30: 39-45, 1983.
30. Ramsey RG, et al: Cancer Res 42: 2909-2912, 1982.
31. Smith PJ, et al: Carcinogenesis 4: 911-917, 1983.
32. Perera MIR, et al: Clin Res 31: 595A, 1983.
33. Howell JN, et al: Proc Natl Acad Sci USA 81: 1179-1183, 1984.
34. Fraser MC: Cancer Nursing 5: 351-360, 1983.
35. Greene MH, et al: Lancet 1: 166-167, 1984.
36. Kraemer KH, et al: Lancet 2: 1076-1077, 1983.

THE ROLE OF HUMAN RAS PROTO-ONCOGENES IN CANCER

Steven R. Tronick, Alessandra Eva, Shiv Srivastava,
Matthias Kraus, Yasuhito Yuasa, and Stuart Aaronson

Laboratory of Cellular and Molecular Biology, National
Cancer Institute, Bethesda, MD 20205

Acute transforming retroviruses have arisen in nature by
recombination of replication competent type C retroviruses
with evolutionarily well conserved cellular genes, termed proto-
oncogenes. When incorporated by the retrovirus, such transduced
cellular (onc) sequences confer properties essential for the
induction and maintenance of virus induced transformation (Weiss
et al., 1982; Duesberg, 1983; Bishop, 1983). Recent studies have
provided evidence that proto-oncogenes can be activated as
oncogenes by other mechanisms as well. Of particular importance
in this regard is accumulating evidence that proto-oncogenes may
be frequent targets for genetic alterations involved in neoplastic
processes affecting human cells. In the present review, we
describe investigations of a family of proto-oncogenes, designated
ras, which has been strongly implicated in processes leading to
malignancy in a wide variety of human cell types.

IDENTIFICATION OF RAS GENES

Studies on the Kirsten and Harvey strains of murine sarcoma
viruses (Kirsten-MSV, Harvey-MSV) led eventually to the identification of a small group of highly conserved cellular oncogenes,
designated as the ras family. Early research on Harvey-MSV and
Kirsten-MSV, both isolated from rats infected with either Moloney
or Kirsten leukemia viruses, demonstrated that each were genetically
related in non-helper virus-derived regions of their genomes (Shih
et al., 1978). With the advent of molecular cloning techniques, it
was possible to demonstrate that most of the non-helper derived
sequences were contributed by endogenous rat retroviral information
(Ellis et al., 1981). However, an additional set of sequences

225

in each viral genome, designated ras, was shown to be derived from the cellular genome and was not homologous to any known viral sequences. The ras sequences in Kirsten-MSV and Harvey-MSV were found to be only partially related and thus represent different members of a gene family (Ellis et al., 1981).

Subsequent to the isolation of Kirsten-MSV and Harvey-MSV, two other murine sarcoma viruses, BALB-MSV and Rasheed-MSV, were shown to contain ras oncogenes derived from the BALB/c mouse and Fisher rat, respectively (Andersen et al., 1981; Gonda et al., 1982). Another ras family member, designated N-ras, has been identified in mammalian cells but has not been identified to date as a transforming gene of any known retrovirus (Shimizu et al., 1983a; Eva et al., 1983; Hall et al., 1983).

RAS PROTO-ONCOGENES OF HUMAN CELLS

Three ras genes of human cells have been molecularly cloned and characterized in detail. The organization of their coding sequences is similar in that each gene contains four exons; however, the exons are distributed over a region anywhere from 4.8 kbp (H-ras) to 45 kbp (K-ras) in length (Chang et al., 1982; Santos et al., 1982; Shimizu et al., 1983b). Pseudogenes of H-ras and K-ras have also been identified (designated H-ras-2 and K-ras-1) (Chang et al., 1982). The molecular cloning and nucleotide sequence analysis of ras genes of yeast has demonstrated a remarkable degree of evolutionary conservation of ras gene structure (DeFeo-Jones et al., 1983; Powers et al., 1984).

RAS GENES ARE FREQUENTLY DETECTED AS HUMAN TRANSFORMING GENES

The involvement of the ras gene family in naturally occurring malignancies came to light in studies in which investigators asked whether DNAs of animal or human tumor cells possessed the capacity to directly confer the neoplastic phenotype to a susceptible assay cell. Some human tumor DNAs were shown to induce transformed foci in the continuous NIH/3T3 mouse cell line (Jainchill et al., 1969), which is highly susceptible to the uptake and stable incorporation of exogenous DNA (Cooper, 1982; Weinberg, 1982).

The first molecularly cloned human transforming gene, whose source was the T24 bladder carcinoma cell line, was demonstrated to be the activated homologue of the normal H-ras gene (Goldfarb et al., 1982; Pulciani et al., 1982a; Santos et al., 1982; Shih and Weinberg, 1982). Subsequent analysis of oncogenes detected by transfection assays has established that the majority of such transforming genes belong to the ras family. Thus, K-ras oncogenes have been detected at high frequency in lung and colon carcinomas (Pulciani et al., 1982b). Carcinomas of the digestive tract, including pancreas, and gall bladder, as well as genitourinary tract tumors, and sarcomas have also been shown to contain ras oncogenes. N-ras appears to be the most frequently activated ras transforming gene in human hematopoietic neoplasms (Eva et al., 1983). These results are summarized in Table 1.

Not only can a variety of tumor types contain the same activated ras oncogene, but the same tumor type can contain different activated ras oncogenes. Thus, in hematopoietic tumors, we have observed different ras oncogenes (K-ras, N-ras) activated in lymphoid tumors at the same stage of hematopoietic cell differentiation, as well as N-ras genes activated in tumors as diverse in origin as acute and chronic myelogenous leukemia (Eva et al., 1983) (Table 1). These findings suggest that ras oncogenes detected in the NIH/3T3 transfection assay are not specific to a given stage of cell differentiation or tissue type.

Retroviruses that contain ras-related onc genes are known to possess a wide spectrum of target cells for transformation in vivo and in vitro. In addition to inducing sarcomas and transforming fibroblasts (Gross, 1970), these viruses are capable of inducing tumors of immature lymphoid cells (Pierce and Aaronson, 1982). They also can stimulate the proliferation of erythroblasts (Hankins and Scolnick, 1981) and monocyte/macrophages (Greenberger, 1979), and can even induce alterations in the growth and differentiation of epithelial cells (Weissman and Aaronson, 1983). Thus, the wide array of tissue types that can be induced to proliferate abnormally by these onc genes may help to explain the high frequency of detection of their activated human homologues in diverse human tumors.

It should be noted that not all oncogenes detected by NIH/3T3 transfection analysis are related to known retroviral oncogenes. For example, Cooper and coworkers have identified and molecularly cloned an oncogene, B-lym, from a B-cell lymphoma (Goubin et al., 1983). B-lym appears to be activated in a large proportion of tumors at a specific stage of B-cell differentiation (Diamond et al., 1983). Studies to date indicate that this oncogene is relatively small in size (<600 bp), and sequence analysis indicates that it possesses distant homology to transferrin (Goubin et al., 1983). These investigators have also detected oncogenes which appear to be specifically activated in tumors at other stages of lymphoid differentiation (Lane et al., 1982) or in mammary carcinomas (Lane et al., 1981). None of these transforming genes appear to possess detectable homology with known retroviral onc sequences.

MECHANISM OF ACTIVATION OF RAS ONCOGENES

The availability of molecular clones of the normal and activated alleles of human ras proto-oncogenes made it possible to determine the molecular mechanisms responsible for the malignant

Table 1. Detection of ras oncogenes in human tumors

Tumor source	Percent Positive	ras oncogene activated		
		H-ras	K-ras	N-ras
Carcinoma	10-30	4/12	6/12	2/12
(lung, gastrointestinal, genitourinary)				
Sarcoma	~ 10	0/2	0/2	2/2
(fibrosarcoma, rhabdomyosarcoma)				
Hematopoietic	10-50	0/9	1/9	8/9
(AML, CML, ALL, CLL)				

conversion of these genes. The genetic lesions responsible for activation of a number of ras oncogenes have been localized to single base changes in their p21 coding sequences. In the T24/EJ bladder carcinoma oncogene, a transversion of a G to a T causes a valine residue to be incorporated instead of a glycine into the 12th position of the predicted p21 primary structure (Tabin et al., 1982; Reddy et al., 1982; Taparowsky et al., 1983b; Capon et al., 1983a). During our analyses of human cells for transforming DNA sequences, we were able to isolate and molecularly clone an oncogene from a human lung carcinoma, designated Hs242 (Yuasa et al., 1983). This gene was also identified as an activated H-ras (human) proto-oncogene, making it possible to compare the mechanisms by which the same human proto-oncogene has been independently activated in human tumor-derived cells.

The Hs242 transforming sequence was isolated and subjected to restriction enzyme analysis in order to compare its physical map with that of the previously reported T24/EJ bladder tumor oncogene (Yuasa et al., 1983), as well as c-H-ras cloned from a normal human fetal liver library (Santos et al., 1982). The restriction map of the Hs242 oncogene closely corresponded with both, diverging only outside the region previously shown to be required for the transforming activity of the T24 ocogene.

To map the position of the genetic lesion in Hs242 leading to its malignant activation, recombinants were constructed in which fragments of the Hs242 oncogene were substituted by the homologous sequences of H-ras (human). By this analysis the genetic alteration that activated the Hs242 oncogene was localized to a 0.45-kbp region that encompassed its second coding exon. Nucleotide sequence analysis of this region revealed that the Hs242 oncogene and H-ras (human) differed at a single base within codon 61. The change of an A to a T resulted in the replacement of glutamine by leucine in this codon. Thus, a single amino acid substitution seems sufficient to confer transforming properties on the product of the Hs242 oncogene. These results also established that the site of activation in the Hs242 oncogene was totally different from that of the T24/EJ oncogene (Yuasa et al., 1983).

In subsequent studies, we have assessed the generality of point mutations as the basis for acquisition of malignant properties by ras proto-oncogenes by molecularly cloning and analyzing other activated ras oncogenes. Activation of an H-ras transforming gene of the Hs578T human breast carcinosarcoma line has been localized to a point mutation at position 12 changing glycine to aspartic acid in the amino acid sequence (Kraus et al., 1984). Recently Wigler and co-workers (Taparowsky et al., 1983a) reported that the lesion leading to activation of the N-ras oncogene in a neuroblastoma line was due to the alteration of codon 61 from CAA to AAA causing the substitution in this case of lysine for glutamine. Another N-ras transforming gene, this one isolated from a human lung carcinoma cell line, SW1271, has been shown to result from a single point mutation of an A to a G at position 61 in the coding sequence resulting in the substitution of arginine for glutamine (Yuasa et al., 1984).

Investigators analyzing K-ras oncogenes (Shimuzu et al., 1983b, Capon et al., 1983b) have achieved strikingly similiar results. In two K-ras transforming genes so far analyzed, single point mutations in the 12th codon have been shown to be respon-' sible for acquisition of malignant properties. Thus, mutations at positions 12 or 61 appear to be the genetic lesions most commonly responsible for activation of ras oncogenes under natural conditions in human tumor cells (Table 2).

IMPLICATIONS

The very high frequency of detection of ras oncogenes in human tumors strongly suggests but does not prove that these genes play a role in the processes leading to the formation of a tumor. More recently it has been possible to ascertain that in patients whose tumor cells possess an activated ras oncogene, the activating lesion is not found in the ras alleles of normal cells (Kraus et al., 1984). Furthermore, analysis of biologically cloned tumor cells from such a patient showed that all tumor cells contained

Table 2. Genetic lesions that activate ras oncogenes of human tumors

ras oncogene	Tumor	Base/amino acid change	Codon no.	Reference
H-ras				
T24	Bladder carcinoma	GlyγVal (GGCγG<u>T</u>C)	12	Tabin et al., 1982 Reddy et al., 1982 Taparowsky et al., 1983b Capon et al., 1983a
Hs0578	Mammary carcinoma	GlyγAsp (GGCγG<u>A</u>C)	12	Kraus et al., 1984
Hs 242	Lung carcinoma	GlnγLeu (CAGγC<u>T</u>G)	61	Yuasa et al., 1983
K-ras				
Calu-1	Lung carcinoma	GlyγCys (GGTγ<u>T</u>GT)	12	Shimizu et al., 1983b Capon et al., 1983b
SW480	Colon carcinoma	GlyγVal (GGTγG<u>TT</u>)	12	Capon et al., 1983b
SK-N-SH	Neuroblastoma	GlnγLys (CAAγ<u>A</u>AA)	61	Taparowsky et al., 1983a
SW1271	Lung carcinoma	GlnγArg (GGTΓG<u>TT</u>)	61	Yuasa et al., 1984

the activated allele. These findings establish that mutations that activate ras oncogenes occur somatically and that these events are powerfully selected for within the tumor. All of the above findings, taken together, imply that the activation of these oncogenes is part of the cause, rather than a result of the neoplastic process.

The normal function(s) of ras proto-oncogenes have not been delineated, nor is it known how the mutations at the position 12 and 61 "hot spots" in ras p21s so dramatically alter their biologic functions. However, it may be possible to determine whether these changes are predictive of a particular clinical course by utilizing currently available biochemical and immunological techniques to specifically recognize altered p21 proteins, transcripts, or alleles.

REFERENCES

Andersen, P. R., Devare, S. G., Tronick, S. R., Ellis, R. W., Aaronson, S. A., and Scolnick, E. M., 1981, Generation of BALB-MuSV and Ha-MuSV by type C virus transduction of homologous transforming genes from different species, Cell, 26:129.

Bishop, J. M., 1983, Cellular oncogenes and retroviruses, in: "Ann. Rev Biochemistry., Vol. 52," E. E. Snell, P. D. Boyer, A, Meister, C. C. Richardson, ed., Academic Press, Palo Alto.

Capon, D. J., Chen, E. Y., Levinson, A. D., Seeburg, P. H., and Goeddel, D. V., 1983a, Complete nucleotide sequences of the T24 human bladder carcinoma oncogene and its normal homologue, Nature, 302:33.

Capon, D. J., Seeburg, P. H., McGrath, J. P., Hayflick, J. S., Edman, U., Levinson, A. D., and Goeddel, D. V., 1983b, Activation of Ki-ras 2 gene in human colon and lung carcinomas by two different point mutations, Nature, 304:507.

Chang, E. H., Gonda, M. A., Ellis, R. W., Scolnick, E. M., Lowy, D. R., 1982, Human genome contains four genes homologous to transforming genes of Harvey and Kirsten murine sarcoma viruses, Proc. Natl. Acad. Sci. USA, 79:4848.

Cooper, G. M., 1982, Cellular transforming genes, Science, 218:801.

DeFeo-Jones, D., Scolnick, E. M., Koller, R., and Dhar, R., 1983, Ras-related gene sequences identified and isolated from Saccharomyces cerevisiae, Nature, 306:707.

Diamond, A., Cooper, G. M., Ritz, J., and Lane, M. A., 1983, Identification and molecular cloning of the human blym transforming gene activated in Burkitt's lymphomas, Nature, 305:112.

Duesberg, P. H., 1983, Retroviral transforming genes in normal cells?, Nature, 304:219.

Ellis, R. W., DeFeo, D., Shih, T. Y., Gonda, M. A., Young, H. A., Tsuchida, N., Lowy, D. R., and Scolnick, E. M., 1981, The p21 src genes of Harvey and Kirsten sarcoma viruses originate from divergent members of a family of normal vertebrate genes, Nature, 292:506.

Eva, A., Tronick, S. R., Gol, R. A., Pierce, J. H., and Aaronson, S. A., 1983, Transforming genes of human hematopoietic tumors: frequent detection of ras-related oncogenes whose activation appears to be independent of tumor phenotype, Proc. Natl. Acad. Sci. USA, 80:4926.

Goldfarb, M., Shimizu, K., Perucho, M., and Wigler, M., 1982, Isolation and preliminary characterization of a human transforming gene from T24 bladder carcinoma cells, Nature, 296:404.

Gonda, M. A., Young, H. A., Elser, J. E., Rasheed, S., Talmadge, C. B, Nagashima, K., Li, C. C., and Gilden, R. V., 1982, Molecular cloning, genomic analysis, and biological properties of rat leukemia virus and the onc sequences of Rasheed rat sarcoma virus, J. Virol., 44:520.

Goubin, G., Goldman, D. S., Luce, J., Neiman , E., and Cooper, G. M., 1983, Molecular cloning and nucleotide sequence of a transforming gene detected by transfection of chicken B-cell lymphoma DNA, Nature, 302:114.

Greenberger, J. S., 1979, Phenotypically distinct target cells for murine sarcoma virus and murine leukemia virus marrow transformation in vitro., J. Nat. Cancer Inst., 62:337.

Gross, L., 1970, Oncogenic Viruses, 2nd edit., Pergamon Press., Oxford.

Hankins, D. W., and Scolnick, E. M., 1981, Harvey and Kirsten sarcoma viruses promote the growth and differentiation of erythroid precursor cells in vitro, Cell, 26:91.

Hall, A., Marshall, C. J., Spurr, N. K., and Weiss, R. A., 1983, Identification of transforming gene in two human sarcoma cell lines as a new member of the ras gene family located on chromosome 1. Nature, 303:396.

Jainchill, J. L., Aaronson, S. A., and Todaro, G. J., 1969, Murine sarcoma and leukemia viruses: assay using clonal lines of contact inhibited mouse cells, J. Virol., 4:549.

Kraus, M., Yuasa, Y., and Aaronson, S. A., 1984, A position 12-activated H-ras oncogene in all HS578T mammary carcino-sarcoma cells but not normal mammary cells of the same patient, Proc. Natl. Acad. Sci. USA, 81:5384.

Lane, M. A., Sainten, A., and Cooper, G. M., 1981, Activation of related transforming genes in mouse and human mammary carcinomas, Proc. Natl. Acad. Sci. USA, 78:5185.

Lane, M. A., Sainten, A., and Cooper, G. M., 1982, Stage-specific transforming genes of human and mouse B- and T-lymphocyte neoplasms, Cell, 28:873.

Pierce, J. H., and Aaronson, S. A., 1982, BALB- and Harvey-murine sarcoma virus transformation of a novel lymphoid progenitor cell, J. Exp. Med., 156:873.

Powers, S., Kataoka, T., Fasano, O., Goldfarb, M., Strathern, J., Broach, J., and Wigler, M., 1984, Genes in S. cerevisiae encoding proteins with domains homologous to the mammalian ras proteins, Cell, 36:607.

Pulciani, S., Santos, E., Lauver, A. V., Long, L. K., Robbins, K. C., and Barbacid, M., 1982a, Oncogenes in human tumor cell lines: molecular cloning of a tranforming gene from human bladder carcinoma cells, Proc. Natl. Acad. Sci. USA, 79:2845.

Pulciani, S., Santos, E., Lauver, A. V., Long, L. K., Aaronson, S. A., and Barbacid, M., 1982b, Oncogenes in solid human tumors, Nature, 300:539.

Santos, E., Tronick, S. R., Aaronson, S. A., Pulciani, S., and Barbacid, M., 1982, T24 human bladder carcinoma oncogene is an activated form of the normal human homologue of BALB- and Harvey-MSV transforming genes, Nature, 298:343.

Shih, C., Weinberg, R. A., 1982, Isolation of a transforming sequence from a human bladder carcinoma cell line, Cell, 29:161.

Shih, T. Y., Williams, D. R., Weeks, M. O., Maryak, J. M., Vass, W. C., and Scolnick, E. M., 1978, Comparison of the genomic organization of Kirsten and Harvey sarcoma viruses, J. Virol., 27:45.

Shimizu, K., Goldfarb, M., Perucho, M., Wigler, M., 1983a, Isolation, and preliminary characterization of the transforming gene of a human neuroblastoma cell line, Proc. Natl. Acad. Sci. USA, 80:383.

Shimizu, K., Birnbaum, D., Ruley, M. A., Fasano, O., Suard, Y., Edlund, L., Taparowsky, E., Goldfarb, M., Wigler, M., 1983b, Structure of the Ki-ras gene of the human lung carcinoma cell line Calu-1, Nature, 304:497.

Taparowsky, E., Shimizu, K., Goldfarb, M., Wigler, M., 1983a, Structure and activation of the human N-ras gene, Cell, 34:581.

Taparowsky, E., Suard, Y., Fasano, O., Shimizu, K., Goldfarb, M., Wigler, M., 1983b, Activation of the T24 bladder carcinoma transforming gene is linked to a single amino acid change, Nature, 300:762.

Weinberg, R. A., 1982, Fewer and fewer oncogenes, Cell, 30:3.

Weiss, R. A., Teich, N., Varmus, H., and Coffin, R. J., 1982. "Molecular Biology of Tumor Viruses, RNA Tumor Viruses. 2nd edit.," Cold Spring Harbor, New York.

Weissman, B. E., and Aaronson, S. A., 1983, BALB and Kirsten murine sarcoma viruses alter growth and differentiation of EGF-dependent BALB/c mouse epidermal keratinocyte lines, Cell, 32:599.

Yuasa, Y., Srivastava, S. K., Dunn, C. Y., Rhim, J. S., Reddy, E. P., and Aaronson, S. A., 1983, Acquisition of transforming properties by alternative point mutations within c-bas/has human proto-oncogene, Nature, 303:775.

Yuasa, Y., Gol, R. A., Chang, A., Chiu, I.-M., Reddy, E. P., Tronick, S. R., and Aaronson, S. A., 1984, Mechanism of activation of an N-ras oncogene of SW-1271 human lung carcinoma cells, Proc. Natl. Acad. Sci. USA, 81:3670.

HEREDITARY AND FAMILIAL DISORDERS LINKING CANCER PRONENESS

WITH ABNORMAL CARCINOGEN RESPONSE AND FAULTY DNA METABOLISM

M.C. Paterson, N.E. Gentner, M.V. Middlestadt,
R. Mirzayans and M. Weinfeld

Health Sciences Division
Chalk River Nuclear Laboratories
Chalk River, Ontario, Canada K0J 1J0

INTRODUCTION

Insight into cancer, one of the principal scourges of modern man, has increased slowly but steadily over the years. Epidemiologists concur that most human malignancies are caused, at least in part, by environmental determinants over which an individual can exercise some control; in principle then, the disease is preventable to some extent (Doll and Peto, 1981). In practice, however, the goal of cancer prevention by large-scale efforts to minimize exposure to the causal agents would seem to be unattainable, as judged by societal experience with two major 'life-style' factors, habitual tobacco usage and sunbathing. Although an ultimate aim is to develop other more socially acceptable prevention strategies, there exists in the interim a requirement for improved diagnostic techniques and more rational treatment protocols. Each of these approaches to cancer control will almost certainly necessitate clearer understanding of the fundamental mechanisms underlying the etiology and pathogenesis of the disease.

One burgeoning line of exploration into the carcinogenic process is the investigation of human genetics as it pertains to mankind's susceptibility to cancer. Although as many as 90% of all human malignant neoplasms are said to have environmental causes (Higginson and Muir, 1979), by far the most potent risk factor is the genetic component. There exists a repertoire of loci in the human genome, any one of which, in its mutated form, can confer a marked increase in cancer risk (Mulvihill, 1980). In fact, ecogenetics, involving the study of individual variation in response to an environmental factor (Mulvihill, 1980), is rapidly emerging as a profitable experimental approach for unravelling the origins of cancer.

A particularly enlightening ecogenetic inquiry concerns the application of laboratory models (derived primarily from microbial systems) to the in vitro investigation of cells from patients in whom astute clinicians have noted an untoward response to a recognized carcinogen (Miller, 1980). These patients, for the most part, are afflicted with Mendelian monogenic traits characterized by a propensity to develop malignancy. Cultured cells from subjects with many of these rare hereditary disorders display enhanced sensitivity to inactivation by the pertinent etiological agent; in several syndromes, this carcinogen hypersensitivity is, in turn, associated with anomalies in the enzymatic processes that repair, replicate past, or otherwise tolerate lesions introduced into DNA by the same carcinogenic agent (Friedberg et al., 1979; Kraemer, 1983; Paterson et al., 1984b). Such correlations provide telling evidence that fully functional DNA metabolic systems form an integral part of the host machinery which *Homo sapiens* routinely marshals in defence against the development of cancer.

EXPERIMENTAL STRATEGIES AND PRIMARY AIMS

This chapter describes our own particular laboratory studies into the various molecular mechanisms that underlie the predisposition to cancer seen in certain hereditary and familial conditions. In each of these undertakings, primary emphasis has been placed on evaluating the role of carcinogen-induced injury to cellular DNA and the faulty enzymatic repair of this damage as a contributing factor in the multistep process whereby a normal somatic cell may undergo malignant conversion.

In general, our experimental approach has entailed subjecting dermal fibroblast strains, derived from selected donors, to a battery of assays which are designed to detect specific biological and/or biochemical abnormalities following exposure to an etiologically relevant carcinogen. Normally a given fibroblast strain was monitored first for reproductive survival, as judged by retention of colony-forming ability (CFA), in response to a panel of appropriate carcinogens; if a strain responded abnormally to any of these agents, a search was then undertaken for anomalies in either the initial induction or the subsequent metabolic processing of specific lesions induced in DNA by the pertinent agent(s). Two disorders -- xeroderma pigmentosum (XP), a skin disease characterized by striking sensitivity to solar ultraviolet (UV) light, and ataxia telangiectasia (AT), its ionizing radiation-sensitive, neurovascular counterpart, served as archetypes for our investigations. Both of the foregoing are rare, autosomal recessively inherited syndromes in which cancer proneness and carcinogen hypercytotoxicity have been closely linked with defects in lesion processing (for review, see Kraemer, 1983 and Paterson et al., 1984b). In charting this experimental course, our intent has been three-fold: (i) to extend current knowledge of known DNA repair deficiency disorders; (ii) to identify other cancer-prone ecogenetic traits, and then to define their molecular basis; and (iii) to utilize these mutant strains to assist in delineating the normal sequence of reactions in different DNA repair processes and in other cellular processes germane to carcinogenesis.

STATUS REPORT ON OUR OWN ECOGENETIC STUDIES

Our progress thus far in six specific ecogenetic investigations is now summarized (for background information, see Paterson et al., 1983, 1984a and b). Space restrictions necessarily preclude all but cursory reference to parallel studies in other laboratories.

1. New Insight into the Molecular Defect in XP

A major breakthrough in our understanding of environmental-hereditary interactions in cancer causation occurred when Cleaver (1968) provided evidence that dermal fibroblasts from XP patients are defective in handling cyclobutyl pyrimidine dimers. These DNA lesions, which are formed by the covalent joining of adjacent intrastrand pyrimidine bases upon absorption of UV radiation, are believed to be largely responsible for the lethal, mutagenic and carcinogenic effects of sunlight (McCormick et al., 1981; Robbins, 1983). Since Cleaver's seminal disclosure some 17 years ago, many advances have been made in defining the DNA repair deficiencies displayed by cultured XP cells after exposure to UV rays and certain chemical carcinogens (for details regarding the overall laboratory picture in XP, including the impairments in post-UV colony survival and DNA metabolism typical of cells from affected donors, see Friedberg et al., 1979; Cleaver, 1980; Kraemer, 1983; Paterson et al., 1984b). In this characterization, fibroblast strains from 119 unrelated XP patients have been allocated to nine genetically distinct groups on the basis of a biochemical complementation test, using a conventional somatic cell fusion technique. As can be seen in Table 1, 98 of the strains have been assigned to eight mutually complementing groups, designated A-H. The primary biochemical anomaly in each of these strains is apparently a deficiency in the ability to execute the nucleotide mode of excision repair. The remaining 21 XP strains have been pooled together to form the ninth complementation group, the so-called variant. The most striking anomaly in these latter strains appears to be a marked deficiency in performing post-replication or daughter-strand repair, an ill-defined process that is

Table 1. DNA Repair Properties of Xeroderma Pigmentosum Complementation Groups[a]

Group	No. of Cases	Excision Repair (% of normal) as judged by		Postreplication Repair
		UV Endonuclease Site Removal	UV-induced Repair Synthesis	
A	49	~0	<5[b]	partly deficient
B	1	<10	3-7	partly deficient
C	32	15-35	10-25	partly deficient
D	9	~0	20-55	partly deficient
E	1	60	40-60	proficient
F	3	70	10-20	?[c]
G	2	~0	<5	partly deficient
H	1	?	30	partly deficient
Variant	21	100	60-100	markedly deficient
Total	119			

[a] Adapted from Paterson et al. (1984b)

[b] One strain (XP8LO) displays 30% of normal repair synthesis

[c] Unknown

presently thought to be instrumental in permitting the *de novo* DNA synthesis machinery to replicate past pyrimidine dimers and other non-coding alterations in template DNA.

The current model for the nucleotide excision repair process has been derived principally from the more extensive and sophisticated studies possible in simple prokaryotes (see Haseltine, 1983; Friedberg et al., 1981; Sancar and Rupp, 1983; Paterson and Gentner, 1984). As shown schematically in Fig. 1, two distinct pathways for this intricate multienzymatic process have been identified to date. The first pathway, originally described in *Escherichia coli* almost two decades ago, is composed of the following sequential reactions: (i) the damage-containing strand is incised upstream from (i.e., on the 5'-side of) the lesion by a damage-recognizing endonuclease (e.g., a so-called UV endonuclease in the case of the pyrimidine dimer); (ii) a second nick is made downstream from (i.e., on the 3'-side of) the lesion by an exonuclease, facilitating the release of the lesion within a short oligonucleotide (in *E. coli*, at least, these first two steps are, in fact, performed in concert by an 'exinuclease complex' and may be followed by 5'⟶3' exonucleolytic removal of 5'-deoxyribonucleoside monophosphates); (iii) the resultant gap is filled in with nucleotides complementary to those in the opposite, intact stand by a DNA polymerase, in a procedure termed repair synthesis; and finally (iv) the pre-existing and newly synthesized strand termini are covalently joined by a DNA ligase.

The second pathway by which nucleotide excision repair may proceed is found in, for example, *Micrococcus luteus* and bacteriophage T4. Their 'UV endonucleases' accomplish incision at a dimer-containing site by the sequential action of a pyrimidine dimer DNA-glycosylase activity and an apyrimidinic/apurinic (AP) endonuclease activity. The former cleaves the N-glycosyl bond between the 5'-pyrimidine member of a dimer pair and and its corresponding deoxyribose, and the latter then hydrolyzes a phosphodiester bond 3' to the newly formed AP site. In all probability, the incised site is subsequently mended as in the first nucleotide excision pathway -- that is, site removal, repair synthesis and strand ligation.

By virtue of their abnormality in excision repair, XP strains belonging to groups A-H are also inept, where tested, in handling a variety of other bulky lesions, such as those induced by reactive metabolites of the following potent chemical carcinogens: benzo[α]-pyrene, N-acetoxy-2-acetylaminofluorene and 4-nitroquinoline 1-oxide (4NQO) (Kraemer, 1983; Paterson et al., 1984b). What is more, these eight genetic forms of the disease all seem to be blocked, inexplicably, at the same stage (incision step) in the excision repair process.

In general, strains belonging to a given excision repair-defective complementation group display a similar degree of repair

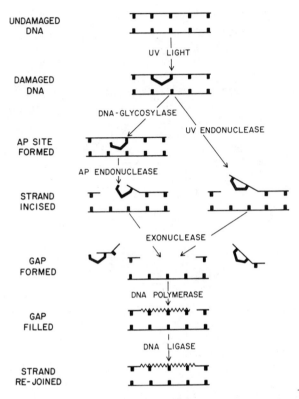

Fig. 1.   Proposed model for the two distinct mechanisms by which
the nucleotide mode of excision repair is known to occur
in different microbial systems. In this mode a carcinogen-
induced defect (illustrated here as a cyclobutyl pyrimidine
dimer) in either chain of the double helix is excised within an oligonucleotide, as detailed in the text. The des-
ignation nucleotide excision distinguishes it from another
general excision repair mode termed base excision.   (In
the latter, a carcinogen-damaged or nonconventional base
is released by a highly specific DNA glycosylase, after
which the resultant AP site is restored by co-ordinated
strand incision/AP site excision/repair synthesis/strand
ligation reactions [for details, consult Friedberg et al.,
1981; Lindahl, 1982].)

deficiency. This holds irrespective of the particular DNA repair assay used, including those presumed to monitor early or late reactions in the excision-repair process. As a case in point, group A strains appear to be severely defective in executing dimer repair, as exemplified by the following two deficits: (i) negligible ability to perform the initial incision event in the removal of dimer-containing sites (detected as UV-induced sites susceptible to subsequent strand incision in vitro by the action of a UV endonuclease contained in a crude protein extract of *M. luteus*, and hereafter referred to as UV endonuclease-sensitive sites); and (ii) pronounced impairment in the capacity to carry out UV-induced repair synthesis (measured as unscheduled DNA synthesis [UDS] or DNA repair replication) (see Table 1). In several other excision repair-defective groups (e.g., C), although a reduced ability to perform dimer repair is apparent, a significant residual level clearly remains; this is true for both assays in Table 1.

XP group D, however, constitutes a glaring exception to the inter-assay uniformity in quantitating the residual repair capacity of representative strains from patients with the disorder (see Table 1). Strains assigned to this group are markedly, if not totally, impaired in effecting the elimination of UV endonuclease-sensitive sites, but nonetheless manage to carry out a substantial amount of UV-induced repair synthesis, ranging from 20-55% of normal, depending upon which laboratory's results are cited. (A second exception is evident in another group, namely, F; in contradistinction to group D, strains in this group appear to act on many more UV endonuclease-sensitive sites than expected from their repair synthesis deficiency.)

One possible explanation for the peculiar excision repair properties of group D fibroblasts is that, following UV exposure, these mutant cells may act in an aberrant manner on a fraction of the dimer-containing sites, inserting repair patches while failing to excise the photoproducts themselves. To test whether some of the dimers are modified but not removed in group D strains, we measured the photoreactivability (a well-documented diagnostic probe of dimer authenticity [Harm, 1976]) of UV endonuclease-sensitive sites in extracted DNA from normal and group D strains as a function of cell incubation time after exposure to 15 $J \cdot m^{-2}$ of far UV (chiefly 254 nm) light. Our assay protocol is depicted in Fig. 2. Following post-UV incubation, each cell culture was lyzed; the extracted DNA was subjected to exhaustive enzymatic photoreactivation (PR) treatment (using highly purified *Streptomyces griseus* photolyase which, in the presence of fluorescent light, simply ruptures the cyclobutane ring of a pyrimidine dimer, thereby regenerating two normal monomeric pyrimidines *in situ* without any additional modification to the site), and was then probed by incubation with an *M. luteus*

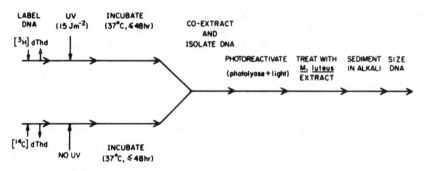

Fig. 2.   Experimental scheme designed to detect aberrant repair of
           UV-induced pyrimidine dimers in XP group D fibroblasts.
           The treatment protocol was virtually identical to that
           followed in a conventional enzymatic assay for dimer quan-
           tification (Paterson et al., 1981b), except for the intro-
           duction of an enzymatic PR step (thus converting remaining
           dimers back to normal monomers *in situ*) prior to treatment
           of the naked DNA with an *M. luteus* protein extract con-
           taining dimer-recognizing UV endonuclease. The ^{14}C-label-
           led DNA from non-UV-irradiated cultures served as an in-
           ternal control which permitted correction for non-specific
           strand breakage stemming from the various physical manip-
           ulations and enzymatic treatments prescribed in the assay.

extract containing UV endonuclease activity. In short, this series
of treatments was expected to detect any dimer-containing sites
which had been altered so as to render them refractory to photoenzymatic monomerization but still susceptible to incision by UV
endonuclease. Lastly, the number of extract-induced single-strand
breaks, and thus the incidence of apparently unrepaired sites remaining in the DNA, was determined by velocity sedimentation in alkaline sucrose gradients.

     Our results, presented in Fig. 3, demonstrated the appearance
of altered sites in the DNA of XP group D (XP2NE) cells specifically
with incubation after UV exposure (also see Paterson, 1982). These
sites did not arise in similarly treated control (GM38) cells, suggesting that their occurrence in the XP strain arose from unsuccessful attempts to repair UV-induced pyrimidine dimers. These novel
sites in the DNA of XP2NE fibroblasts reached an incidence approaching 8 per 10^8 daltons by 48 hrs; this number was equivalent to ~15%
of the dimers initially introduced, and was similar in magnitude to
the residual level of UV-stimulated repair synthesis (15-20% of
normal) arising in the XP strain. Accumulation of novel sites after
UV irradiation was not confined to XP group D. As illustrated in

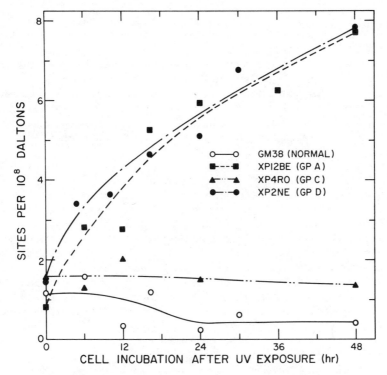

Fig. 3. Incidence of novel sites accumulating in the DNA of normal
and XP strains as a function of post-UV incubation time.
The experimental protocol is outlined in Fig. 2. Each
datum point is the mean of multiple determinations (SE<15%).

Fig. 3, sites also appeared in the UV-damaged DNA of incubated group
A (XP12BE) cells, with kinetics very similar to those in group D
cells. On the other hand, a representative group C strain, XP4RO,
behaved very much like the normal GM38 strain.

In both XP groups A and D strains, there was no decrease (compared to the number originally induced) in total UV endonuclease-
sensitive sites or in the number of dimers actually remaining in
DNA (Gentner et al., 1981), but there was an apparent decrease in
the number of UV endonuclease-sensitive sites subject to restoration
by enzymatic PR (Fig. 3). One interpretation of these findings is
that the photoenzymatic treatment gives rise to strand breaks at

these seemingly metabolically modified dimer-containing sites (that is, the same sites that are normally recognized by UV endonuclease). If so, then these sites should be detectable as frank single-strand breaks if extracted DNA was subjected to enzymatic PR alone (that is, without ensuing *M. luteus* extract treatment). We have now demonstrated that this is indeed the case. This intriguing observation is consistent with the notion that during post-UV incubation of group A and D fibroblasts, a phosphodiester bond between the two dimer-forming pyrimidines may be cleaved, and that at these modified sites individual DNA chains are then held together solely by the cyclobutane ring (i.e., -p-T̂-p-T̂-p- ⟶ -p-T̂ p-T-p- or -p-T̂-p T-p-). It seems that the excision repair process tends to abort at this stage in group A cells since they carry out little repair synthesis, whereas in group D cells the intradimer backbone cleavage is apparently accompanied by aberrant insertion of a repair patch, presumably proximal to the unexcised photoproduct. To test this hypothesis, we performed photochemical reversal on the dimer-containing excision fragments isolated from post-UV incubated normal cells, and were able to observe the release of both free thymidine and thymidine monophosphate molecules. Their combined yield proved to be essentially stoichiometric with the number of dimers photoreversed, signifying that most of the excised oligonucleotide fragments did indeed contain a dimer at one end, with an internal phosphodiester break (e.g., T̂ p-T-p-N- and p-T̂ p-T-p-N- ⟶ T, pT and p-T-p-N-) (Gentner et al., 1984).

Our inability to detect the release of free thymine upon direct photoreversal of dimer-containing excision products corroborates the earlier report by LaBelle and Linn (1982) that human cells do not initiate dimer excision by hydrolysis of the N-glycosyl bond of one member of the dimer pair, as do *M. luteus* and bacteriophage T4. Rather, cleavage of the intradimer phosphodiester linkage would seem to be the first step in the human nucleotide excision repair process, followed by classical strand incision/lesion excision/repair synthesis/strand ligation steps. In this new mode, depicted in Fig. 4, the proposed function of the putative pyrimidine dimer-DNA phosphodiesterase is to induce a localized structural change at the dimer-containing site such that the site is then recognizable by a generalized 'bulky lesion-repair complex', perhaps analogous to the UVRABC exinuclease complex which is active in *E. coli* on a host of chemically disparate lesions (Sancar and Rupp, 1983). Breakage of the phosphodiester bond between dimerized pyrimidines in human cells may additionally serve to relieve regional conformational stress imparted by the intradimer cyclobutane bridge, thus restoring hydrogen bonding to adjoining base pairs in the double-stranded helix and, in so doing, presumably enhancing the fidelity of *de novo* DNA synthesis on a UV-damaged template. Investigation into these and other ramifications of the new model are in progress.

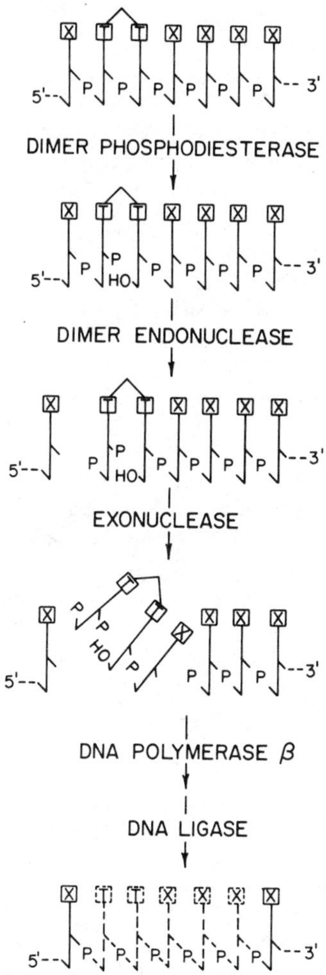

Fig. 4. New model for the nucleotide mode of excision repair operating on UV-induced cyclobutyl pyrimidine dimers in cultured human skin fibroblasts. Note that only the dimer-
containing strand of the DNA duplex is shown here. The
essential difference between this model and that for prokaryotes in Fig. 1 is that here the initial reaction is
catalyzed by a putative pyrimidine dimer-DNA phosphodiesterase rather than by either a dimer-DNA glycosylase, as
in *M. luteus* and phage T4, or an 'exinuclease' complex, as
in *E. coli*. In the scheme shown here, the dimer is depicted at the 5'-end of the excision fragment and the
cleavage of the intradimer phosphodiester linkage is assumed to yield 3'-P and 5'-OH termini. Other possibilities
clearly exist and the exact location and nature of the
breaks associated with dimer removal await determination.

2. Defective Repair of 4NQO Lesions in AT Cells

A considerable portion of our research effort over the past decade has been devoted to elucidating the primary biochemical defect(s) in ataxia telangiectasia (reviewed in Paterson et al., 1983, 1984a and b). Persons inheriting this complex neurovascular and immunological disorder are prone to lymphoproliferative neoplasia and react adversely (sometimes fatally) to conventional radiotherapy. Cultured cells from these patients also exhibit enhanced radiosensitivity, as judged by impaired CFA and elevated levels of chromosomal aberrations after X irradiation. In our studies fibroblasts from most AT donors were found to be defective in the ability to repair certain (as of yet chemically undefined) types of alkali-stable DNA radioproducts, as indicated by (i) a deficiency in executing γ ray-stimulated DNA repair synthesis and (ii) a reduced capacity to remove radiogenic DNA lesions (assayed as sites sensitive to damage-recognizing endonucleases and DNA glycosylases in a crude *M. luteus* extract). These data led us to propose that such AT strains may harbor an anomaly in an excision repair pathway operating on particular classes of alkali-stable radioproducts (e.g., altered base or sugar residues); these strains have consequently been designated exr⁻. However, other AT strains, although themselves as radiosensitive as the exr⁻ strains and established from donors presenting typical hallmarks of the disease, exhibited no demonstrable deficiency in repairing radiogenic damage to their DNA; they have accordingly been denoted exr⁺.

Two independent lines of evidence from other investigators have substantiated our division of AT strains into two major classes (exr⁻ and exr⁺) on the basis of DNA repair capability. Firstly, Scudiero (1980) has convincingly demonstrated that the capacity of AT strains to undertake DNA repair synthesis after treatment with the alkylating agent N-methyl-N'-nitro-N-nitrosoguanidine (MNNG) mimics that observed after γ ray exposure -- that is, exr⁻ strains are deficient and exr⁺ strains are proficient. Secondly, Jaspers and Bootsma (1982) have made the intriguing observation that, whereas in normal cells pretreatment with X radiation has no effect on the amount of DNA repair synthesis induced by subsequent exposure to UV light, the same preirradiation of AT cells serves to modify the level of UV-induced repair synthesis, acting as an inhibitor in exr⁻ strains and as a stimulus in exr⁺ strains.

An earlier study in our laboratory provided one of the first pieces of evidence that the putative DNA repair deficiency may not be confined to damage introduced by ionizing radiation (Smith and Paterson, 1980). A class of guanyl adducts induced by 4NQO was shown to be removed more slowly in two AT strains -- namely, AT2BE and AT4BI -- than in a normal control, a finding consistent with

the hypersensitivity of these two particular AT strains to the cytotoxic effect of this chemical carcinogen.

In a current follow-up study, we have used 1-β-D-arabinofurano-
sylcytosine (araC), a metabolic inhibitor of DNA synthesis, to in-
tentionally block completion of the excision repair process operating
on 4NQO-purine adducts in DNA. In this approach, which has been
popularized by Collins and Johnson (1981), the extent of strand
break accumulation during post-4NQO incubation with araC becomes a
measure of the efficiency of the excision repair process. As depicted in Fig. 5, the level of araC-detectable sites that were
repaired during 2 hr after treatment with different 4NQO concentrations proved to be significantly higher in GM38 (normal) cells than
in AT2BE and AT4BI cells. This observation provides additional
proof that at least two AT strains are indeed faulty in processing
4NQO-purine adducts in DNA.

Since the four major reaction products formed in DNA by 4NQO
can be readily detected by various chromatographical methods (Ikenaga
et al., 1981), we are presently assaying the normal and AT strains
for their ability to excise these chemically distinct adducts. This
strategy should permit us to confirm, and extend in a more direct
and detailed manner, this specific DNA repair anomaly associated
with certain AT genotypes. In view of the disturbing interlaboratory
discrepancies in the DNA repair properties of cultured AT fibroblasts
(for review, see Lehmann et al., 1982), such confirmation would be
a welcome addition to the literature.

3. Faulty Repair of O^6-Methylguanine Lesions in Nontransformed Cells from Cancer Patients

Of the reaction products formed in DNA by MNNG and N-methyl-N-
nitrosourea (MNU), O^6-methylguanine (O^6-MeGua) residues in particular
have been strongly implicated in the mutagenic, carcinogenic and
possibly lethal potency of these two methyl-N-nitroso compounds
(Singer, 1979; Lindahl, 1982). These guanyl adducts are repaired
in cultured human fibroblasts in the same manner as initially proposed in $E.\ coli$ (Olsson and Lindahl, 1980), i.e., by the direct
transfer of the offending methyl group from the O^6-position of the
purine base to a cysteine residue in the protein, termed O^6-methyl-
guanine-DNA transmethylase (Pegg et al., 1982). The reaction is
highly unusual among recognized DNA repair processes, being stoichiometric and suicidal, rather than catalytic and regenerating. That
is, each transmethylase molecule is consumed in the reaction as its
activity is exhausted upon S-alkylation of its acceptor cysteine
residue.

Approximately 20% of all established human tumor cell strains
are said to display the Mer⁻ phenotype, as defined by the following

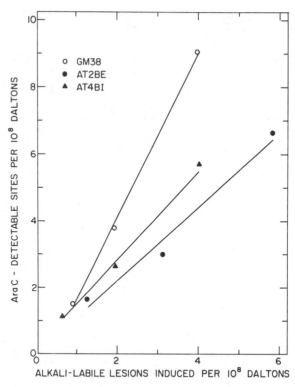

Fig. 5.   4NQO dose-dependent incidence of strand breaks accumulating in the DNA of normal and AT strains due to araC-
induced abortive repair during post-treatment incubation.
The experimental protocol was patterned after that of
Mirzayans and Waters (1981). 4NQO treatments (≤10 μM)
were administered for 30 min at 37°C in serum-free growth
medium. Note that the doses received by each strain have
been expressed in terms of alkali-labile lesions formed
in DNA from cultures which were allowed no time for repair,
thereby normalizing for any interstrain differences in
lesion formation.

criteria: (i) reduced capacity to support the growth of MNNG-treated
adenovirus; (ii) enhanced susceptibility to MNNG-induced cell inactivation; (iii) increased sensitivity to MNNG-induced production of
sister chromatid exchanges; and (iv) depressed constitutive levels
of O^6-methylguanine-DNA transmethylase (Day et al., 1980; Sklar and
Strauss, 1981; Yarosh et al., 1983). The remaining tumor lines are
similar to all nontransformed human fibroblast strains reported to
date, and are thus designated Mer[+] (Scudiero et al., 1984).

In collaboration with Dr. D.M. Parry and her colleagues in the Clinical and Environmental Epidemiology Branches of the U.S. National Cancer Institute in Bethesda, MD, we have recently identified a number of *nontransformed* fibroblast strains that display impaired CFA in response to MNU treatment (see Table 2). Included are strains from the following subjects, all of whom are either afflicted with or predisposed to neoplasia: (i) three affected members of a family with Gardner syndrome (GS), an autosomal dominant trait characterized by premalignant colonic polyps, soft tissue tumors, and cystic lesions of the skin (McKusick, 1978); (ii) a patient suffering from acquired immune deficiency syndrome (AIDS), which manifests itself as life-threatening opportunistic infections and/or malignancies, especially Kaposi sarcoma (Center for Disease Control, 1982); and (iii) a patient with Hodgkin's disease (HD) who developed multiple primary neoplasms subsequent to receiving conventional chemotherapy (D.M. Parry, personal communication). We present here a brief description of the in vitro properties of these strains.

Gardner Syndrome Family. In our search for environmental-hereditary interactions predisposing to gastrointestinal cancer, we previously reported MNNG hypercytotoxicity in vitro in one of four GS families studied (Paterson et al., 1981a). Surprisingly, this defect in post-MNNG CFA was observed, without exception, in strains from affected females whereas strains from affected males were indistinguishable from clinically normal donors. To confirm this apparent sex-dependent variability in cellular expression of enhanced susceptibility to an N-methyl-N-nitroso chemical, we have measured loss of colony-forming ability as a function of MNU treatment (1 hr at 37°C in serum-free, HEPES-buffered Ham's F12 medium) in strains from five affected core members of the MNNG-hypersensitive GS family and from two healthy volunteers. The CFA assay practised by us was essentially that described by Paterson and coworkers (1982). Our findings, summarized in Table 2, indicated that strain GM3314, derived from the proband in the family, was markedly sensitive to MNU, as reflected by a dose reduction factor (DRF) of ~6 (using D_{10}, i.e., dose that reduces colony survival to 10%, as the quantitative measure of a given strain's response to the cytotoxic agent). Strains GM3944 (proband's affected sister) and GM3946 (proband's affected daughter) also displayed impaired post-MNU CFA; however, their impairment (DRF ~2) was considerably less than in GM3314. On the other hand, the two remaining strains (GM3948 and GM3954), one of which was obtained from an afflicted female, formed colonies at normal rates after MNU treatment (Table 2).

To investigate a probable biochemical basis for the observed cellular chemosensitivity segregating in family members presenting the affliction, we measured constitutive levels of O^6-methylguanine-DNA transmethylase in sonicates of cultured fibroblasts from these individuals. The assay adopted by us was an adaptation of that

Table 2. Relation between Post-MNU Survival and O^6-Methylguanine-DNA Transmethylase Activity in Strains from Normal or Cancer-Predisposed Subjects

| Strain | Donor | | | | MNU $D_{10} \pm SE$[b] (mM·hr) | O^6-MeGua-DNA Transmethylase Activity[c] ($\times 10^{-5}$) |
	Clinical Status[a]	Age	Sex	Relation		
GM38	normal	9	female	proband	1.31 ± 0.05	1.3 ± 0.13
GM969	normal	2	female	proband	1.57 ± 0.04	1.3 ± 0.14
GM3314	GS	48	female	proband	0.23 ± 0.08 (S)[d]	0.069 ± 0.018
GM3944	GS	38	female	sib	0.68 ± 0.06 (S)	0.63 ± 0.027
GM3946	GS	22	female	child	0.63 ± 0.07 (S)	0.57 ± 0.027
GM3948	GS	30	female	child	1.15 ± 0.07	1.2 ± 0.037
GM3954	GS	24	male	child	1.33 ± 0.04	1.2 ± 0.045
3638T	HD, tonsilar & colonic carcinoma	65	male	proband	0.90 ± 0.41 (S)	0.52 ± 0.026
3652T	AIDS	32	male	proband	0.69 ± 0.14 (S)	0.32 ± 0.063

[a] GS, Gardner syndrome; HD, Hodgkin's disease; AIDS, acquired immune deficiency syndrome

[b] Dose reducing survival to 10% ± standard error of the mean

[c] Methyl acceptor sites per cell

[d] Sensitive, using the two-tail t test of Tarone et al. (1983) to compare the D_{10} of the indicated strain to the mean (1.44 ± 0.08) of the two normal strains and taking p = 0.05 as the level of significance

described by Olsson and Lindahl (1980). The data, given in Table 2, indicated that the level of transmethylase protein in GM3314 was only ~5% (6.9×10^3 molecules per cell) of that present in the two normal controls. The other two MNU-hypersensitive strains (GM3944 and GM3946) each possessed ~50% of the normal complement, implying a possible gene dosage effect. In these three GS strains, then, the deficiency in the methyl-acceptor protein correlated closely with the impairment in post-MNU colony survival. Parallel experiments also demonstrated that the five GS strains examined here all had normal amounts of DNA glycosylase activities for 7-methylguanine and 3-methyladenine, two other major reaction products formed by methyl-N-nitroso compounds. We thus propose that a malfunction in the repair of O^6-MeGua residues may be largely, if not completely, responsible for the MNU hypersensitivity exhibited by strains from certain affected members of this GS family.

Other Cancer-Prone Patients. Cell sonicates of strains 3638T and 3652T, derived from the HD and the AIDS patient, respectively, contained reduced quantities of O^6-methylguanine-DNA transmethylase (Table 2). As seen previously in the GS family, the residual methyl-acceptor protein in these strains was consistent with their moderate susceptibility to MNU-induced killing; again, a transmethylase deficiency offers a likely explanation for the observed hypercytotoxicity to MNU.

Follow-up studies are currently underway to determine (i) if other factors, in addition to reduced constitutive levels of transmethylase activity, contribute to the chemosensitivity seen in these two strains (as well as in the three MNU-hypersensitive GS strains discussed above), and (ii) if there is complementation among the various mutant strains with respect to transmethylase expression.

4. Fetal Strain Displaying Age-Dependent Increase in MNU Toxicity

Our laboratory has discovered yet another nontransformed fibroblast strain which displays defective colony-forming ability upon exposure to MNU (Middlestadt et al., 1984). The strain, GM11, was originally derived from an eight-week-old fetus; it was described as apparently normal in the supplier's current catalog (NIGMS Human Genetic Mutant Cell Repository, 1984). Our discovery was made fortuitously when the strain was selected as one of the normal controls in our investigation into the post-MNU CFA of the GS strains summarized previously. GM11 cells proved to be exquisitely sensitive to MNU compared to control (GM10) cells, age-matched in vivo and in vitro (see Fig. 6). Moreover, the magnitude of the enhancement in chemosensitivity was dependent upon the age of the cells in culture, increasing from a DRF of approximately 2 at passage 6 to greater than 10 at passage 23. Of additional significance was the

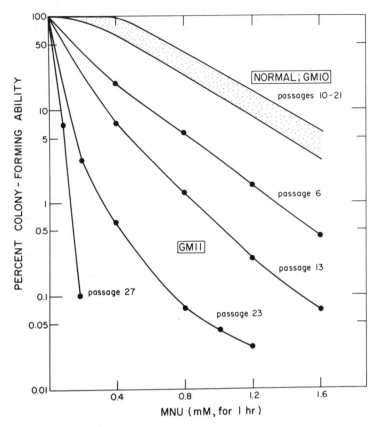

Fig. 6.   MNU dose-response curves for two age-matched fetal fibroblast strains as a function of culture age. The stippled
area is bounded by the steepest and shallowest curves obtained for normal (GM10) cultures ranging from passages
10-21.

fact that the dose-response curve generated for GM11 at passage 23,
for example, was clearly nonlinear, as typified by a steep initial
slope (at low concentrations of MNU) which tailed off to a more
gradual decline at higher concentrations; the final slope closely
paralleled the survival response of normal cells. We interpret
such biphasic curves as reflecting the presence of two cell populations, one hypersensitive to MNU and the other normal. The former

population appears to increase from ~25% of the total culture at passage 6 to >99% by passage 23.

This age-dependent increase in MNU-induced cytotoxicity contrasted sharply with the 1.6-fold hypersensitivity, irrespective of culture age, to killing by methyl methanesulfonate (MMS). Since MNU produces considerable quantities of 0^6-MeGua adducts in DNA, whereas MMS forms relatively little (Margison and O'Connor, 1979), we assayed cell sonicates of GM11 for 0^6-methylguanine-DNA transmethylase content. Reduced amounts of 0^6-methyl-acceptor protein, but normal levels of DNA glycosylases active on 3-methyladenine and 7-methylguanine, were found. In fact, at passage 10 or greater, sonicates of all GM11 cultures possessed negligible capacity to accept methyl groups from a test DNA substrate containing donor 0^6-MeGua residues. At earlier culture ages, however, appreciable amounts of transmethylase protein were present; for example, sonicates from passage 4 cultures, the youngest assayed to date, contained approximately 25-30% of the level found in age-matched controls.

We are currently extending these studies to the youngest cultures available (passage 2) in order to quantitate accurately the in vitro age-dependent decrease in 0^6-methylguanine-DNA transmethylase activity vis-à-vis changes in colony-forming ability and mutation induction after MNU treatment. This may possibly enable us to correlate a deficiency in the removal of 0^6-MeGua adducts with specific lethal and mutagenic events. Furthermore, aside from providing new insight into the genetic control of transmethylase expression, this intriguing fetal strain may ultimately assist in clarifying the role of the Mer⁻ phenotype in the transformation process.

5.   Other Conditions Linking Cancer Proneness with Carcinogen Hypersensitivity

Using the clinical pictures in XP and AT as paradigms, we have uncovered a number of additional Mendelian single-gene disorders in which cancer predisposition evident in the clinic is similarly associated with carcinogen hypercytotoxicity observable in the laboratory. Examples of these newly described ecogenetic traits (with the pertinent carcinogen[s] given in brackets) include: Rothmund Thomson syndrome (γ rays; Smith and Paterson, 1982); combined hereditary cutaneous malignant melanoma/dysplastic nevus syndrome (UV rays and 4NQO; Smith et al., 1982 and 1983); and tuberous sclerosis (γ rays; Paterson et al., 1982). Thus far, only in the first syndrome has the observed carcinogen susceptibility been linked with a biochemical anomaly, namely, a particular malfunction in an excision-repair pathway acting on base/sugar radioproducts.

The preceding disorders are characterized by a well-defined genetic etiology. Our search for new human models of nature-nurture interactions in the genesis of neoplastic transformation has not been restricted to such source material, however. In the course of our six-year collaboration with U.S. NCI, we have assessed the post-carcinogen CFA and DNA repair properties of fibroblast strains from an assortment of cancer-prone subjects; these include special patient groups, unusual individual patients, and, in particular, members of 'cancer families' (summarized in Paterson et al., 1983 and 1984a). These latter families have been so designated because of an excessive occurrence of neoplasia, generally of specific histologic types, in kindred related by blood or environment. In many of these kinships, cancer has developed following documented exposure to a known biospheric, occupational or therapeutic carcinogen, raising the possibility that the individual may be genetically predisposed to the neoplastic effects of the agent. Two notable associations disclosed thus far between predisposition to familial malignancy and cellular hypersensitivity to an etiologically relevant carcinogen are the following:

(a) A 42-year-old woman, who lost four of her six offspring (two daughters and two sons) and several blood relatives to acute myelogenous leukemia, presented rectal carcinoma 14 years following radiotherapy for uterine cervical cancer. Dermal cells from the woman and her two leukemic daughters exhibited impaired colony survival in response to γ rays, whereas those from her husband, the two remaining unaffected sons, and a sister with breast cancer displayed normal γ ray tolerance (Bech-Hansen et al., 1981b). Consequently, in this family there is a good correlation between cancer occurrence in vivo and elevated radiosensitivity in vitro. The latter trait may therefore be a direct cellular expression of a 'leukemogenic factor' segregating through the maternal side of the family.

(b) A 30-year-old male with bilateral gynecomastia (and a well-documented family history of diverse malignancies) presented adenocarcinoma of the breast three decades following irradiation for an enlarged thymus. Cultured fibroblasts from the patient displayed diminished colony survival after exposure to either γ rays or bleomycin, a free radical-generating (and hence radiomimetic) chemical (Greene et al., 1983). Elevated radiosensitivity in cells from the patient's normal mother and hypersensitivity to bleomycin in cells from his unaffected sister add support to the suspicion that genetic susceptibility contributed to an increased risk of radiogenic neoplasia in the patient.

6. Conditions Linking Cancer Predisposition with Carcinogen Hyperresistance

While the foregoing clinical-laboratory investigations have demonstrated that enhanced sensitivity to carcinogen-induced cell killing may often be correlated with propensity to develop specific malignancies, we have also observed just the converse -- that is, *enhanced resistance* to carcinogen toxicity in fibroblasts from persons at high risk of familial malignancy. We now outline our findings to date on two cancer families in which this unprecedented correlation has been made.

In Vitro Radioresistance in a Family Prone to Diverse Cancers. The first family is characterized by an unusual clustering of divergent types of malignancies, such as bone and soft-tissue sarcomas, breast and brain cancers, and leukemia (see Fig. 7 for an abridged pedigree; Blattner et al., 1979). The distribution of neoplasms observed is not unlike that seen in the Li-Fraumeni familial syndrome of breast cancer and soft-tissue sarcoma (Li and Fraumeni,

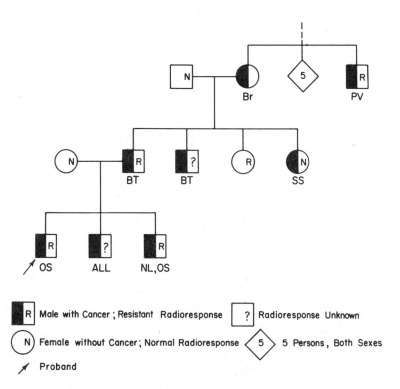

Fig. 7. Abridged pedigree of a cancer family with diverse malignancies (including two of possible radiogenic origin). The clinical status and cellular radioresponse are compared for each member. Abbreviations used: OS, osteosarcoma; ALL, acute lymphoblastic leukemia; NL, neurilemoma; SS, soft-tissue sarcoma; BT, brain tumor; Br, breast cancer; and PV, polycythemia vera.

1969). The cancers in this first family have appeared over six generations in a pattern explicable by transmission of a partially penetrant, autosomal dominant gene with pleiotropic effects. The family was of particular significance because two members presented clinical abnormalities attributable to previous radiation exposure: (i) an adolescent brother of the proband developed a vertebral osteosarcoma in the field of radiotherapy administered 12 years earlier for bilateral malignant neurilemomas; and (ii) his paternal great-uncle contracted polycythemia vera five years after occupational exposure to radioactive heavy water.

Pertinent clinical and laboratory characteristics are indicated in Fig. 7 for various members in this cancer family (for details, see Bech-Hansen et al., 1981a). Of eight family members assayed by us for post-γ ray CFA, significantly increased radioresistance (RR) was seen in four members with neoplasia (including the two having a history of radiation exposure) and a fifth without, but not in a member with leiomyosarcoma or in two normal spouses. In brief, the RR phenotype was detected in five of the six members in the cancer-prone lineage, but not in two spouse controls, implying that increased tolerance to the lethal effects of radiation may be a cellular manifestation of a genetically determined susceptibility factor common to diverse forms of cancer.

Biochemical delineation of this novel RR trait may possibly uncover a new mechanism of carcinogenesis underlying a number of common malignancies. On this premise, conventional DNA repair assays have been performed on the following RR strains: 2675T (proband with osteosarcoma), 2673T (his father with astrocytoma), 2674T (his brother with malignant neurilemoma and radiogenic osteosarcoma) and 2800T (his paternal great-uncle with radiogenic polycythemia vera). To determine intrinsic cellular capacity to repair radiogenic DNA damage in general, we measured the amount of DNA repair synthesis performed by these four RR strains in the 2-hr period following exposure to 500 Gy of γ radiation (Paterson et al., 1983). The amount of repair synthesis induced in these strains did not differ significantly from that occurring in normal controls. Likewise, both the initial yield and the subsequent rate of disappearance of single-strand breaks and of *M. luteus* extract-sensitive sites proved to be similar in an RR (2674T) compared to a control (GM38) strain. Together, these combined data imply strongly that RR strains both sustain and repair radiogenic DNA damage at normal rates.

To characterize further the DNA metabolic properties of representative RR strains, DNA replicative synthesis was monitored in 2675T and 2800T fibroblasts after γ ray exposure. As demonstrated in Fig. 8, both the extent of initial inhibition of *de novo* synthesis induced by the radiation treatment and the time interval before

256

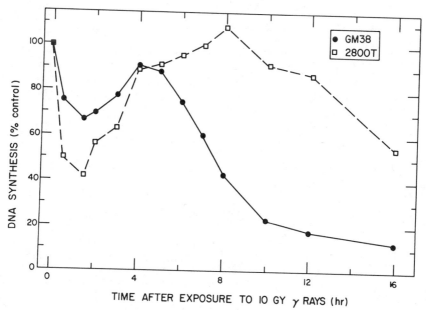

Fig. 8. γ Ray-induced inhibition and recovery of DNA replicative synthesis in normal (●) and RR (□) fibroblasts. Exponentially growing cultures were prelabelled with ^{14}C-thymidine (dThd) and divided into two groups; one received 10 Gy of γ rays while the other received none. At each indicated time during subsequent incubation, a culture from each group was labelled with ^{3}H-dThd for 10 min and then lyzed, after which the DNA was collected and its radioactivity counted. The ratio of ^{3}H/^{14}C values for corresponding irradiated and non-irradiated cultures served as a measure of the extent of radiogenic inhibition of *de novo* DNA synthesis in each strain.

its subsequent recovery were much greater in 2800T cells than in normal (GM38) cells. Furthermore, the degree of recovery was more extensive and was maintained for longer times in the RR strain than in the normal control. A similar pattern of post-radiation DNA replication has also been observed in 2675T (data not shown). The increased and protracted depression in replicative synthesis after γ ray treatment in RR strains may promote cellular recovery by 'buying additional time' during which repair processes can act on potentially lethal radioproducts and, by so doing, may leave an exceptionally low number of noncoding lesions for the replication machinery to navigate past.

It is noteworthy perhaps that the abnormality in radiation-induced depression of DNA semi-conservative synthesis observed in the RR strains is the exact opposite of that universally displayed by radiosensitive AT strains. In the latter, the extent to which ionizing radiation inhibits *de novo* DNA synthesis is appreciably diminished compared to that arising in similarly treated normal cells (see, e.g., Houldsworth and Lavin, 1980).

We have previously proposed that the RR phenotype may result from an increased activity of an error-prone DNA metabolic process which facilitates elevated survival but at the expense of an increased mutation load (Bech-Hansen et al., 1981a). To test this working hypothesis, our laboratory is in the process of measuring the frequency of γ ray-induced 6-thioguanine-resistance in RR compared to normal strains.

In Vitro Resistance to MMC in a Multiple Polyposis/Sarcoma Family. The cardinal features of the second family are colonic polyps prone to malignant transformation in coexistence with malignant extra-alimentary sarcomas (Fraumeni et al., 1968). The pattern of malignant involvement in the kinship is compatible with autosomal dominant inheritance of a single mutant, pleiotropic gene of high penetrance. Our initial interest in the family was stimulated in part by the appearance of a suspected cytotoxic drug-induced cancer in a 28-year-old female member who had undergone combined therapy for a glioblastoma three years earlier. Following treatment, which included 1,3-bis(2-chloroethyl)-1-nitrosourea, the patient developed a fatal nonlymphocytic leukemia, a recognized sequela of alkylating agent therapy. Consequently, strain 3437T from this patient along with strains from four other family members were assayed for colony-forming ability upon exposure to the model alkylating agent MNU and other DNA-damaging agents.

As shown in Table 3, all five strains responded normally to the lethal action of MNU. Somewhat surprisingly, however, three of the strains -- namely 3701T, 3704T and 3437T -- exhibited *enhanced resistance* to the inactivating effects of another antineoplastic chemical, mitomycin C (MMC). 3437T cells proved to be especially drug resistant, yielding a D_{10} value for post-MMC CFA which was ~5.5 times greater than that found for normal controls. It is noteworthy that all three MMC-resistant strains were derived from family members either with or at high risk of cancer (i.e., in the cancer-prone lineage). Of the remaining two strains, which displayed normal levels of post-MMC colony survival, one of the donors served as a spouse control while the other was asymptomatic. Thus, in this kinship, there was complete concordance between cancer predisposition in vivo and cellular hyperresistance to MMC in vitro.

Table 3. Post-Carcinogen Colony-Forming Ability of Skin Fibroblasts from Normal Subjects and Members of a Multiple Polyposis/Sarcoma Family

| Strain | Donor | | | | MNU D_{10} ± SE[a] (mM·hr) | MMC D_{10} ± SE[a] (µg/ml·hr) |
	Clinical Status	Age	Sex	Relation		
"Normal"[b]	normal	2-83	male/female		1.37 ± 0.03	0.420 ± 0.038
3437T	glioblastoma, ANL[c]	26	female	proband	1.34 ± 0.03	2.36 ± 0.23 (R)[d]
3701T	endometrial carcinoma	75	female	paternal aunt	1.40 ± 0.35	1.06 ± 0.12 (R)
3702T	normal	66	male	paternal uncle	1.36 ± 0.06	0.526 ± 0.42
3703T	normal	60	female	mother	1.27 ± 0.13	0.414 ± 0.043
3704T	normal	52	female	paternal aunt	1.26 ± 0.27	0.823 ± 0.149 (R)

[a] Dose reducing survival to 10% ± standard error of the mean

[b] Average survival response of 15 control strains from unrelated normal donors

[c] Acute nonlymphocytic leukemia

[d] Reistant, using the two-tail t test of Tarone et al. (1983) to compare the D_{10} of the indicated strain to that of the "Normal" and taking p = 0.05 as the level of significance

MMC is a potent inducer of cross-links between the complementary strands of the double helix (see, e.g., Fujiwara, 1982). These cross-links, and not the numerically greater monoadducts, appear to be the prime contributors to the cytotoxic, and perhaps the carcinogenic, potential of this agent. On *a priori* grounds, such interstrand cross-links are expected to constitute an effective block to *de novo* replicative synthesis and (unless successfully circumvented by repair processes) should therefore be tantamount to reproductive death. To determine whether an enhanced ability to repair specifically this class of lesions was responsible for the MMC-resistant phenotype, colony survival of 3437T versus normal cells was compared after treatment with two other well-known DNA cross-linking agents, *cis*-diamminedichloroplatinum II (*cis*-DDP) and 8-methoxypsoralen (activated by UV-A light). For both agents, the post-treatment CFA for 3437T cells was similar to that exhibited by control cells, indicating that 3437T did not owe its MMC hyperresistance to any 'super-proficient' ability to repair DNA cross-links. This strain has also been shown to be ~5 times more resistant than normal controls to the lethal effects of 4NQO, another agent which, like MMC, requires metabolic reduction for activation (Tada and Tada, 1975; Tomasz and Lipman, 1981). Hence these survival experiments raised the possibility that 3437T cells were resistant to MMC- and 4NQO-induced cytotoxicity because they lacked the normal complement of reductases responsible for the conversion of these compounds to activated intermediates capable of damaging DNA. (An alternative explanation, namely, reduced capacity to take up drugs, seemed remote in view of the normal response of 3437T cells to inactivation by MNU, *cis*-DDP and photoactivated psoralen.) That diminished bioreduction might indeed account for most, if not all, of the cross-resistance to MMC and 4NQO has been surmised from the following three observations:

(a) Using the alkaline elution method, we have demonstrated that 3437T cells must be exposed to ~5 times as much MMC as GM38 cells in order to sustain comparable levels of interstrand cross-linking (see Fig. 9).

(b) Following identical 4NQO treatments, the incidence of both alkali-labile and alkali-stable adducts (a measure of drug dosimetry) was at least three times lower in 3437T cells than in normal cells.

(c) Extracts of 3437T cultures have been shown to contain only about 15% of the 4NQO reductase activity that is present in normal cell extracts.

It is known that enzyme-mediated bioreduction reactions may be directed towards the destruction or the activation of potential genotoxins, depending upon the particular chemical (Wright, 1980). It is quite conceivable then, that under certain conditions individuals with a specific bioreductive enzyme deficiency may carry an

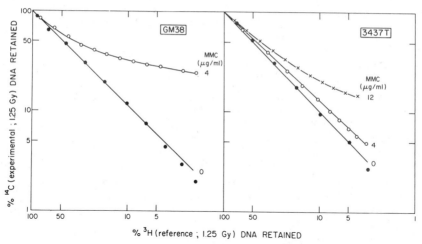

Fig. 9. Assay by alkaline elution of the interstrand cross-links
induced by MMC in the DNA of normal cells (left panel)
and MMC-hyperresistant cells (right panel). Experimental
cultures, labelled with ^{14}C-dThd, were treated (1 hr,
37°C) with serum-free growth medium containing the indicated concentrations of MMC. Following MMC treatment,
the cells were collected and exposed to 1.25 Gy of ^{60}Co
γ rays, and each cell sample was mixed with an equal
number of reference ^{3}H-labelled cells that had received
the same γ ray exposure. Cell mixtures were then lyzed
on filters and their DNAs were assayed by alkaline elution
for rate of unwinding, as detailed in van der Schans et
al. (1983). For each elution point, the percentage of
total ^{14}C-experimental DNA retained on the filter was
plotted versus the percentage of ^{3}H-reference DNA retained.
As expected, in the absence of interstrand cross-links in
the experimental DNA, a slope of -1 was found. Cross-links
induced in the ^{14}C-experimental DNA by the MMC treatment
resulted in a diminished rate of ^{14}C-DNA compared to ^{3}H-
DNA elution. A 'cross-link factor' may be calculated (not
shown) which suggests that ~20 µg/ml MMC treatment would
be required with 3437T to achieve the same level of cross-
linking as results from 4 µg/ml MMC administered to GM38.

amplified 'carcinogen load' compared to the general population.
Furthermore, changing cellular biochemistry has been implicated in
the stepwise development of cancer. In particular, Farber (1984)
has championed a resistant hepatocyte model for liver carcinogenesis
in which an initiated cell, due to altered enzymology, acquires
resistance to the genotoxic effects of various carcinogens. We are
presently examining the similarities, if any, between their findings

261

and ours, to determine if carcinogen resistance may have played a role in cancer development in the polyposis/sarcoma family.

CONCLUSION

The take-home message is clear. By studying the biochemical basis for abnormal carcinogen responsiveness in rare individuals who are at increased risk of cancer because of some peculiarity in their personal or familial medical history, we are attempting to gain new insight into the origins of human neoplasia and, more importantly, into fundamental mechanisms of carcinogenesis such as may apply to common malignancies in society-at-large. Continued studies along the lines of those outlined here promise to assist in predicting and treating, and eventually in preventing, neoplastic transformation in man.

ACKNOWLEDGMENTS

Our research was financed in part by U.S. NCI Contracts NOl-CP-21029 (Basic) and NOl-CP-9100 with the Clinical and Environmental Epidemiology Branches, National Cancer Institute, Bethesda, MD. We are most grateful to L.D. Johnson, S.J. MacFarlane, R.S. McWilliams, G.M. Norton, and B.P. Smith for excellent technical assistance; and to A. Stewart for her patience and persistence in the preparation of the camera-ready manuscript. The senior author wishes to express his sincere thanks to Drs. W.A. Blattner, J.F. Fraumeni, Jr., M.H. Greene, F.P. Li, R.W. Miller, J.J. Mulvihill, D.J. Tollerud and especially D.M. Parry of the Clinical and Environmental Epidemiology Branches of the U.S. National Cancer Institute for their wise counsel and unfailing encouragement during the course of the studies described here.

REFERENCES

Bech-Hansen, N.T., Blattner, W.A., Sell, B.M., McKeen, E.A., Lampkin, B.C., Fraumeni, J.F., Jr., and Paterson, M.C., 1981a, Transmission of in-vitro radioresistance in a cancer-prone family, Lancet, 1:1335.
Bech-Hansen, N.T., Sell, B.M., Mulvihill, J.J., and Paterson, M.C., 1981b, Association of in vitro radiosensitivity and cancer in a family with acute myelogenous leukemia, Cancer Res., 41:2046.
Blattner, W.A., McGuire, D.B., Mulvihill, J.J., Lampkin, B.C., Hananian, J., and Fraumeni, J.F., Jr., 1979, Genealogy of cancer in a family, JAMA, 241:259.
Center for Disease Control, 1982, Opportunistic infections and Kaposi's sarcoma among Haitians in the United States, Morbid. Mortal. Weekly Rep., 31:353.

Cleaver, J.E., 1968, Defective repair replication of DNA in xeroderma pigmentosum, Nature, 218:652.

Cleaver, J.E., 1980, DNA damage, repair systems and human hypersensitive diseases, J. Environ. Pathol. Toxicol., 3:53.

Collins, A.R.S., and Johnson, R.T., 1981, Use of metabolic inhibit-
ors in repair studies, in "DNA Repair: A Laboratory Manual of
Research Procedures, Vol. 1, Part B", E.C. Friedberg and P.C.
Hanawalt, eds., p. 341, Marcel Dekker, Inc., New York.

Day, R.S., III, Ziolkowski, C.H.J., Scudiero, D.A., Meyer, S.A.,
Lubiniecki, A.S., Girardi,A.J., Galloway, S.M., and Bynum, G.D.,
1980, Defective repair of alkylated DNA by human tumor and SV40-
transformed human cell strains, Nature, 288:724.

Doll, R., and Peto, R., 1981, The causes of cancer, J. Natl. Cancer
Inst., 66:1191.

Farber, E., 1984, Cellular biochemistry of the stepwise development
of cancer with chemicals: G.H.A. Clowes Memorial Lecture,
Cancer Res., 44:5463.

Fraumeni, J.F., Jr., Vogel, C.L., and Easton, J.M., 1968, Sarcomas
and multiple polyposis in a kindred: A genetic variety of
hereditary polyposis?, Arch. Intern. Med., 121:57.

Friedberg, E.C., Bonura, T., Love, J.D., McMillan, S., Radany, E.H.,
and Schultz, R.A., 1981, The repair of DNA damage: Recent developments and new insights, J. Supramolec. Struct. Cell. Biochem.,
16:91.

Friedberg, E.C., Ehmann, U.K., and Williams, J.I., 1979, Human
diseases associated with defective DNA repair, Adv. Radiat.
Biol., 8:85.

Fujiwara, Y., 1982, Defective repair of mitomycin C crosslinks in
Fanconi's anemia and loss in confluent normal human and xeroderma pigmentosum cells, Biochim. Biophys. Acta, 699:217.

Gentner, N.E., Rözga, B., Smith, B.P., Paterson, M.C., and Cadet,
J., 1981, Proc. 9th Ann. Meeting Am. Soc. Photobiol., p.164
(abstr.).

Gentner, N.E., Weinfeld, M., Johnson, L.D., and Paterson, M.C.,
1984, Incision of the phosphodiester bond internal to the pyrimidine dimer-forming bases may occur during excision repair
of UV-induced damage in human fibroblasts, Env. Mutag., 6:429
(abstr.).

Greene, M.H., Goedert, J.J., Bech-Hansen, N.T., McGuire, D., Paterson, M.C., and Fraumeni, J.F., Jr., 1983, Radiogenic male breast
cancer with *in vitro* sensitivity to ionizing radiation and
bleomycin, Cancer Invest., 1:379.

Harm, H., 1976, Repair of UV-irradiated biological systems: Photoreactivation, in: "Photochemistry and Photobiology of Nucleic
Acids, Vol. 2", S.Y. Wang, ed., p.219, Academic Press, New York.

Haseltine, W.A., 1983, Ultraviolet light repair and mutagenesis
revisited, Cell, 33:13.

Higginson, J., and Muir, C.S., 1979, Environmental carcinogenesis:
Misconceptions and limitations to cancer control, J. Natl.
Cancer Inst., 61:1291.

Houldsworth, J., and Lavin, M.F., 1980, Effect of ionizing radiation on DNA synthesis in ataxia telangiectasia cells, Nucleic Acids Res., 8:3709.

Ikenaga, M., Tada, M., and Kawazoe, Y., 1981, Measurement of base damage caused by 4-nitroquinoline 1-oxide, in: "DNA Repair: A Laboratory Manual of Research Procedures, Vol. 1, Part A", E.C. Friedberg and P.C. Hanawalt, eds., p.187, Marcel Dekker, Inc., New York.

Jaspers, N.G.J., and Bootsma, D., 1982, Abnormal levels of UV-induced unscheduled DNA synthesis in ataxia telangiectasia cells after exposure to ionizing radiation, Mutat. Res., 92:439.

Kraemer, K.H., 1983, Heritable diseases with increased sensitivity to cellular injury, in: "Update: Dermatology in General Medicine", T.B. Fitzpatrick, A.Z. Eisen, K. Wolff, I.M. Freedberg, and K.F. Austen, eds., p. 113, McGraw-Hill Book Co., New York.

LaBelle, M., and Linn, S., 1982, In vivo excision of pyrimidine dimers is mediated by a DNA N-glycosylase in Micrococcus luteus but not in human fibroblasts, Photochem. Photobiol., 36:319.

Lehmann, A.R., James, M.R., and Stevens, S., 1982, Miscellaneous observations on DNA repair in ataxia telangiectasia, in: "Ataxia-telangiectasia -- A Cellular and Molecular Link between Cancer, Neuropathology and Immune Deficiency, B.A. Bridges and D.G. Harnden, eds., p.347, John Wiley & Sons, Chichester.

Li, F.P., and Fraumeni, J.F., Jr., 1969, Soft-tissue sarcomas, breast cancer, and other neoplasms: A familial syndrome?, Ann. Intern. Med., 71:747.

Lindahl, T., 1982, DNA repair enzymes, Ann. Rev. Biochem., 51:61.

Margison, G.P., and O'Connor, P.J., 1979, Nucleic acid modification by N-nitroso compounds, in: "Chemical Carcinogens and DNA, Vol. 1", P.L. Glover, ed., p.111, CRC Press, Florida.

McCormick, J.J., Silinskas, K.C., Kateley, S.A., Tower, J.E., and Maher, V.M., 1981, The induction of anchorage independent growth and tumor formation of diploid human fibroblasts by carcinogens, Proc. Am. Assoc. Cancer Res., 22:122 (abstr.).

McKusick, V.A., 1978, "Mendelian Inheritance in Man: Catalogs of Autosomal Dominant, Autosomal Recessive, and X-linked Phenotypes (Fifth Ed.)", The Johns Hopkins University Press, Baltimore.

Middlestadt, M.V., Norton, G., and Paterson, M.C., 1984, Absence of O^6methylguanine-DNA methyltransferase activity in a nontransformed human fetal fibroblast line, Env. Mutag., 6:430 (abstr.).

Miller, R.W., 1980, Clinical clues to interactions in carcinogenesis, in: "Genetic and Environmental Factors in Experimental and Human Cancer", H.V. Gelboin et al., eds., p.351, Japanese Scientific Societies Press, Tokyo.

Mirzayans, R., and Waters, R., 1981, DNA damage and its repair in human normal or xeroderma pigmentosum fibroblasts treated with 4-nitroquinoline 1-oxide or its 3-methyl derivative, Carcinogenesis, 2:1359.

Mulvihill, J.J., 1980, Clinical observations of ecogenetics in human cancer, Ann. Intern. Med., 92:809.

NIGMS Human Genetic Mutant Cell Repository (Eleventh Ed.), 1984, U.S. Department of Health and Human Services, Bethesda.

Olsson, M., and Lindahl, T., 1980, Repair of alkylated DNA in *Escherichia coli:* Methyl group transfer from O^6-methylguanine to a protein cysteine residue, J. Biol. Chem., 255:10569.

Paterson, M.C., 1982, Accumulation of non-photoreactivable sites in DNA during incubation of UV-damaged xeroderma pigmentosum group A and group D cells, Prog. Mutat. Res., 4:183.

Paterson, M.C., Bech-Hansen, N.T., Blattner, W.A., and Fraumeni, J.F., Jr., 1983, Survey of human hereditary and familial disorders for γ ray response in vitro: Occurrence of both cellular radiosensitivity and radioresistance in cancer-prone families, in: "Radioprotectors and Anticarcinogens", O.F. Nygaard and M.G. Simic, eds., p.615, Academic Press, New York.

Paterson, M.C., Bech-Hansen, N.T., Smith,P.J., and Mulvihill, J.J., 1984a, Radiogenic neoplasia, cellular radiosensitivity and faulty DNA repair, in: "Radiation Carcinogenesis: Epidemiology and Biological Significance", J.D. Boice, Jr., and J.F. Fraumeni, Jr., eds., p.319, Raven Press, New York.

Paterson, M.C., and Gentner, N.E., 1984, Introduction: Environmentally induced DNA lesions and their biological consequences, in: "Repairable Lesions in Microorganisms", A. Hurst and A. Nasim, eds., p.1, Academic Press, New York.

Paterson, M.C., Gentner, N.E., Middlestadt, M.V., and Weinfeld, M., 1984b, Cancer predisposition, carcinogen hypersensitivity, and aberrant DNA metabolism, J. of Cell. Physiol. Suppl., 3:45.

Paterson, M.C., Sell, B.M., Smith, B.P., and Bech-Hansen, N.T., 1982, Impaired colony-forming ability following γ irradiation of skin fibroblasts from tuberous sclerosis patients, Radiat. Res., 90:260.

Paterson, M.C., Smith, B.P., Krush, A.J., and McKeen, E.A., 1981a, *In vitro* hypersensitivity to N-methyl-N'-nitro-N-nitrosoguanidine in a Gardner syndrome family, Radiat. Res., 87:483.

Paterson, M.C., Smith, B.P., and Smith, P.J., 1981b, Measurement of enzyme-sensitive sites in UV- or γ-irradiated human cells using *Micrococcus luteus* extracts, in: "DNA Repair: A Laboratory Manual of Research Procedures, Vol. 1, Part A", E.C. Friedberg and P.C. Hanawalt, eds., p.99, Marcel Dekker, Inc., New York.

Pegg, A.E., Roberfroid, M., von Bahr, C., Foote, R.S., Mitra, S., Bresil, H., Likhachev, A., and Montesano, R., 1982, Removal of O^6-methylguanine from DNA by human liver fractions, Proc. Natl. Acad. Sci. U.S.A., 79:5162.

Robbins, J.H., 1983, Hypersensitivity to DNA-damaging agents in primary degenerations of excitable tissue, in: "Cellular Responses to DNA damage", E.C. Friedberg and B.A. Bridges, eds., p.673, Alan R. Liss, Inc., New York.

Sancar, A., and Rupp, W.D., 1983, A novel repair enzyme: UVRABC
excision nuclease of *Escherichia coli* cuts a DNA strand on both
sides of the damaged region, Cell, 33:249.

Scudiero, D.A., 1980, Decreased DNA repair synthesis and defective
colony-forming ability of ataxia telangiectasia fibroblast cell
strains treated with N-methyl-N'-nitro-N-nitrosoguanidine,
Cancer Res., 40:984.

Scudiero, D.A., Meyer, S.A., Clatterbuck, B.E., Mattern, M.R.,
Ziolkowski, C.H.J., and Day, R.S., III, 1984, Relationship of
DNA repair phenotypes of human fibroblast and tumor strains to
killing by N-methyl-N'-nitro-N-nitrosoguanidine, Cancer Res.,
44:961.

Singer, B., 1979, N-nitrosoalkylating agents: Formation and persistence of alkyl derivatives in mammalian nucleic acid as contributing factors in carcinogenesis, J. Natl. Cancer Inst.,
62:1329.

Sklar, R., and Strauss, B., 1981, Removal of 0^6-methylguanine from
DNA of normal and xeroderma pigmentosum-derived lymphoblastoid
lines, Nature, 289:417.

Smith, P.J., Greene, M.H., Adams, D., and Paterson, M.C., 1983,
Abnormal responses to the carcinogen 4-nitroquinoline 1-oxide
of cultured fibroblasts from patients with dysplastic nevus
syndrome and hereditary cutaneous malignant melanoma, Carcinogenesis, 4:911.

Smith, P.J., Greene, M.H., Devlin, D.A., McKeen, E.A., and Paterson,
M.C., 1982, Abnormal sensitivity to UV-radiation in cultured
skin fibroblasts from patients with hereditary cutaneous malignant melanoma and dysplastic nevus syndrome, Int. J. Cancer,
30:39.

Smith, P.J., and Paterson, M.C., 1980, Defective DNA repair and
increased lethality in ataxia telangiectasia cells exposed to
4-nitroquinoline 1-oxide, Nature, 287:747.

Smith, P.J., and Paterson, M.C., 1982, Enhanced radiosensitivity
and defective DNA repair in cultured fibroblasts derived from
Rothmund Thomson syndrome patients, Mutat. Res., 94:213.

Tada, M., and Tada, M., 1975, Seryl-tRNA synthetase and activation
of the carcinogen 4-nitroquinoline 1-oxide, Nature, 255:510.

Tarone, R.E., Scudiero, D.A., and Robbins, J.H., 1983, Statistical
methods for in vitro cell survival assays, Mutat. Res., 111:79.

Tomasz, M., and Lipman, R., 1981, Reductive metabolism and alkylating
activity of mitomycin C induced by rat liver microsomes, Biochemistry, 20:5056.

van der Schans, G.P., Paterson, M.C., and Cross, W.G., 1983, DNA
strand break and rejoining in cultured human fibroblasts exposed to fast neutrons or gamma rays, Int. J. Radiat. Biol.,
44:75.

Wright, A.S., 1980, The role of metabolism in chemical mutagenesis
and chemical carcinogenesis, Mutat. Res., 75:215.

266

Yarosh, D.B., Foote, R.S., Mitra, S., and Day, R.S., III, 1983, Repair of O^6-methylguanine in DNA by demethylation is lacking in Mer⁻ human tumor cell strains, Carcinogenesis, 4:199.

APPLICATION OF STATISTICAL METHODS TO EXPERIMENTAL

RADIATION STUDIES AND TO RADIATION EPIDEMIOLOGY

Albrecht M. Kellerer

Institut für Medizinische Strahlenkunde
der Universität Würzburg
Versbacher Straße 5
D-8700 Würzburg

INTRODUCTION

Epidemiological studies of radiation carcinogenesis suffer commonly - if not always - from dosimetric uncertainties and from incompleteness of data. The dosimetric problems can be complex and, as pointed out in several of the present lectures, they always require substantial efforts even for approximate solutions. The problems of data censoring are often far less intractable and, as they are not specific to radiation studies, they can be solved by the established mathematical tools of epidemiology. It is, therefore, surprising that too many studies of radiation epidemiology - and even experimental radiation studies - are still performed without correction for competing risks. This lecture is introductory in nature and intended to further the application of the proper statistical methods by a survey of basic definitions and concepts, and by an illustration of numerical procedures in terms of selected epidemiological studies and animal experiments.

The survey can be brief, as the reader can consult not only the original contributions and several excellent monographs (e.g. 1,2), but also summaries that have been addressed specifically to the non-mathematical user (e.g. 3,4). The examples, too, are given in brief form with the intent to present essentials; for details of the data and the numerical methods the original works have to be consulted. While the examples have been selected according to current and past involvements of the author, other examples from radiation studies - and more detailed statistical treatments - are found, for example, in a recent   symposium (5).

The Notion of Censored Data

In radiation studies one deals often with a   multiplicity of parameters. Tumor rates, for example,   are studied as a function of dose and time after exposure. Information may also be required on the influence of   factors   such   as age at exposure or   of   various   physical   parameters   that determine the quality of   the   radiation   or   its   mode   of application. For the definition of the basic quantities   it is required to disregard, first, most of these complexities and   to   consider   simplified   cases.   In   particular,   a distinction will be   made   between   uncensored,   right-censored, and double-censored data. While the   definitions   of basic quantities refer equally to   these   cases,   different mathematical methods are   required   to   obtain   statistical estimates under the various conditions of censoring.

The simplest case is that of uncensored data.   It   is, however, a condition that never occurs   in   epidemiological or in experimental studies of radiation carcinogenesis, and it is referred to merely for   comparison   with   the   common conditions. The term uncensored means that the observations are complete, and this imposes two   conditions: First   the individuals must remain at risk and under observation until the specified effect occurs, i.e. there must be   no   competing risks. Secondly it is assumed, that one deals   with   a manifest disease, i.e. a disease   that   is   either   rapidly lethal or otherwise readily discovered. Examples   of   manifest diseases are leukemias, osteosarcomas   or,   among   the non-lethal examples, mammary neoplasms in the rat.

One speaks of right-censored data, when   the   observed effect is manifest, and there are competing risks. One   can then either have   exact   or   incomplete   observations.   The former are the times to the tumor. The latter are times   of censoring, i.e.   times   where   individuals   disappear   from observation   for   reasons   unrelated   to   the   tumor.   The hypothetical time to the effect is then merely known to   be larger than the observed time of censoring. It is   critical that censoring must occur   for   reasons   unrelated   to   the tumor. If this condition is   not   met,   complexities   arise that are not dealt with in the present   survey.   Mathematical methods to correct for competing risks are   straightforward, and there is little justification that their application is not yet common practise in radiation studies.

A more complex situation is that of double-censored data. It arises when there are competing risks, and the effect is non-manifest. In this case one has never the exact time to the effect. The individuals are at risk up to a time which can be predetermined, for example when animals are sacrificed at selected times, or can be a random variable determined by death occurring for reasons unrelated to the tumor. The tumor can only be observed incidentally, i.e., the exact time to the tumor is never known. If the tumor is present, the time of death is an upper bound of the time to the tumor. If the tumor is not present, the time of death is a lower bound of the hypothetical time to the tumor. Double censored data permit a straightforward analysis in experiments with systematic serial sacrifices; however, this can be a very expensive procedure. In survival experiments more sophisticated methods can be applied, and examples will be given.

Definition of Basic Quantities

The most fundamental quantity, although one that can not always be estimated conveniently, is the tumor rate, $r(t)$, at specified time. It is equal to the probability for the occurrence of the tumor per unit time interval and per individual still at risk. For the purpose of the present discussion, occurrence of a manifest tumor is equated with the time when it is first observed. Added complexities that arise from the consideration of the unobservable monocellular or oligocellular initiation and the later manifestation are here disregarded.

Age and sex dependent spontaneous tumor rates are a familiar and commonly utilized notion. However, one requires large collectives to obtain estimates of tumor rates with adequate resolution in time. It is therefore more convenient to consider the time integral of the tumor rate which is called the cumulative tumor rate:

$$R(t) = \int_{o}^{t} r(t')dt' \tag{1}$$

In many instances the tumor rates are sufficiently small that the cumulative tumor rates remain substantially less than 1. In principle, however, the cumulative tumor rates can exceed 1. For leukemias in certain strains of mice, or mammary tumors in rats the cumulative tumor rates, even of unirradiated animals, can be considerably larger than 1 towards the end of the life time (see Example 4, below). The notion of the cumulative tumor rate can be understood in analogy to the cumulative mortality rate for a human population. The latter also assumes values beyond 1 for the old age groups; for example, the cumulative mortality rate is 1 for a 77 year old man (FRG, population statistics 1978) and for a 83 year old woman. It is 3.1 for a man and 2.2 for a woman at age 90. The general term hazard function is familiar in mathematical statistics and comprises the notions of tumor rates, mortality rates, or similar quantities. In analogy one can also use the term cumulative hazard function.

Instead of the cumulative tumor rate one can consider the cumulative incidence. This is the probability, corrected for competing risks, to incur the tumor up to the specified time. The cumulative incidence is related to the cumulative tumor rate by the equation:

$$I(t) = 1 - \exp(-R(t)) \qquad (2)$$

Crude cumulative incidences, i.e., incidences not corrected for competing risks, are not infrequently utilized in radiation studies. They are substantially smaller than the cumulative incidence, whenever there are competing risks. This can lead to fallacious conclusions. For example, it is widely held that the frequency of radiation induced tumors decreases at high doses. However, much of the evidence rests on inadequate analyses based on crude cumulative incidences. There are few - if any - studies where the observation has been reliably confirmed in terms of competing risk corrected incidences.

It is not uncommon to consider the complement of the cumulative incidence. This is usually called the survival function, whether one deals, in fact, with survival or with the absence of a specified effect of any type. The survival function, in this sense, is:

$$S(t) = 1 - I(t), \quad \text{or} \quad -\ln(S(t)) = R(t) \qquad (3)$$

It follows that the common semi-logarithmic plot of the survival function is identical with the linear plot of the cumulative rate. It is also evident from Eqs(2) or (3) that cumulative incidence and tumor rate are identical whenever they are much smaller than 1. In many studies, and in particular in epidemiological studies of radiation carcinogenesis, I(t) and R(t) are, therefore, interchangeable.

ANALYSIS OF RIGHT-CENSORED DATA

Estimates of the Cumulative Incidence and the Cumulative
Tumor Rate

The cumulative incidence is estimated in terms of an equation that is commonly termed the Kaplan-Meier (6) formula, although it has also been utilized by less recent authors, among them D. Bernoulli (7):

$$I(t) = 1 - \prod_{t_i < t} (1 - 1/N(t_i)) \qquad (4)$$

In this equation $N(t)$ is the number of individuals still at risk before time t, and t are the times when tumors occur. The formula is here given for the case when the tumor times are exact. The extension to observations in discrete time intervals is straightforward.

The standard deviation is given by the equation (6):

$$\sigma(t) = (1 - I(t)) \sqrt{\sum_{t_i < t} 1/N(t_i)^2} \qquad (5)$$

The cumulative tumor rate can be estimated by the following equation (see (8), and (9) for a utilization in a radiation study):

$$R(t) = \sum_{t_i < t} 1/N(t_i) \qquad (6)$$

With the standard deviation:

$$\sigma(t) = \sqrt{\sum_{t_i < t} 1/N(t_i)^2} \qquad (7)$$

For small samples the product-limit estimate (Eq(4)) of $I(t)$ and the value $1 - \exp(-R(t))$ from the sum-limit estimate (Eq(6)) can differ substantially. For large samples the two estimates are closely equivalent.

Example 1: Radium-224 Osteosarcoma Data of Spiess

Several decades ago at a German private clinique, children with tuberculosis and adults with ankylosing spondylitis were treated inappropriately with excessive doses of radium-224, an alpha-emitter with a half life of 3.5 days which is deposited mainly on the surface of bones. Spiess, who had warned against this treatment very early,

273

Table 1: Separation of the radium-224 patients (data by Spiess) into dose groups (13).

Group number	Dose classes (gray)	Mean skeletal doses ± st.dev. in group (gray)	Number of patients	Number of osteo-sarcomas
Adults				
1	D <1	.58 ± .21	214	1
2	1≤ D <2	1.43 ± .26	189	2
3	2≤ D <4	2.82 ± .58	163	6
4	4≤ D	5.79 ± 1.33	83	5
Juveniles				
5	D <4	2.40 ± 1.1	34	1
6	4≤ D <8	5.95 ± 1.1	63	5
7	8≤ D <12	9.95 ± 1.1	52	8
8	12≤ D <16	13.9 ± 1.2	30	7
9	16≤ D	26.5 ± 11	32	14

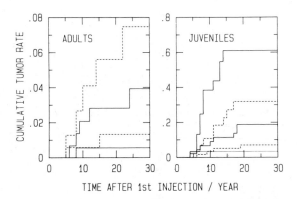

Fig. 1: Sum-limit estimates of the cumulative osteosarcoma rates in the radium-224 patients (13). The curves correspond, in ascending order, to the dose groups in Table 1.

and Mays have later followed the patients and have analysed the resulting osteosarcoma rates (10,11).

Utilizing the estimated mean skeletal doses and separating the juvenile and the adult patients into several dose classes (see Table 1) one obtains with the sum-limit estimate (Eq.(6)) the cumulative tumor rates shown in Fig.1. The standard deviations are not inserted, to keep the figure readable; in line with the relatively small number of observed cases in the individual dose classes they are substantial. Nevertheless, one obtains, even from these simple estimates, the general trend of the incidence of osteosarcomas vs. skeletal dose.

With only a few dose groups of limited size the individual estimates will usually not permit quantitative statements on the dose-effect relation. For a more coherent treatment one must utilize models that constrain the set of possible solutions. The most common non-parametric approach is the proportional hazards model. In this model the time dependence of the tumor rates or cumulative tumor rates is expressed by a base-line function, say $R_o(t)$, and according to the model the base-line function is increased in a treated group by a constant factor which depends on dose and, possibly, on other parameters of the treatment:

$$R(t,D) = \beta(D) \; R_o(t) \qquad\qquad (8)$$

No a priori assumption is made on the shape of the base-line function. The numerical procedure searches for that function and those proportional hazards factors that fit the data best in terms of maximum likelihood. This model, which is also called the Cox model (13), utilizes a relatively simple algorithm (see for example the program listed in (2)), and appears to be consistent with the data obtained in many epidemiological studies, as well as animal experiments.

Example 2: Radium-224 Osteosarcoma data of Spiess (cont'd)

The data have been treated in terms of the proportional hazards model, again with the subdivision of the juveniles and adults into dose groups according to Table 1. Fig.2 gives, as plain lines, the results of a separate analysis for the two collectives. Similar base-line functions and similar proportional hazards factors are obtained in the groups of juveniles and of adults with similar mean skeletal doses. This sugests a joint application of the proportional hazards model. The results of the joint analysis are given as dotted lines. One concludes that the results are not substantially different with the two approaches. This leads to the surprising conclusion that, in this important collective of persons submitted to the effects of an internal alpha-emitter, one can not see the increased sensitivity of the juveniles that one would expect on general biological and medical grounds.

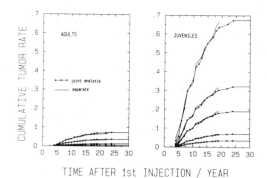

TIME AFTER 1st INJECTION / YEAR

Fig. 2: Cumulative osteosarcoma rates for the German radium-224 patients (data by Spiess, see dose groups in Table 1) according to the proportional hazards model (12). The separate analysis for the adult and the juvenile patients in the joint analysis agree closely.

The proportional hazards analysis, applied to a number of dose groups, yields the dose-effect relation in terms of the proportional hazards factors at the discrete dose values. A modified approach is required to avoid the loss of information and the degree of arbitrariness that is caused by pooling individuals into a few dose groups.

The Cox algorithm, in its normal form, treats the proportional hazards coefficients as products of exponential functions of the various parameters that are considered. This is adequate for a determination of trends. However, it is characteristic for radiation studies, that one wishes to go a step further and to consider different analytical dose effect relations, for example a linear-quadratic dose dependence or such a dependence modified by a saturation term:

$$R(t,D) = (aD-bD^2) \exp(-cD) R_o(t) \qquad (9)$$

One needs then certain modifications in the numerical procedure. They are based on standard non-linear optimization algorithms which are applied to the expression for the likelihood. In the present survey it is not necessary to write out the formulae for the likelihood; it is sufficient to note that the modified proportional hazards analysis is feasible.

Example 3: Radium-224 Osteosarcoma Data of Spiess (cont'd)

In an additional step of the analysis the data have been subjected to the proportional hazards analysis in terms of Eq(9), and the relation in Fig.(3) has been obtained as the maximum likelihood solution. The resulting risk estimates at low doses are smaller by a factor of 2 than earlier estimates based on a linear regression. A current follow-up (14) of ankylosing spondylitis patients treated with much smaller doses of radium-224 will ultimately be compared to the present risk estimate.

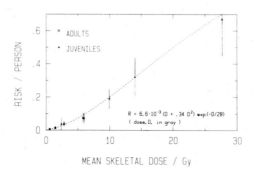

Fig. 3: Final value of the cumulative osteosarcoma rate (25 years after treatment) according to the proportional hazards model with Eq(9). Standard errors are obtained by a bootstrap method (12).

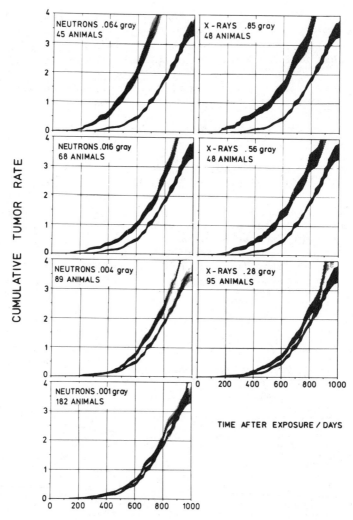

Fig. 4: Cumulative mammary tumor rates in Sprague-Dawley rats exposed to different doses of x-rays and of 340 keV-neutrons at age 60 days. The control incidence with standard deviations is repeated in each panel (15).

The proportional hazards model is a familiar tool, applied, for example, in various studies on the survivers of the atomic bomb explosions. However, it must be kept in mind that it is based on a specific assumption and that it may be incompatible with certain data. An alternative to the proportional hazards model is the accelerated failure-time model that is expressed by the assumption:

$$R(t,D) = R_o(a(D) \cdot t) \tag{10}$$

Another alternative is the time shift model:

$$R(t,D) = R_0(t+s(D)) \tag{11}$$

These models, too, can be employed in non-parametric form, i.e. with no a priori assumptions on the base line function (see also (2)). However, there seem to be no published accounts of such approaches in the literature in radiation studies with right censored data. The reason may be the inconvenience of an algorithm that is less simple and elegant than that for the proportional hazards model. This technical aspect should, however, not prejudice against these models.

Example 4: Mammary Tumors in Sprague-Dawley Rats. Data by Shellabarger

Experiments with female Sprague-Dawley rats exposed to x-rays and neutrons have shown the high relative biological effectiveness of neutrons at low doses for the induction of mammary tumors (15). Fig.4 represents the observations in terms of the sum-limit estimates with standard deviations. It illustrates that the data are consistent with the assumption of a dose dependent forward shift of the high spontaneous incidence in time. It is less certain, although a quantitative analysis has not yet been performed, whether the data could also be described adequately in terms of the proportional hazards model.

The experiment is based on relatively large groups of animals with high cumulative tumor rates. This has obviated the need for an analysis in terms of the different models. The separate sum-limit estimates suffice to show dose and time dependences.

In studies with limited data sets one may often want to go a step further, and utilize a fully parametric approach. A variety of analytical models offer themselves, and have been employed on occasions. It goes beyond the present survey to weigh their relative merits or limitations. However, a few of the more commonly invoked relations will be mentioned.

One model which is familiar in toxicology and which has also been invoked in various radiation studies (see, for example (16,17)) is the postulate of a cumulative incidence that equals the log-normal distribution. The analysis is usually performed by utilizing a log-probit plot of the Kaplan-Meier estimates. In principle, it is also possible to derive the maximum likelihood solution numerically. In a joint analysis of several dose groups one has, in principle, 2 parameters for each group, the mean and the variance of the logarithmic variable, time. However, for the model to be entirely consistent, the variance has to be the same for the different dose groups. Different variances correspond to curves that insersect, i.e., that do not correspond to a consistent dose dependence. In practise the intersection point may be too early or too late to be of concern, and differing values of the second parameter may then be considered.

An alternative is the Weibull-model:

$$R(t) = k \cdot (t-w)^P \qquad (12)$$

In the Weibull-model the coefficient k and the latent period, w, can be assumed to be a function of dose. The exponent, however, has to be a common parameter for different dose groups; the reason is - as with the log-normal model - that one obtains otherwise intersecting curves.

The Weibull-model is often utilized without the additional parameter w. In this form it is a special case of the proportional hazards and of the accelerated time model. One can then not decide on the basis of the model, whether - as is sometimes said - "one has more tumors at specified times, or the same number of tumors earlier."

Example 5: Radium-224 Osteosarcoma Data of Luz et al.

Luz et al. have performed an extensive study of osteosarcoma induction by radium-224 in different strains of mice (16,17).

Fig.5 gives results for an experiment that has demonstrated the increased tumor rates with reduced dose rates. The authors have mainly employed the log-normal

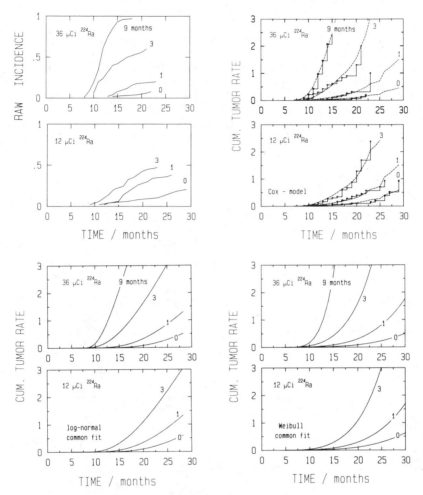

Fig. 5: Induction of osteosarcomas in mice by radium-224 in an experiment by Luz et al. (16,17). The curves in the double panels correspond to the activities 12 and 36 µCi, and to different protraction times (instantaneous application to 9 months). - Results are given for crude incidences (top left panels), for the sum-limit estimates (step functions in the top right panels), and for a joint analysis in terms of the Cox, the log-normal, and the Weibull model.

model. However, to compare different models, a variety of approaches has been applied (18), and Fig.5 gives a synopsis of the results. One notes that — with the exception of the crude incidences — they are largely equivalent.

It is of interest to compare the induction of osteo-sarcomas by the short-lived radium-224 with the effect of the long-lived radium-226 in the data of Mays on beagles which have been treated thoroughly in terms of the Weibull and the Cox-model (5). A further application of the Weibull model is made in the current large scale study at TNO (19) of the synergism of hormones and ionizing radiations in producing mammary tumors in various strains of mice.

Analysis of Double-Censored Data

Only the simple case of double-censored data will be considered, i.e. it is assumed that a tumor is non-manifest and non-lethal. In actual cases one deals, frequently, with in-between situations where tumors are partly lethal. One must then utilize an approximative treatment by judging, for every tumor, whether it has been found incidentally, or in lethal context, or whether the context must be left undecided (1,3). As will be seen, even double-censored data in their simple form present mathematical problems that are more difficile than those for right-censored data.

In most radiation studies with non-manifest tumors sacrifices at one specified time or serial sacrifices are performed. The estimate of the prevalence is then simply the fraction of animals with tumor in a group of sacrificed animals. The standard deviations are those of the binomial distribution. However, this approach can be prohibitive whenever one requires the time dependence of the pre-valence, i.e. when serial sacrifices are necessary. It is, therefore, important to apply more general methods.

Hoel and Walburg (20) have pointed out, a considerable time ago, that isotonic regression (21) can, for double-censored data, take the place of the Kaplan-Meier estimate. Isotonic regression is slightly more complicated than the Kaplan-Meier formula. However, the algorithm that is required is straightforward (see, also (22)). The result of isotonic regression is a maximum likelihood solution, i.e. the procedure applies even to small samples. It is, how-ever, difficult to obtain standard errors for the result.

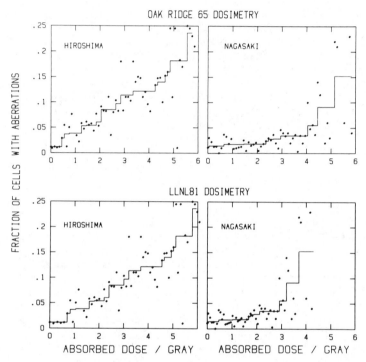

Fig. 6: Fraction of cells with chromosome aberrations in the adult health study sample for Hiroshima and Nagasaki for the T65 dosimetry and the Livermore 1981 dosimetry.

The dots are the data according to Otake (23), the lines are the results of an isotonic regression on these data.

Example 6: Chromosome Aberrations in the Atomic Bomb
Survivers

In the Adult Health Study Sample survivers of the
atomic bomb explosions are regulary examined, and there
have also been repeated analyses of persistent chromosome
aberrations. Otake (23) has published the data that are
represented by the scattered points in Fig.6. These points
result when the fraction of cells with chromosome aberrations is plotted for relatively fine dose classes. In
Otake's work and in later analyses power functions of
absorbed dose have been fitted to the data. Isotonic
regression can provide a non-parametric maximum likelihood
fit, i.e. that monotoneous dependence of prevalence on
absorbed dose that is associated with the highest
likelihood. The resulting curves are also given in the
figure. The upper panels utilize the former Oak Ridge T65
dosimetry, the lower panels are based on a a transformation
according to the change of air kerma values from the Oak
Ridge T65 to the Livermore 1981 dosimetry. The example
serves as illustration. A final analysis will have to await
the final consensus on the new dosimetry and derivation of
new personal shielding factors.

There is no simple numerical procedure, for double-
censored data, that corresponds to the Cox algorithm for
the proportional hazards model. Solutions can, nevertheless, be obtained by applying standard non-linear
optimization procedures to the equations for the partial
likelihood. In the same way, one can obtain maximum
likelihood solutions for the time-shift or the accelerated
time model. There are, in some cases, numerical problems of
convergence; this is a technical inconvenience, but it can
be overcome by utilizing different initial estimates.

Example 7:

Pulmonary carcinomas in Sprague-Dawley rats have been
induced in various inhalation studies by Lafuma et al.
(24). A maximum likelihood analysis has been applied to the
radon-daughter inhalation experiments, and the proportional
hazards model, the time-shift, and the accelerated time model have been compared. The fits obtained with the various
models were not substantially different although the accelerated failure-time model gave the best likelihood (25).

In a recent study the induction of lung carcinomas by
fission neutrons was compared to the yields obtained by

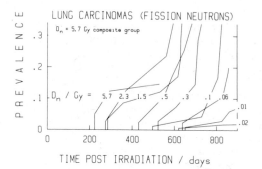

Fig. 7: Isotonic regression for the prevalence of lung carcinomas in Sprague Dawley rats exposed to fission neutrons in an experiment by Lafuma et al. (25).

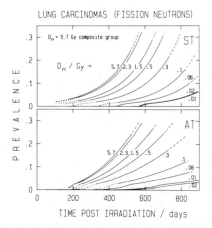

Fig. 8: Results of a joint maximum likelihood analysis of the same data as in Fig.7 in terms of the time-shift model (ST) and the accelerated time (AT) model (26).

radon inhalations (26). Fig.7 gives the isotonic regression for the different dose groups in the neutron experiments. Fig.8 shows, for comparison, the results of the accelerated time model and the time-shift model for the same data.

From the results of isotonic regression in Fig.7 one can understand why the proportional hazards model is not applicable to the neutron data. There is little or no temporal overlap in the observations of tumors in the high and the low dose groups. This is due to the very substantial life shortening after high neutron doses. Without temporal overlap no meaningful results can be obtained for the proportional hazards model. A different experimental design, including early sacrifices for the low dose groups, would be required, if one were to attempt a proportional hazards analysis. However, as seen in the earlier study with radon daughters, the results are largely equivalent for the three models. It appears that any of the three models leads to reliable risk estimates.

CONCLUSIONS

In certain studies of radiation epidemiology and in experimental radiation-carcinogenesis analyses corrections for competing risks are still insufficiently applied. The need for the correct procedures must, therefore, be emphasized.

The Kaplan-Meier estimate, and the largely equivalent sum-limit estimate, are familiar. Isotonic regression, which serves the same function for double-censored data, is less well known and deserves to be utilized more extensively in radiation studies.

The most commonly employed approach is the proportional hazards analysis for right-censored data. Other models require more complex numerical methods, but they are alternatives to the proportional hazards model that deserve to be considered. For double-censored data all three models require complex numerical procedures. Although this is an inconvenience, it should not limit the application of the models.

When one studies multiple small samples, it can be necessary to utilize analytical models. Often the approach is empirical rather than an attempt to identify mechanisms.

286

In this case there is freedom in the choice of the analytical expression. Knowledge on radiation carcinogenesis has to rely on the synthesis of information from animal studies with various tumors systems and from epidemiology. It is, therefore, desirable that comparable models be used. The Weibull-model may be most suitable for such intercomparisons.

The preceding examples and considerations have been confined to the relatively simple cases of right-censored and double-censored data. In practise one often deals with more complex situations which require modified solutions.

This survey has dealt with estimates of basic quantities, such as tumor rate, cumulative tumor rate, cumulative incidence, or prevalence. It has not dealt with tests. In concluding one may note that with the logrank test, and with the various other generalized rank tests one has suitable procedures for right censored data, but that there are no corresponding tests for double-censored data. For sufficiently large data sets certain tests can always be constructed, but there appears to be no test, as yet, that permits the non-parametric comparison of prevalences in two groups of moderate size with double-censored data. The case of double-censored data, i.e., of non-manifest diseases, has comparatively less interest in epidemiology, but it is important in the context of experimental studies, and it deserves, therefore, added attention.

Acknowledgement

This work has been partly supported by EURATOM research contract BIO 461 D.

REFERENCES

1. N. E. Breslow and N. E. Day, Statistical Methods in Cancer Research, Vol.1 - The Analysis of Case-Control Studies. IARC Scientific Publications No.32, IARC, Lyon, 1980.

2. J. D. Kalbfleisch and R. L. Prentice, The Statistical Analysis of Failure Time Data, Wiley, New-York, 1980.

3. R. Peto, Guidelines on the Analysis of Tumor Rates and Death Rates in Experimental Animals. Br.J.Cancer 29:101 (1974).

4. R. Peto, M. C. Pike, P. Armitage, N. E. Breslow, D. R. Cox, S. V. Howard, N. Mantel, K. McPherson, J. Peto, and P. G. Smith, Design and Analysis of Randomized Clinical Trials Requiring Prolonged Observation of Each Patient. I. Introduction and design,Br.J.Cancer 34:585 (1976), II. Analysis and examples, Br.J.Cancer 35:1 (1977).

5. Symposium: Extrapolation to Low Doses of Ionizing Radiation, Radiat.Res.90:33 (1982), (Contributions by A. M. Weinberg, P. G. Groer, R. E. Barlow, A. S. Whittemore, A. McMillan, R. L. Prentice, A. V. Peterson, P. Marek).

6. E. L. Kaplan and P. Meier, Non-parametric Estimation from Incomplete Observations, J.Amer.Stat.Assoc.53:457 (1958).

7. D. Bernoulli, Essai d'une nouvelle analyse de la mortalite causee par la petite verole, et des avantages de l'inoculation pour la prevenir. Memoires de Math.et de Phys.de l'Acad.Roy.des Sciences, 1-45, Paris 1766.

8. W. Nelson, Theory and applications of hazard plotting for censored failure data, Technometrics 14:945 (1972).

9. C. J. Shellabarger, R. D. Brown, A. R. Rao, J. P. Shanley, V. P. Bond, A. M. Kellerer, H. H. Rossi, L. J. Goodman, and R. E. Mills, Rat mammary carcinogenesis following neutron or x-radiation, Symp.on the Effects of Neutron irradiation upon Cell Function, Munich, 1973, in: "Biological Effects of Neutron Irradiation", 391-401, IAEA-SM-179/26, Vienna (1974).

10. C. W. Mays and H. Spiess, Epidemiological Studies of German Patients Injected with Ra-224, in: Proc.of the 16th Midyear Topical Meeting of the Health Physics Society, NTIS CONF 830101, Springfield, VA, 1983.

11. C. W. Mays and H. Spiess, Bone Sarcomas in Patients Given Radium-224 Radiation Carcinogenesis: Epidemiology and Biological Significance, J. D. Boice,Jr. and J. F. Fraumeni, Jr. eds, Raven Press, New York, 1984.

12. H. Spiess, C. W. Mays, D. Chmelevsky, and A. M. Kellerer, A Proportional Hazards Analysis of the Osteosarcoma Rates in German 224-Radium Patients, to appear, Proc.Symp."The Radiobiology of Radium and Thorotrast", Munich, CEC, 1984.

13. D. R. Cox, Regression Models and Life Tables (with discussion), J.R.Stat.Soc.B, 34:187 (1972).

14. R. R. Wick and W. Gössner, Incidence of Tumours of the

Skeleton in 224-Ra-Treated Ankylosing Spondylitis Patients, in: "Biological Effects of Low-Level Radiation", 281-288, IAEA-SM-266/15, Vienna, 1983.

15. C. J. Shellabarger, D. Chmelevsky, and A. M. Kellerer, Induction of Mammary Neoplasms in the Sprague-Dawley Rat by 430-keV Neutrons and X-Rays, J.Natl.Cancer Inst.64:821, 1980.

16. A. Luz, W. A. Müller, W. Gössner, and O. Hug, Estimation of Tumour Risk at Low Dose from Experimental Results after Incorporation of Short-Lived Bone-Seeking Alpha Emitters 224-Ra and 227-Th in Mice, in: "Biological and Environmental Effects of Low-Level", Radiation 11:171, IAEA-SM-202/406, Vienna, 1976.

17. A. Luz, Zur Pathogenese des strahleninduzierten Osteosarkoms, GSF-Berich B 1387, ISSN 0721-1694, 1980.

18. D. Chmelevsky, et al., Comparison of Models for the Time Dependence of Tumor rates - A study of osteosarcoma induction in mice by 224-Radium, in preparation.

19. J. J. Broerse, L. A. Hennen, M. J. van Zwieten, and C. F. Hollander, Mammary Carcinogenesis in Different Rat Strains after Single and Fractionated Irradiations, in: Proc. "European Seminar on Neutron Carcinogenesis", J. J. Broerse and G. B. Gerber, eds., 155-168, EUR 8084 EN, Luxembourg, 1982.

20. D. G. Hoel and H. E. Walburg,Jr.,Statistical Analysis of Survival Experiments. J.Natl.Cancer Inst. 49:361 (1972).

21. R. E. Barlow, D. J. Bartholomew, J. M. Bremner, and H. D. Brunk, Statistical Inference under Order Restrictions; The Theory and Application of Isotonic Regression, New-York: John Wiley & Sons, 1972.

22. A. M. Kellerer and D. Chmelevsky, Analysis of Tumor Rates and Incidences - A Survey of Concepts and Methods -, in: Proc. "European Seminar on Neutron Carcinogenesis", J. J.Broerse, G. B. Gerber, eds., 209-231, EUR 8084 EN, Luxembourg, 1982.

23. M. Otake, Dose-Response Relationship of Neutron and Gamma Rays to Chromosomally Aberrant Cells among Atomic Bomb Survivors in Hiroshima and Nagasaki, J.Radiat.Res. 20:307 (1979).

24. J. Lafuma, Cancers pulmonaires induits par differents emetteurs alpha inhales: Evaluation de l'influence de divers parametres et comparaison avec les donnees obtenues chez les mineurs d'uranium, in: "Late Biological Effects of Ionizing Radiation", Vol.II, 531, IAEA-SM-224/109, Vienna, 1978.

25. D. Chmelevsky, A. M. Kellerer, J. Lafuma, and J. Chameaud, Maximum Likelihood Estimation of the Prevalence of Non-Lethal Neoplasms - An Application to Radon Daughter Inhalation Studies -, Radiat.Res.91:589 (1982).

26. D. Chmelevsky, A. M. Kellerer, J. Lafuma, M. Morin, and R. Masse, Comparison of the Induction of Pulmonary Neoplasms in Sprague-Dawley Rats by Fission Neutrons and Radon Daughters, Radiat.Res.98:519 (1984).

BIOLOGICAL MONITORING STUDIES IN OCCUPATIONAL AND ENVIRONMENTAL

HEALTH

Reinier L. Zielhuis

Chair of occupational and environmental health
University of Amsterdam
Academic Medical Center
Meibergdreef 15, 1105 AZ Amsterdam, The Netherlands

TERMINOLOGY

In the last two decades Biological Monitoring (BM)-programs
have rapidly expanded, in addition to and sometimes as an alternative to environmental monitoring (EM). However, enthusiastic acceptance of a new approach may easily lead to confusion, e.g. in definitions and consequently in practice.

In 1980 the NIOSH, the OSHA and the CEC-Health and Safety Di-
rectorate organized a Symposium on "Assessment of toxic agents at
the workplace; roles of ambient (environmental) and biological monitoring" (Berlin et al, 1984). Although this meeting was limited
to occupational health, the definitions agreed upon also apply to
environmental health.

The symposium defined and accepted the following terminology:

Monitoring is a systematic continuous or repetitive health-related
activity, designed to lead if necessary to corrective actions. Three
relevant types of monitoring may be defined:

Ambient (environmental) monitoring (EM) is the measurement and assessment of agents at the workplace (or general environment) and
evaluates ambient exposure ánd health risk compared to an appropriate reference.

Biological monitoring (BM) is the measurement and assessment of
agents or their metabolites either e.g. in tissues, secreta, excreta, expired air or any combination of these to evaluate exposure ánd
health risk compared to an appropriate reference.

Health surveillance (or Health effects monitoring, HEM) is the periodic medico-physiological examination of exposed subjects with
the objective of protecting health and preventing occupationally
(environmentally) related disease. The detection of established disease is outside the scope of this definition.

I emphasize some aspects:
- The three definitions may also apply to animals; however, discussion of this is outside the scope of this paper.
- The term "biomonitoring" or "biologic monitoring" still is often
  loosely applied as "a mixture" of BM and HEM. A recent example
  gives the ACGIH (1984), which recently decided to propose "Biological Exposure Indices" (BEI's) as supplementary to TLV's. BEI's
  are suggested to furnish information on individual response (HEM)
  ánd of individual overall exposure (BM). However, this denies an
  essential difference in objective: BM assesses exposure and health
  risk, i.e. the probability of impairment of the state of health,
  whereas HEM assesses the state of early impairment of health itself.
- Both EM and BM assess exposure ánd health risk; BM measures man
  (internal) and EM the outside environment (external).
- The findings of EM and BM should always be compared to appropriate reference levels, based upon a non-exposure situation or upon
  non-exposed subjects, or compared to established chemical quality
  limits.
- Although monitoring involves continuous or at least repetitive
  measurement, in practice it may also be carried at one point of
  time. However, repetitive measurement has a great advantage: the
  trend adds an additional significance to the data measured.
- Clinical medicine also incresingly applies BM to assess therapeutic drug levels in blood, spinal fluid, etc.; moreover, BM may
  aid in diagnosing an alleged clinical intoxication.
- In recent years BM of breast milk has become an important topic.
  This assesses exposure to the lactating mother (BM), but at the
  same time it can also be regarded as EM in respect of the suck-
  ling infant. One example: in the USA Pellizari et al (1982) investigated whether breast milk could be used as an indicator of
  occupational/environmental pollution with volatile organic solvents. Milk was collected from 48 women, living in urban areas.
  The authors detected int. alia 26 halogenated compounds, 17 alde-
  hydes, 20 ketones, 10 alcohols, 6 esters, 2 ethers, 14 furanes,
  13 alkanes, 7 alkynes, 11 cyclic and 14 aromatic compounds, i.e.
  in total over 100 xenobiotic compounds.
- In practice mostly urine, blood and expired air are used as sample specimen; however, hair, nails, saliva, deciduous teeth, placenta and subcutaneous fat may also be applied. It should be realized that increased levels in hair may be largely due to direct
  contamination from polluted air, soildust/hands. Externally deposited metals may become bound to SH-groups. Endogeneously absorbed
  and exogeneously absorbed metals can often not be distinguished.

Moreover, in a recent autopsy study in the Netherlands no relation was observed between levels of Cd, Cu, Mn, Pb, Fe, Mg or Zn
with levels in various body tissues (Aalbers, 1984). Therefore,
BM of hair may also be regarded as indirect EM, except when the
agent is only ingested (e.g. methylmercury).
- A few (bio)chemical effects, which are more or less agent-speci-
fic, may also be applied within the context of a BM-program, e.g.
inhibition of the activity of cholinesterase enzymes in total
blood or plasma/serum in exposure to some (mostly organophosphate)
pesticides, zinc protoporphyrin levels in blood in exposure to inorganic lead.
- In recent years non-invasive physical techniques for BM have been
developed, e.g. "magnetopneumography" to assess the Fe-burden in
the lungs (Kalliomäki et al, 1981) and "partial body neutron activation" to assess the cadmium burden in liver and kidney, measurement of lead in deciduous teeth or in bone (X-fluorescence technique), metallic mercury in superficial tissues in the head (review
by Lauwerys, 1983a).
- There exists also an other approach in both EM and BM: specimen
banking (Luepke, 1979), i.e. systematic sampling and storage of
environmental or biological samples for deferred examination, analysis and evaluation. Measurement may be deferred for a period of
years, even decades after collection. Studies of metal levels in
archeological bones can be regarded as specimen banking "avant la
lettre". Because this paper only refers to BM in ambulant workers
or members of the general public, specimen banking will not be
discussed.

ASSESSMENT OF EXPOSURE AND OF HEALTH RISKS

As outlined in my first paper, we may distinguish different
concepts of exposure: (1) "external exposure in general sense" (concentrations, duration, frequency); (2) "external exposure in a narrow sense" (amount of intake, external load); (3) "internal exposure" (amount of uptake, body burden, internal load) and (4) internal exposure to the critical effector organ.

EM measures concentrations in air, food, water, soil, etc. The
human body is regarded as a "black box"; the toxicokinetics are not
taken into account. BM measures agents and/or its metabolites in
biological samples. It is easily understood that, even although
actual exposure of the critical effector organ can usually not be
measured as such, BM permits a more appropriate estimate than EM.
Because BM indirectly takes into account the toxicokinetics of the
agent and also biological variation in kinetics, it also assesses
individual differences both in internal exposure and in health risks.
Therefore, from the viewpoint of health protection BM approximates
actual internal exposure and health risk better than EM.

Most animal experiments permit to establish exposure-response relationships, based upon the concentration inhaled or the dose ingested; from this one has to extrapolate to man. However, by taking into account the toxicokinetics and by measuring the toxic agent or metabolite in animal tissues/excreta/secreta a more valid extrapolation can be made. Two examples may illustrate this. Gehring et al (1979) showed that the incidence of liver angiosarcoma in rats was a function of the ug equivalents of vinylchloride metabolites formed; this model predicted the observed risk in humans better than when extrapolating from the EM-parameters. Sato et al$_3$(1975) exposed male and female volunteers for 2 h to 75 mg benzene/m^3; the benzene content of blood and of expired air was measured. During exposure the benzene level in blood was highest in the male volunteers, but after exposure the level in blood and expired air was higher and decreased more slowly in the female volunteers. This sex-dependent difference in kinetics can be explained by the difference in relative free fatty mass which on the average is two times higher in women than in men. This study in humans was supported by studies in fat and lean rats. Moreover, a decrease of the number of leucocytes occurred in the fat rats earlier than in the lean rats.

ADVANTAGES AND LIMITATIONS OF BM

In addition to the advantage mentioned above, other well-known advantages of BM over EM exist: (1) assessment of total exposure simultaneously from different sources and through different pathways; (2) indirect estimate of total amount inhaled/ingested/dermally absorbed, taking into account the impact of physical activity on respiratory intake and the impact of heat load on dermal absorption. (3) biochemical/haematological effect parameters in blood and urine may be measured at the same time and also BM-parameters of several agents. (4) Moreover, BM may be more cost effective than EM.

However, emphasis upon the present limitations provides a more forceful stimulus to promote research and development than uncritical enthusiasm over the advantages. The present limitations can largely be overcome in the not too distant future.

The first drawback is that BM may carry some inconvenience to subjects examined. This particularly applies to sampling of blood, more so in repetitive measurements. Also sampling of urine, hair, expired air, placenta, saliva, etc. requires at least coöperation and expenditure of time. This inconvenience will be percieved less when those responsible for BM work from a basis of mutual confidence, which may be more readily achieved in occupational health than in environmental health.

BM is essentially a method to be applied by physicians and paramedical personel, trying to prevent as much as possible inconvenience, loss of time, etc. BM should also be accompanied by an ongoing health education program. Moreover, each subject has to be fully informed on his/her personel data which have to be treated as confidential. In my first paper I have already emphasized that clients/patients do not easily recognize the difference between BM and HEM; this should always be made clear. The group data should also be reported to representatives of workers and of the general public, and not only to management or governmental authorities.

The most serious drawback, which gradually may be overcome, is that at the present moment routine BM-programs only exist for a limited number of chemicals, albeit most of them widely encountered during work, at home and/or in the ambient environment. However, there certainly is a rapid expansion in the number of chemicals which can be monitored. The 1977-CEC/EPA/WHO symposium on "The use of biological specimens for the assessment of human exposure to environmental pollution" (Berlin et al, 1979) summarized the state of the art. The experts concluded that for 7 metals and for 13 other compounds reasonably valid routine BM methods existed by analyzing 12 tissues/excreta/secreta, which can be sampled in ambulant clients/ patients without much inconvenience. In 1983 our laboratory was invited by the WHO (Dept. Environmental Health) to prepare an update of the 1977-review (Zielhuis et al, 1984a). We reviewed the literature extensively, and we concluded that the present state of the art allows a much wider application than in 1977. Sampling and analysis of blood, plasma/serum, urine, breast milk, placenta, hair/ nails, expired air or faeces permits routine BM-programs for assessing exposure and health risk for 12 metals (elements, inorganic or organic compounds), 5 organochlorine pesticides, 4 polyhalogenated hydrocarbons of low volatility, 6 volatile halogenated hydrocarbons, 5 aromatic and aliphatic hydrocarbons, 18 other organic compounds and 3 internal asphyxiants. Concluding: in 1977 for 20, in 1983 for 53 compounds. The criterion for acceptance was: application in the ambulant general population and availability of quantitative reference levels in non-exposed subjects. Moreover, also the quality of BM-programs has considerably increased. There certainly is still a long way to go, but there certainly has been a rapid expansion within the last 5-10 years. This is also illustrated in several recently published books on BM, e.g. Baselt (1983), CEC (1983), Lauwerys (1983b), Aitio (1984).

We should, however, recognize that in the case of exposure to chemicals, which exclusively or mainly exert effects on the mucosae of eyes, respiratory tract or on the skin and which are not or hardly absorbed by the body, valid BM-methods cannot be developed. Neither can BM be applied afterwards in incidental exposure to chemicals with a short half life.

ASPECTS OF STRATEGIES FOR BM

In my first paper I defined strategy as: "the logical sequence of steps to achieve a valid answer to a specified question". BM for assessment of exposure and of health risk may replace qualitative assessment of the sources of exposure (step 3) and quantitative EM-assessment of exposure (step 5). Assessment of health risk (step 6) can be based directly on the BM parameters in the group at risk and in the control group. However, where specific preventive technical measures have to be taken, e.g. in controlling emissions from specified sources of exposure. EM-assessment of exposure certainly is also needed. BM cannot replace the full sequence of steps, outlined in the first paper, but it may provide cost-effective short cuts within the complete sequence of steps.

Three objectives of a BM-program

The design of a BM-program depends first of all on the specific objective of the study, within the framework of cause-directed (B) or situation-directed (C)-studies.

It is important to distinguish three objectives:
(1) To assess whether overexposure does (not) exist. I proposed to the CEC (Zielhuis, 1974) a socalled "Biological Quality Guide" (BQG) for assessment of exposure and health risk in regard to inorganic lead among the general population. I concluded that no actual over-exposure and increased health risk needs to be expected in a certain area, irrespective of the source of exposure, when in a representative group of the general population, living in that area the blood lead levels (PbB) do not exceed in 98% of subjects 350 µg Pb/1, in 90% 300 µg Pb/1 and in 50% 200 µg/1. When this BQG is not exceeded, EM of the many potential sources of exposure is not necessary. This proposal was accepted by the Council of Ministers of the CEC, and it became the basis for the 1977-Directive to carry out population studies in the nine countries in 1979 and 1981. Later on (Zielhuis et al 1979) we proposed a more restricted BQG for 4-6 years old Kindergarten children (95% < 300 µg Pb/1, 90% < 250 µg Pb/1, 50% < 200 µg Pb/1), because of their greater susceptibility. This proposal was only accepted by the Dutch government and not by CEC.

In occupational health one may advise a somewhat different approach (Zielhuis and Wibowo, 1978): when the zinc protoporphyrin level does not exceed 2.5-3 µg ZPP/g Hb in workers regularly exposed to inorganic lead for at least a few months, one should hardly expect that the PbB-levels exceed 400 µg Pb/1 in male workers. Only when the ZPP exceeds this level, PbB has to be measured. Measurement of ZPP in blood cannot be applied in general population studies, because the increase of ZPP is not sensitive enough to assure that the BQG for PbB is not exceeded.

Similar negative BM-approaches can be carried out in exposure to most other chemicals, at least when reasonably established biological guidelines exist. This "negative" approach allows to establish non-risk situations, and is more cost-effective than EM-assessment.

(2) Assessment of overexposure in groups of subjects. Assessment of overexposure and maybe of increased health risks may require a more elaborate BM-program. One may also add a few more or less effect-specific biochemical HEM-parameters (e.g. for renal function: Retinol Binding Protein, β_2Microglobulin, total protein in urine). When in workers exposed to trichloroethene (TRI) the urinary levels of trichloroacetic acid (TCA) exceed 50 mg/g creat, then more BM-parameters should be examined (Monster 1984a): in exposure to e.g. 50 ppm (270 mg/m^3) one may expect at the end of an 8 h exposure shift in alveolar air about 50-80 µg/m^3, in blood 0.9 mg trichloroethylene/1, 5 mg trichloroethanol/1 or 60-70 mg trichloroacetic acid/1, and for both metabolites respectively in urine about 100 mg/g creat and 100 mg/g creat. By increasing the number of parameters measured, one is able to assess the extent of overexposure more adequately.

I emphasized already in my first paper that most parameters are not normally distributed in exposure to xenobiotic agents. Frequency distributions permit to pinpoint subgroups or individuals most at risk. When the distribution is reasonably log-normal (which often is not the case), one may also calculate geom. averages and the 95% geom. confidence interval.

(3) Assessment of individual exposure. In overexposed individuals one should establish exposure and health risk as accurately as possible. Particularly in the case of praeclinical intoxication BM may approximate BM in clinical medicine. Moreover, HEM may also have to be carried out.

In our laboratory Monster et al (1983) studied the individual relationship between parameters of internal exposure and of external (EM) exposure to tetrachloroethene (PERC). The regression equation was: Ln TWA (µmol PERC/m^3=2.78 + 0.708 Ln PERC (alv.air). R^2= 0.93, geometric residual error = 1.43, n=21. When 8.3 µmol PERC/1 blood, 20 µmol TCA/1 blood, 515 µmol/m^3 exhaled air and 3.0 µmol TCA/mmol creat is not exceeded, exposure does not exceed 2050 µmol PERC/m^3 (50 ppm) during the work week (1 µmol PERC/m^3=0.166 mg/m^3).

In exposure to 1,1,1,-trichloroethane (methylchloroform, MC) Monster (1984b) also studied the impact of measuring two BM-parameters simultaneously on the accuracy of the estimate of individual exposure to MC as t.w.a. over the 40 h workweek: the geom. residual error was lowest (g.r.e. 1.30; r=0.97), when measuring both MC and TCA in blood at Friday at the end of the workshift or at Monday morning before work (g.r.e. 1.28; r=0.98), whereas measurement of only one of these parameters yielded a g.r.e. between 1.39 and 1.46 and r=0.95 and 0.94. In the above mentioned PERC-study the residual error was also lowest when measuring both PERC and TCA in blood at Friday at the end of the workshift, g.r.e.=1.19, r=0.98. Measurement of several parameters may increase the specificity of measurement. This approach needs certainly further research and development.

Sampling points of time

In assessment of exposure the points of time of sampling for BM may be very critical. In exposure to trichloroethene (TRI) the most important metabolites are trichloroethanol (TCE, $T_{\frac{1}{2}}$=10-15 h) and tri-chloroacetic acid (TCA, $T_{\frac{1}{2}}$=70-100 h). TCE reaches its maximum level in blood, expired air and urine very quickly, and it has a short $T_{\frac{1}{2}}$. However, TCA continues to rise until about 20-40 h after exposure and accumulates in repeated exposure. Therefore, in assessing short term exposure and health risks one should measure TCE during the course of or at the end of the workshift. When one wants to assess overall ex-posure and health risks due to longterm exposure, one has to measure TCA levels in blood or urine. In exposure for 6-8 h the TRI-level in alveolar air decreases quickly from about 6.5% of the inhaled concen-tration at $\frac{1}{2}$h after exposure to 0.65% at 16 h (the following morning). In consecutive exposure especially the percentages at 16 h and 64 h increase (Monster 1984a).

In exposure to metals, e.g. lead with a $T_{\frac{1}{2}}$ for PbB of 2-4 wk, Cd in urine with a $T_{\frac{1}{2}}$ up to several years, the time of sampling is less critical. Nevertheless, the Pb and Cd-levels in blood only estimate total exposure over the last weeks/months whereas CdU estimates Cd-exposure accumulated over years. When one wants to as-sess the mobile lead body burden in subjects not exposed any longer for several months, then measurement of PbB has not much value, whereas the ZPP level in blood still remains high over a long period of time. In that case one may have to measure chelatable Pb in urine (EDTA-injection).Alessio et al (1976) showed that chelatable Pb in urine and ZPP are still highly correlated also many months after oc-cupational exposure.

Biological monitoring of carbon monoxide (CO) is carried out by measuring the HbCO-level in blood or the CO-level in expired air; the $T_{\frac{1}{2}}$ is about 5 h. However, in exposure to dichloromethane (me-thylene chloride), which is metabolized into CO, the $T_{\frac{1}{2}}$ is about twice as long, because biotransformation still goes on after expo-sure. Therefore, the maximum %HbCO is achieved after exposure. In exposure to methylenechloride for 2-3 h, BM should assess exposure to the agent itself in expired air or in blood; the critical effect is narcosis due to methylene chloride. In exposure for more than 3 h the critical health risk is due to CO, and BM of CO has to be car-ried out.

BM assesses total exposure: during work, at home, in the ambient environment. In the Rotterdam seaport Coret et al (1974) measured the %HbCO in drivers, who took autocars ashore; smoking was forbidden. During the nightshift previously smoking drivers started work with an increased %HbCO; this even decreased during the night shift, although they were exposed to CO. During the dayshift, smokers started with a low %HbCO, which increased during work with av. 4% HbCO.

Twenty years ago Curphey et al (1965) measured for six months the CO-levels in ambient air and the CO-level in blood of the general population in Los Angeles. There was a good correlation between both levels in non-smokers (high in winter, decreasing to low levels in june), but not at all in smokers. The personal life style overruled ambient exposure.

In exposure to agents with a short half life, one may have to compromise between the optimal sampling time and practical feasibility. In our experience, in occupational health one usually has to choose between (1) during or at the end of the work shift, (2) the following morning before work (at 16 h) or (3) after the weekend before work (at 60-64 h). One should realize, however, that the parameters to be measured will not always be the same at these three practical sampling points of time.

This discussion of sampling points of time emphasizes that the actual strategy of measurement may to a large extent be determined by the specified objective of the study, the type of exposure, the agent, the life style of the population examined and by the health risk to be assessed.

Chemical analysis

It is beyond the scope of this paper to discuss the analytical aspects of BM. One warning may suffice: never rely on quantitative data, when analytical accuracy and precision is not known, and when the analytical laboratory does not participate in interlaboratory comparison studies. No consistent strategy is possible, when appropriate quality control of EM-, BM- and HEM-data is not carried out.

Another aspect of analysis is the detection limit. Ongoing analytical research may considerably decrease the detection limit, maybe by applying more sophisticated techniques. It depends upon the specific objective of a BM-study and the availability of established acceptable biological guidelines, whether one has to apply highly sensitive analytical methods. When the TLV-MAC for occupational exposure is expressed in many mg/m^3, then in many cases one may have not to measure in $\mu g/m^3$ in expired air, in $\mu g/l$ in blood or urine.

However, in cause-directed studies (study B, first paper), which aim
at expanding knowledge on exposure-response relationships, one shall
try to cover the whole range of internal exposure. Moreover, in
environmental health one usually encounters much lower exposure levels than in occupational health, not always to be assessed with
methods appropriate for higher occupational exposure. In the study
on occupational exposure to tetrachloroethene, discussed before
(Monster et al, 1983) the detection level was 0.1 mg/m^3 (0.6 μmol/m^3).
However, we also carried out studies on exposure to tetrachloroethene
in the general population. In 1978 we carried out a study among
subjects living at short distance from dry-cleaning shops in the
inner city of Amsterdam (Verberk and Scheffers, 1980); alveolar concentrations up to 37 mg/m^3 could be measured in adult not occupationally exposed residents, with a distinct gradient proportionate
to the distance (up to about 30 m) from the sources of emission. We
could still apply the method with a detection level of 0.1 mg/m^3.
In 1980-1981 we lowered the detection level down to 1 μg/m^3 in alveolar air. We were then able with this more advanced method to assess
exposure in 4 and 5 year old children, attending a kindergarten
situated near a factory and in old aged subjects living in an old
folk's home near a former chemical waste dump. In the non-exposed
subjects we measured 2 to 5 μg/m^3 in exhaled air, in the exposed
children 24 ± 7 μg/m^3, in the old aged subjects up to about 20 μg/
m^3 (in many subjects below 2-3 μg/m^3) (Monster et al 1984c). In the
first study we observed a considerable overexposure in adult inhabitants of houses living above and next to dry-cleaning shops; however, an increased health risk did probably not exist. In the second
and third study exposure was only slightly increased. On the basis
of the study in the old aged subjects a proposal to demolish the
recently built old folk's home was not carried out.

Although strictly speaking in the last two studies we also
could have used the less sensitive method, which might have suffered
to conclude that the acceptable limits were not exceeded, we could
not have been able to establish the extent of exposure in comparison to controls. In this study we even observed in one old subject
a level of 27 μg/m^3 in her alveolar air, probably due to the presence of recently dry-cleaned clothes in her room.

At this moment we are carrying out studies in patients who
have been exposed for at least several months to tetrachloroethene
(PERC) during work in dry cleaning shops, but who had temporarily
to stop working because of not work-related diseases. We determined
the concentration of PERC in expired air several times, starting 4
to 7 days after stopping work. The patients were still exhaling
PERC at least up to 8-12 weeks after occupational exposure. The
study is still going on. The $T\frac{1}{2}$=5-7 days proved to be about the
same as we had determined in short term (30-60 min) experimental
exposure of volunteers in the late post exposure period. This study
shows that in the case of volatile solvents with a long $T\frac{1}{2}$ it is

still possible to assess previous occupational exposure, even when the levels in expired air have become very low.

The application of increasingly sensitive methods, however, is criticized by some experts because this might create unwarranted fear among the population: when laymen do not understand the difference between assessment of exposure and of health risk and assessment of the state of health, they may regard any established exposure as evidence of actual impairment of health. However, we have to explain the scientific facts time and again; we cannot omit studies because of the fear of unwarranted conclusions.

Further development of analytical methods leads to decreasing detection limits; this has been already the case for many compounds. We should not distrust this development, but we should apply these sensitive methods when the aim is to assess actual total exposure, and particularly when the study objective is to establish exposure-response-relationships.

Another aspect of analysis is speciation. This is increasingly applied in EM, but in BM the development of speciation is still in an early phase. In 1983 we discussed the importance of metal speciation in total exposure and risk assessment for the CEC/WHO/EPA Conference on Heavy Metals in the Environment, in Heidelberg (Zielhuis 1983) and in the Dahlem Conference on Changing Metal Cycles and Human Health in Berlin (Zielhuis and Wibowo, 1984b).BM of metals is still mainly based upon measurement of metal element levels in biological specimens, whereas the metal species determines both toxicokinetics and health risks. Most occupational and environmental studies on exposure to arsenic, on which the present exposure response-relationships have been based, rely on measurement of total As in urine. However, we should at least distinguish between three groups of As-compounds: (1) inorganic high solubility compounds, which may cause effects on nervous system, liver and skin (int. alia carcinoma) after systemic absorption; these compounds are metabolized into monomethyl arsonic acid and dimethyl arsinic acid; (2) inorganic low solubility As-compounds which may induce lung cancer; BM of As in urine will only to a limited extent assess external exposure and health risk; (3) organic As-compounds in marine food; they do not cause cancer, and are quickly excreted unchanged. Depending upon the industrial process workers may be exposed to different As-compounds, which differ in solubility and health risk. In ambient exposure the general public and workers may ingest marine food, but also mineral water (in France about 100 times higher consumption per caput than in the Netherlands, with average about 20 µg inorganic As/l). Relying on total As in urine data leads to inadequate assessment of actual exposure and health risk. Nevertheless, the ADI was recently only based upon the element As as such; the CEC and WHO drinking water standards only mention arsenic as such; the OSHA-proposal for the MAC for workroom air is mainly built upon studies, which rely on total As in urine. In recent years it has become possible to apply BM-methods which assess exposure to inorganic As and organic marine food As separately (Buchet et al, 1981a, 1981b, Norin and Vahter, 1981). Assessment of exposure to e.g. chromium and nickel meets similar problems. However, speciation is not only relevant in exposure to metals. For instance Noren (1983) measured organochlorine contaminants in human milk; she discovered that the PCB-pattern in human milk differs from that in commercially available mixtures used as standards. This is an other example that BM-speciation may lead to better understanding of actual exposure and health risk.

BIOLOGICAL EXPOSURE LIMITS?

Assessment of health risk by BM is to be preferred above EM. This makes it possible also to propose Biological Exposure Limits to be applied in occupational and environmental health. The German MAK-Commission of the "Deutsche Forschungsgemeinschaft" and the ACGIH and also the WHO and the CEC have started to publish such BEI's for occupational exposure, although particularly workers' unions raise many objection to do so (Berlin et al, 1984).

The WHO has proposed several health-based Occupational Biological Exposure Limits, e.g. for lead, cadmium, a few solvents and pesticides, either as maximum individual limits or as group average limits. The CEC Directives for assessment of population exposure to inorganic lead (CEC, 1977) was based upon a maximal accepted frequency distribution of blood lead levels (CEC, 1977); the CEC-Directive (CEC, 1982) for occupational exposure to lead sets a limit of PbB for male workers; a proposal for a different biological limit for female workers was not accepted by the CEC-Council of Ministers. In his review of BM in occupational health Lauwerys (1983) suggested a large number of Biological Exposure Limits, albeit many of them as "tentative".

Whether biological exposure limits should be treated as regulatory limits, is a matter of policy decisions. However, occupational and environmental health departments should apply non-regulatory biological quality guidelines, even when still "tentative", because they may serve as important signals for action.

CONCLUSION

In my first paper I outlined the overall strategy for assessment of exposure and health risk. Biological monitoring may be of considerable help. In preventing adverse overexposure BM may even be preferred above EM. However, the limitations should be carefully considered; the specific aspects of BM, dependent upon the type

of exposure, the toxicokinetics of the agents under consideration
and the personal life style, age, sex, disposition of subjects,
etc. determine the strategy of assessment. We may expect a rapid
further development and expansion of BM-methods. This will guarantee a better assessment of exposure and of health risk for an increasing number of chemicals, both in occupational and environmental exposure, and in this way it will greatly contribute to the prevention of adverse health effects both in environmental and occupational health.

SUMMARY

Both environmental (EM) and biological (BM) monitoring assess
exposure and health risk. BM has some advantages over EM: (1) it
takes into account total exposure to the same agent from all sources and routes of intake; (2) it approximates better the critical
organ burden; (3) physical activity, dermal absorption and oral ingestion are taken into account; (4) it reflects the toxicokinetics;
(5) biochemical effect parameters may be measured in the same medium;
(6) it may be more cost effective. However, BM has also its limitations: (1) inconvenience to subjects; (2) only available for a number of substances; (3) the points of time of sampling are critical;
(4) for locally acting chemicals BM is not feasible.

Nevertheless, application of BM both in environmental and occupational health offers many possibilities for assessment of exposure and of health risk (not: state of health). There has been a
rapid expansion of BM-methods in the last decade. The operational
BM-program depends upon the specific objective of the study: (1)
assessment of short term or of long term exposure; of exposure ad
hoc or of past exposure; (2) assessment of single or of combined
exposure; (3) cross-sectional study or longitudinal follow up; (5)
the agent(s) under consideration; (6) the at risk groups under consideration; (7) applied to workers or to the general population;
(8) applied to groups or individuals; (9) application in children.

It is important to distinguish three BM-approaches: to assess
(1) whether a "problem" exists in groups; (2) intensity of exposure
and health risk in groups; (3) exposure and health risk in individuals, e.g. cases of poisoning.

Because the distributions of BM-parameters are usually skew,
percentile distributions or geometric averages ($\bar{x}g$) and standard
deviations much better present the actual exposure and health risk
in a group of subjects than arithmetic averages.

Various biological specimens can be used in ambulant "healthy"
subjects, particularly expired air, urine, blood; much less suitable is hair and nails; saliva may be used, but little data are available. Recently some non-invasive physical techniques have come

available, e.g. for Cd (liver and kidney) and Fe (lungs). BM of breast milk receives increasingly attention, more for assessment of the intake of infants than for assessment of exposure of the mother.

In the future BM may also be applied in regulatory standard setting.

REFERENCES

Aalbers, Th. G., 1984, "Cardiovascular diseases and trace elements", Thesis Technical University Delft, The Netherlands

Aitio, A., Riihimaki, V. and Vainio, H. (eds), 1984, "Biological monitoring and surveillance of workers exposed to chemicals", Hemisphere, Washington etc.

Alessio, L., Bertazzi, P.A., Monelli, V. and Toffoletto, F., 1976, Free erythrocyte protoporphyrin as an indicator of biological effects of lead in adult males, III Behaviour of free erythrocyte protoporphyrin in workers with past exposure. Int. Arch. Occup. Environ. Health, 38: 77-88

American Conference Governmental Industrial Hygienists (ACGIH), 1984, Report of ACGIH biological exposure indices committee, Occupational Safety and Health Reports, 5-31, 1376-1378

Baselt, R., C., 1980, "Biological monitoring methods for industrial chemicals", Biomed. Publ., Davis, Calif.

Berlin, A., Wolff, A.H. and Hasegawa, Y. (eds), 1979, "The use of biological specimens for the assessment of human exposure to environmental pollutants", Nijhoff, The Hague, etc.

Berlin, A., Yodaiken, R.E. and Henman, B.A., 1984, "Assessment of toxic agents at the workplace", Nijhoff, The Hague, etc.

Buchet, J.P., Lauwerys, R. and Roels, H., 1981a, Comparison of the urinary excretion of arsenic metabolites after a single oral dose of sodium arsenate, monomethylarsonate or dimethylarsinate in man, Int. Arch. Occup. Environ. Health, 48: 71-79

Buchet, J.P., Lauwerys, R. and Roels, H., 1981b, Urinary excretion of inorganic arsenic and its metabolites after repeated ingestion of sodium metaarsenite by volunteers, Int. Arch. Occup. Environ. Health, 48: 111-118

Commission of the European Communities (CEC), 1977, Directive Biological assessment of exposure of the general public to lead, Council of Ministers, march 29

Commission of the European Communities (CEC), 1982, Directive Protection of workers occupationally exposed to metallic lead and its compounds, Council of Ministers, july 29

Commission of the European Communities (CEC), Alessio, L., Berlin, A., Roi, R. and Boni, M. (eds), 1983, "Human biological monitoring of industrial chemicals series", Office for official publications, Luxembourg

Coret, L., Hoek, C.van de, and Vroege, D., 1974, Carbonmonoxide problems in removing automobiles from carrierships (in Dutch), Tijdschr. Soc. Geneesk., 52: 427-431

Curphey, Th. J., Hood, L. P. L. and Perkins, M. M., 1965, Carboxy-haemoglobin levels in relation to air pollution, Arch. Environ. Health, 10: 179-185

Gehring, P.J., Watanabe, P.G. and Park, C.N., 1979, Risk of angio-sarcoma in workers exposed to vinylchloride as predicted from studies in rats, Toxicol. Appl. Pharmacol., 49: 15-21

Kalliomäki, K., Aittoniemi, K., Kalliomäki, P.L. and Moilanen, M., 1981, Measurement of lung-retained contaminants in vivo among workers exposed to metal aerosols. Am. Ind. Hyg. Assoc. J., 42: 234-238

Lauwerys, R.R., 1983a, In vivo tests to monitor body burdens of to-xic metals in man, in "Chemical toxicology and clinical che-mistry of metals", Proc. 2nd Conf. Montreal, Brow, S.S. and Savory, J. eds, Academic Press, London, 113-121

Lauwerys, R.R., 1983b, "Industrial chemical exposure. Guidelines for biological monitoring", Biomed. Publ., Davis, Calif.

Luepke, N-P. (ed), 1979, "Monitoring environmental materials and specimen banking", Nijhoff, The Hague

Monster, A., Regouin-Peeters, W., Schijndel, A.van and Tuin, J.van der, 1983, Biological monitoring of occupational exposure to tetrachloroethene, Scand. J. Work Environ. Health, 9: 273-281

Monster, A.C., 1984a, Biological monitoring of industrial solvents: trichloroethylene, in: Aitio et al, l.c., p.111-130

Monster, A.C., 1984b, Biological monitoring of exposure to 1,1,1-trichloroethane; paper presented at the American Chemical So-ciety Symposium on "Biological monitoring of organic chemicals", St.Louis, Mo, USA, April, 11+12, 1984; to be published in the Proceedings

Monster, A.C. and Smolders, J.F.J., 1984c, Tetrachloroethene in ex-haled air of persons living near pollution sources. Int. Arch. Occup. Environ. Health, 53: 331-336

Norén, H. and Vahter, M., 1981, A rapid method for the selective analysis of total urinary metabolites of inorganic arsenic, Scand. J. Work Environ.Health, 7: 38-44

Norin, K., 1983, Some aspects of the determination of organochlorine contaminants in human milk, Arch. Environ. Contam. Toxicol., 12: 277-283

Pellizari, E.D., Hartwell, T.D., Harris, B.S.H., Waddell, R.D., Whitaker, D.A. and Erickson, M.D., 1982, Purgeable organic compounds in mothers' milk. Bull. Environ. Contam. Toxicol., 28: 322-328

Sato, A., Nakajima, T., Fujiwara, Y. and Murayama, N., 1975, Kine-tic studies on sex difference in susceptibility to chronic benzene intoxication with special reference to body fat con-tent. Br. J. Ind. Med., 32: 321-328

Verberk, M.M. and Scheffers, T.M.L., 1980, Tetrachloroethene in ex-
    haled air of residents near drycleaning shops. Environ. Res.,
    21: 432-437
Zielhuis, R.L., 1974, Biological quality guide for inorganic lead,
    Int. Arch. Arbeitsmed. 32: 103-127
Zielhuis, R.L. and Wibowo, A.A.E., 1978, Periodic monitoring of
    lead workers (in Dutch), Tijdschr. Soc. Geneesk.,56: 678-681
Zielhuis, R.L., Castilho, P.del, Herber, R.F.M., Wibowo, A.A.E. and
    Sallé, H.J.A., 1979, Contaminations of lead and other metals
    in blood of two and three year old children living near a se-
    condary smelter, Int. Arch. Occup. Environ. Health, 42: 231-239
Zielhuis, R.L., 1983, Total risk assessment for heavy metals, in:
    Proceedings international conference heavy metals in the en-
    vironment, vol.I, CEP Consultants Ltd, Edinburgh, 27-32
Zielhuis, R.L., Wibowo, A.A.E., Herber, R.F.M. and Monster, A.C.,
    1984a,Rationale for interest or concern and considerations for
    specimen collection. Report to the WHO, contract E 15-372-5,
    to be published by WHO, Geneva
Zielhuis, R.L. and Wibowo, A.A.E., 1984b,Standard setting and metal
    speciation: arsenic, in: Niagru, J.O. (ed.) Changing metal cy-
    cles and human health, Dahlem Konferenzen, Life Sciences Re-
    search Report 28, Springer Verlag, Heidelberg etc., 323-344

THE RECOGNITION OF NEW KINDS OF OCCUPATIONAL TOXICITY*

John A.H. Lee, Thomas L. Vaughan, Paula H. Diehr
and Robin A. Haertle

SUMMARY

New and potentially toxic chemicals are constantly being
introduced into industry. New toxic effects occur, and it is not easy
to find them early. There is much evidence from epidemiologic studies
that low risks - a doubling or trebling of the incidence of a common
cancer - are common, and unrecognized.

Recognition is easier if the syndrome produced is unlike any of
the diseases that occur in the community, and may be delayed if it is
clinically indistinguishable from one of them. A system of health
surveillance that made an orderly comparison of the number and type of
sicknesses occurring with the expected numbers would, in large-scale
industry, have adequate statistical power to improve the detection of
episodes of toxicity to a useful extent.

INTRODUCTION

People on occasion do things for amusement that are risky.
Examples include scuba diving and hang gliding (Table 1-1). For
economic reasons, they may take jobs in industries that to this day

---

*From the Departments of Epidemiology and Biostatistics, School of
Public Health, University of Washington, Seattle WA 98195, U.S.A.
This study was partially funded by the U.S.Department of Energy
through sub-contract DE-AC07-761D01570 from EG&G (Idaho), Inc.
The views expressed are those of the authors, and do not necessarily
represent the views of the Department of Energy.

Table 1-1. Some comparative risks for work and leisure*

Annual British Occupational Fatality Rates		Risk of Death in Sporting Activities. Per Participant Year	
Construction Industries	1.5	Scuba Diving	2.0
Railway Staff	1.8	Glider Flying	4.0
Coal Miners	2.1	Power Boat Racing	8.0
Offshore Oil	16.0	Sport Parachuting	20.0

*Rates per 10,000. Adapted from (1).

pose real hazards. For example, the estimated prevalence of coal workers pneumoconiosis today is 4.5%, and some 4,000 deaths each year are attributed to legislatively defined "black lung disease" (2). Risks of this kind in mining, transport, and the construction industries are minimized to the best of everyone's ability, e.g., the black lung problem (3). But they persist.

Further, industry often uses materials that are highly toxic, but in processes that are normally safe. In these circumstances, constant watch has to be kept for breakdown in procedures, containment systems and the like. In spite of this, actual poisoning of workers by known and regulated toxic agents is not uncommon. Both the problems of unavoidable risks, and the prompt removal of accidental ones are the subject of much discussion and effort (e.g., 4-6). However serious they may be, these are known hazards, with know if difficult remedies. Workers may be hurt by unexpected effects of well-known toxins, or by the unpredicted effects of new chemicals to which they are among the first humans exposed. It is the purpose of this paper to examine the problems of new toxic agents, and to suggest what can practically be done.

Unfolding of a Toxin's Capabilities

The potential for damage that toxic agents possess is not revealed all at once. The slow recognition of the true range of effects of some well-known toxins provides a major source of knowledge of new hazards (Table 1-2). Part of this delay is simply a result of the latent period of some pathologic processes, notably cancer. Thus the recognition of radiation-induced skin cancer only 7 years after the discovery of the agent, does not suggest any delay in diagnosis. But it is puzzling that the mesotheliomas associated with asbestos had to be discovered by clinical observation in a mining community. It might have been supposed that the numerous cases of asbestosis under close medical observation for compensation purposes would have had an even higher attack rate, and would have been the group in which relationship of asbestos exposure to mesothelioma was recognized. Declining exposures are probably also likely to be important. Only if the concentration of carbon disulphide is low enough for the workers to avoid brain damage is it likely that the cardio-vascular effects will be recognized. Monitoring limited to the known specific effects of a toxin may not be enough. No industry using a known toxin can be confident that some new effect will not emerge.

New Agents That Are Unexpectedly Toxic

Part of the difficulty in promptly recognizing toxic effects of chemicals is the huge number of chemicals which already exist or are being newly introduced into today's society. In fact, over 4 million

Table 1-2   The Slow Definition of Toxic Capabilities

Toxic Agent	Component of Syndrome	Year of Recognition
Asbestos	Chronic Pulmonary Disease	1906
	Lung Cancer	1935
	Mesothelioma	1960
	Lymphoma	1980
Ionizing Radiation	Dermatitis	1896
	Cataract	1902
	Skin cancer	1902
	Lung Cancer	1935
	Leukemia	?1930's
	Multiple Myeloma	?now
Vinyl Chloride	"Liver Disease"	1949
	Acroosteolysis	1967
	Hepatic Angio-sarcoma	1974
Carbon Disulphide	Psychosis	19th century
	Peripheral Neuropathy	19th century
	Ischemic Heart Disease	1968

Sources: (asbestos, 7-10) (ionizing radiation, 11-15)
(vinyl chloride, 16) (carbon disulphide, 17)

Table 1-3 The Continuing Emergence of Occupational Toxicity

Condition	Agent	Year
Mesothelioma	Asbestos	1960
Nasopharyngeal carcinoma	Woodwork	1965
Lung Cancer	Chloromethyl Ether	1973
Hepatic Angio-sarcoma	Vinyl Chloride	1974
Peripheral Neuropathy	Methyl-butyl-Ketone	1974
Neuropathy	Chlordecone (Kepone)	1974
Endometrial Carcinoma	Estrogen	1975
Male Sterility	DBCP	1977
Melanoma	???	1981

Sources: (9, 27, 28, 25, 16, 29, 30, 31, 24, 32)

chemicals have now been registered by the American Chemical Society, and about 6,000 new ones are being identified every week (18). As many as 50,000 of these are believed to be in everyday use (19-22). Inclusion of pharmaceuticals, pesticides and food additives would add significantly to this total.

As industries change, new toxic chemicals come into use and are recognized as such by their effect on human beings. Table 1-3 gives a partial listing of such documented recent events. The timely recognition of new, and unanticipated, kinds of toxicity from chemicals to which workers are exposed is both necessary and difficult. As an administrator from the Standard Oil Company (Indiana) commented,

> Most preventive medicine programs function
> efficiently in discovering such cases for
> those conditions which we know enough to look
> for. We are utterly incapable, without the
> power of a computer system, to do necessary
> epidemiological studies and statistical
> analyses to discover new "high risk,"
> such as might occur from exposure to chemical,
> physical, and biological hazards.(23)

The next section of this document examines the problem of the recognition of occupational toxicity by agents thought to be harmless, and the performance of current methods.

Before a new kind of occupational toxicity can be recognized, the very idea has to be conceived that among a group of workers, something out of the ordinary is happening. Such an idea can come from outside the work environment - previous experience, animal studies, data from quite different human populations, from the surveillance of national or local data undertaken by governments, and so on. It can come, of course, from the perception that unusual disease exists among the workers, or that there is more than there should be of some common disease. Hypotheses derived from sources outside the health experience of the workers are discussed here first, followed by the clinical recognition of occupational disease.

Hypothesis Generation: Theory and Laboratory Studies

There is no good way of deciding in advance which chemicals will be toxic to human beings. Even when it is known that they are toxic for example, thalidomide, vinyl chloride monomer, or dibromo chloropropane - the reasons for the untoward activity of the particular molecular structures remains unknown. Animal studies are useful, but are done for only a small proportion of the new chemicals introduced into industry (see preceding section). Society is left with the observation of people being poisoned as its principal means of discovering what is poisonous.

Animal studies that can confirm and deepen epidemiologic insights (e.g., the production of liver tumors in rats by vinyl chloride monomer (33, 34) or the production of sterility in male rats by DBCP) have been very useful. A difficulty is that bacterial or animal testing is not directly relevant to human beings; species differences are large, and such differences have no consistent pattern. For one, chemical mice are more like men than cats; for another, the reverse. The cardiovascular toxicity of carbon disulphide is a rare example of the situation where recognition of a substantial occupational hazard depended on animal studies (35). For the foreseeable future, then, epidemiological studies must play a critical role in identifying human toxins and minimizing their impact on society. Much remains to-be done, however, before this role is successfully filled.

Clearly, the task of determining the relative safety of the chemicals in everyday use is a formidable one. Traditional approaches which can identify a chemical's potential for human toxicity include: a) examination of molecular structure for similarity with known carcinogens or teratogens, b) short-term bioassays to screen for mutagenicity or other DNA interactions, and c) animal exposure experiments. Unfortunately, few of the chemicals in everyday use have undergone even these limited screening tests--only about 150 new chemicals are adequately tested in animals and reported each year (36, 37). There is a contrast between attitudes to a new paint, adhesive or lubricant, and those to a new drug. People are expected to take the drug into their bodies, where it is designed to be biologically active. Animal testing is the rule for drugs. Industrial chemicals, even when their carcinogenicity is known, commonly continue to be used in industry without worker surveillance, or an attempt to build up knowledge of the human risk. Thus Karstadt and colleagues comment:

> We studied availability of epidemiologic data for chemicals designated by the IARC as animal carcinogens, but for which published human data were insufficient to permit a firm conclusion as to carcinogenicity, by conducting a survey of U.S. manufacturers, importers, and processors of the chemicals.
>
> We found that manufacturers-importers-processors had performed or contracted for completed epidemiologic studies of 8 of the 75 chemicals about which we inquired; 6 of the studies have been published and studies of 6 more chemicals were in progress at the time of our inquiry (fall 1980). A study of TRIS and ethylene dibromide was reported as going through peer review in fall 1980, and was therefore close to completion at that time. There were medical surveillance programs or reviews of worker health records for 13 chemicals. Allowing for duplication of chemicals in the three categories, 23 different chemicals were reported as being under some sort of formal or informal review. Thus, fewer than one-third of the 75 chemicals about which we inquired have been or are being subjected to study that was, is, or could become an epidemiologic study. (38)

Hypothesis Generation: Other Human Populations

Ideas derived from the experience of one population can be transferred to another. Table 2-1 gives some examples of the successful use of this approach. The transfer of the idea may be across national boundaries - for example, reciprocal transatlantic movement of the ideas for the studies of nasal cancer and bladder cancer, or between different sorts of exposure - for example, the search for leukemia among A-bomb victims after studies of radiologists.

Hypothesis Generation: National Health Surveillance

The occupation of the deceased is recorded on the death certificate, and in a number of populations deaths are systematically related by cause to occupation (e.g. U.S. 1950, England and Wales 1911 - 1970, etc.). These studies have been reviewed and their results consolidated (48) (49). There are problems with such analyses - the occupation on the death certificate may be a recent one, and not the source of the deceased's illness, and the population data is from the

312

Table 2-1. Excess Endemic Disease Found After Directed Research

Condition	Agent	Year	Relative Risk
Bladder Cancer	Beta-Naphthylamine	1954	5.5
Leukemia	Radiation	1957	about 10
Breast Cancer	Radiation	1965	about 5
Lung Cancer	Arsenic	1974	2.1
Nasal Cancer	Wood Dust	1977	4.4
Lymphocytic Leukemia	Benzene & Xylene	1983	4.5

Sources: (46, 40, 41, 39, 42, 43, 44, 45)

census, while the death data uses information provided by the survivors. Nevertheless, over the years, such studies have been immensely useful. They necessarily deal with broad occupational groups and large geographic areas, and their utility is primarily as background material for more focused studies or political discussion. However, they can on occasion pose entirely new hypotheses - for example, the current concern about an elevated risk of lung cancer in butchers (50).

The percentage distribution of deaths in a population by cause (Proportional Mortality Ratios, PMR) may usefully be examined if no information about the population at risk is available. PMR's by occupation have been made for the population of Washington State in the U.S. (51). A proportional analysis relies on the assumption that other causes of death remain equal in the population. In reality, a disease that has an ordinary incidence in a population group with a low death rate from other causes will have an elevated PMR, e.g., Hodgkin's disease in school teachers. Factors that cause several diseases (e.g., asbestos causing chronic pulmonary disease, lung cancer and mesothelioma) will produce less marked effects for each one because of the elevation of the number of deaths used for comparison.

Industry is often localized, and hence location can be used as a surrogate measure for occupation (53, 54). The occupational hazard has to be large enough to increase the death rate for the whole county to a measurable extent. Such hazards can be deliberately sought for. For example, the production of lung cancer by smelters (55), or by shipyards.

313

The Clinical Challenge

It is difficult to step from the presumption that nothing is wrong
to the idea that something might be amiss. The nature of the trouble
is unknown, as is what might be causing it. The problem, as it faces
the clinician, is determined by the relationship between the disease
produced by the toxin and the disease occurring naturally in the
community. If the occupational disease is outside the spectrum of
disease from that community, then the association of several similar
cases of unprecedented disease is the vital event in the recognition
that a problem exists. If the toxin produces extra cases of a
condition already common in the community, a quantitative judgement as
to the size and reality of this excess must be made. In the first
case, the expected number of cases can be taken as zero, and the
problem is to make the observation. In the second, the observation is
straightforward, but computation of the expected numbers is necessary.

The Recognition of Unusual Disease

Any medical practice cares for one or two people whose disorders
defy rational diagnosis. But the clinical findings in each one of
these individuals will be unique. There is no common link. In
contrast, occupational cases, although strange, are likely to be
rather similar. The person who has both full information about
the clinical features of sick people, and is informed by experience of
the ordinary diseases in the community, is obviously the physician.
The recognition of occupational toxicity that produces disease which
does not ordinarily occur depends on the watchfulness of the physician
taking care of the patients.

> The alert clinician remains the most important
> source of leads to occupational cancer. When groups
> of cases occur, particularly of rare tumors among
> relatively young persons, an occupational exposure
> should be suspected.(56)

> Virtually every known human carcinogen and teratogen
> has first been recognized by an alert clinician.(57)

Classic examples of the recognition of unusual disease as being of
toxic origin include the recognition by Sleggs of the link between
asbestos exposure and mesothelioma (9); by Hadfield of the link
between woodworking and nasal carcinoma (27). (Curiously, the
original reporters of an unusual disease may be very conservative -
Slegg collected 60 mesotheliomas, and Hadfield 25 nasal carcinomas,
before reporting). A physician may be suspicious enough to order
unusual laboratory tests for a particular patient. For example:

> On July 11,1975, an internist in Hopewell submitted a
> serum sample on a worker at the LSPC plant with severe

tremors to the Center for Disease Control (CDC)
Toxicology Laboratory for Kepone analysis. The result,
reported on July 19 and transmitted on July 21 to the
Virginia State Department of Health showed a highly
elevated serum Kepone level, 7.5 ppm. Follow-up field
investigations on July 2 and 23 by the Epidemiology
Bureau, revealed massive contamination of the plant site
and a high incidence of unusual illness in workers.(30)

In this example, the essential decision was to keep extra, if very
simple, records:

> In 1971, one of Dr. Creech's patients at the plant
> died with hepatic angiosarcoma, but the etiologic
> significance of the single case was of course, not
> recognized initially. Fortunately, as company physician,
> Dr.Creech received notification of deaths among plant
> employees. For his own interest, he listed the causes of
> mortality in a notebook. In 1973, he noticed a second
> and then a third case of angiosarcoma of the liver among
> the decedents.(58)

Sometimes the effects of a new agent are quite unlike anything that
has been seen before. New drugs particularly do this (e.g., 59). A
less extreme situation is found when a disease exists, but is known to
be rare. If three cases then appear in a small group of workers, as
occurred with the hepatic angio-sarcomas, this was enough for a major
national study to be launched (60). This formal study, in turn led to
substantial modifications of industrial practice. Eight cases of
vaginal adenocarcinoma in young women were collected in one oncologic
service. Seven of them had been treated at the Massachusetts General
Hospital between 1966 and 1969. This concentration of a very rare
tumor indicated clearly that something was amiss. Eventually, the
cause was run down to exposure to diethylstilbestrol in utero, but the
initial perception of the problem hinged on the physician's knowledge
of what to expect (61).

Recognition of Excess Endemic Disease

The recognition of a concentration of unusual disease is likely to
depend heavily on the physician's special knowledge and experience.
However, disease produced by an occupational toxin may be clinically
indistinguishable from cases due to other and non-occupational causes
in the community - bladder cancer; lung cancer; psychosis. The
recognition of an excess risk of a disease that is already rather
common in the community is a difficult clinical problem. It can be
done (e.g., the clinical recognition of an excess risk of bladder
cancer among workers preparing the dye fuchsin (62), of malignant
melanoma at Livermore (32), of lung cancer in workers exposed to
mustard gas (63). Such recognition of an excess of a common disease

does not draw on the physician's unique perspective, and management or workers sometimes make the initial observation. Thus, for example, Whorton, the discoverer of the reproductive effects of DBCP, comments:

> Had it not been for the alert and perceptive observation by the workers themselves, DBCP would still be produced without anyone's realizing it posesses this selective testicular toxicity; nor would the issue of adverse reproductive effect to males caused by workplace environmental contaminants be more than a theoretical possibility. Society owes a large debt to those few men in a California pesticide factory for their independent and courageous action (64).

A formal screening system was apparently responsible for the discovery of the carcinogenicity of chloro-methyl-ether (CME):

> In a chemical manufacturing plant with approximately 2000 employees periodic chest x-ray surveys were carried out for years. In 1962 management became aware that an excessive number of workers suspected of having lung cancer were being reported in one area of the plant, and turned to a chest consultant, who recommended a program to establish the degree of risk by semi-annual screening (28).

Thoughtful civil servants may also play a role. Thus,

> In 1974, the Workmen's Accident Compensation Section of the Tokyo Labour Standards Bureau asked one of the authors whether or not the lung cancer of a worker who had worked in a chemical plant was occupational, because there had been two previous deaths due to lung cancer in this plant...The size of the plant was small, with about 20 workers usually employed (65).

This led to studies that have implicated benzoyl trichloride as a human carcinogen (66).

To find such episodes, the judgement must be made that there is more of some disease in a particular community or group than would reasonably be expected. Examples are given in Table 2-2.

It should not be thought that all the high risks have already been discovered, or that if new ones emerge they are promptly recognized. Systematic study of the distribution by occupation of all the people in a community who develop a particular disease may demonstrate an undiscovered risk that is certainly above the threshold level for clinical detection. Thus, to take two examples from 1983, a ten-fold increase in risk of esophageal carcinoma was reported for workers vulcanizing rubber (67), and a twelve-fold rise in risk of bladder cancer in diesel truck drivers (68). The latter problem was probably missed because the workers were scattered among numerous

316

Table 2-2   Recognition of Excess Endemic Disease

Condition	Agent	Year	Relative Risk
Lung Cancer	Mustard Gas	1968	?10
Lung Cancer	Chloromethyl Ether	1973	8
Endometrial Carcinoma	Estrogen	1975	4.5
Male Sterility	DBCP	1977	*
Melanoma	???	1981	4

* No estimate was given by the authors. Although sterility is common, the extra risk was clearly very large.

Sources: (63, 28, 31, 24, 32)

places of employment. No single physician was providing primary care for a number of truck drivers sufficiently large to make the connection, and bladder cancer is treated in a sufficiently large number of hospitals for the necessary concentration to fail to occur at that level either. The difficulty is sufficiently great for the rather desperate comment to be made (with reference to the link between exposure to mustard gas and lung cancer) that "one of the rules of thumb in defining environmental agents as causes of cancer in man is to evaluate the effect of heavy exposures first, rather than studying lightly exposed persons" (69).

Thus, for an unexpected toxic hazard to be recognized, if it produces unusual disease, the victims must in some way be brought together (e.g., common workplace, common treatment center, shared nationality). If it produces further cases of a disease common in the community, not only must there be concentration, but apparently the community risk must be increased at least 4-fold by the exposure (Table 2-3). Episodes of toxicity that do not meet these modest requirements will not be found by traditional medical and administrative systems. This being so, how much increased but unrecognized hazard might there be?

Hypotheses and Their Need for Validation

Observations of particular people becoming sick lead to hypotheses that such an exposure is linked to a particular sickness. The modern flow of such hypotheses, good and not so good, is a direct effect of increasing sensitivity and sophistication of workers, management, the news media and the informed public. This is right and proper. However, there are difficulties. Hypotheses are expensive to validate. In the United States, the conduct of a well designed case-control study to test an hypothesis about the etiology of human disease costs in the region of $300,000 to $600,000. The loss of money, diversion of scientific manpower, and so on, involved in the testing of hypotheses that do not work out, is considerable.

Further, the time needed to marshall a group of scientific people who are willing to make the appropriate commitment of time, and to collect the funds to support the enterprise, is long. During this interval, the hypothesis is the best approximation that society has to the truth. It is indeed, up to that time, based on the best current data. If the hypothesis is not correct, during the interval required for the validation to be conducted the agency or company may suffer great political damage. The problem is becoming more severe as expectations of safety and longevity in the population rise. Further, for any risk low enough to be the subject of controversy, the public perception of it is likely to be seriously biased.

> People do not have accurate knowledge of the risks they face. As our society puts more and more effort into the regulation and control of these risks (banning cyclamates in food, lowering highway speed limits, paying for emergency coronary-care equipment, etc), it becomes increasingly important that these biases be recognized and, if possible, corrected. Improved public education is needed before we can expect the citizenry to make reasonable public-policy decisions about societal risks (70).

Along with faulty perceptions of risk, anxiety is a factor.

> The workers we interviewed were preoccupied with questions of control. They expressed a sense of powerlessness in the face of uncertainties about exposure and long-term effects on health. Contributing to their sense of impotence was the technical complexity of information about risk and their inability to use what information they received. Concern about control also reflected their lack of confidence in management efforts to minimize hazards. Many factory workers believed that production and profits were given priority over protection of health; many laboratory technicians felt that research was given priority over people (71).

Errors in Hypothesis Formation

Apart from propositions that are obviously sheer speculation, apparently well grounded hypotheses about the causation of disease may turn out to be wrong. The system used for collecting the data on which the hypothesis is based by may be defective. Thus, for example,

318

the postulated excess incidence of leukemia among radiation workers at
the Portsmouth Navy Yard was apparently due to a selective loss of
non-leukemia deaths from the original data collection (72, 73). A
pre-condition for the hypothesis that high fall-out from atmospheric
nuclear tests in Southern Utah was related to the high leukemia rate
among the children living there (74), was found, on measurement, not
to be valid (75). Further, the comparison group (Southern Utah
children before the tests), appears to have behaved anomalously (77).

Errors in Analysis

Sometimes the news media, even among a sophisticated population
such as that of Montreal, can create a perception among the public of
a problem, such as an increased risk of cancer, that has no basis is
reality (77). The suppression of such canards diverts scientific
resources from better things, and distracts attention from real
problems. On occasion, official data can produce a degree of
confusion. This apparently occurred in the U.S. in 1975 when the
unadjusted monthly numbers of deaths from cancer provided in the
Monthly Vital Statistics Report showed a sudden jump. The system was
designed to monitor abrupt changes in infectious disease, and
apparently created an illusion on this occasion. The official report
followed closely on the events (78), and a definitive report of the
whole affair does not seem to have been published.

Doll and Peto, discussing the problem of estimating the effects of
low level radiation, comment that:

> The much larger effects recently suggested by some
> investigators do not stand up to critical examination
> and derive chiefly from an analysis by inappropriate
> statistical methods of the data on the workers at the
> Hanford Nuclear plant. When these data are analysed
> according to standard efficient epidemiological methods
> (Darby and Reissland, 1981) [(79)], there is nothing in
> them to suggest that the estimates of total cancer risk
> made by the committee referred to above need to be revised.

Other Failures of Hypotheses

The translation of an hypothesis from the mode in which it was
developed to a different one seems to be a particularly rigorous test.
Apparently unsuccessful hypotheses derived from animal studies or
quite different sorts of human toxicity include fluoride and its lack
of effect on human cancer rates (81, 82, 86,), and the absence of
carcinogenic effect of asbestos derived from taconite (83, 84).

Sometimes large studies with several data sources can also provide
results which subsequent studies do not validate. Not just clinical
reports, but serious epidemiology may not stand up to testing (e.g.
87, 88, 89). There is thus a continuing need to test and validate

hypotheses about the human toxicity of industrial materials. Such
testing must use data sets that are independent of each other, and be
done in as many and various circumstances as feasible.

THE PREVALENCE OF UNDETECTED HAZARD

The frequency with which new kinds of occupational toxicity are
discovered, and the low sensitivity of current methods for their
detection suggest that there are likely to be a number of occupations
where a substantial but undetected hazard exists. Such a hazard could
be spread rather evenly across groups of workers, with none of those
exceeding a four-fold increase in rise for some condition.
Alternatively, and more commonly, if an agent is not thought to be
toxic, there is no reason to separate the workers exposed to it for
special study. Thus, vinyl chloride and benzoyl chloride are
harmless-looking molecules that have been used for a long time. In
such a situation, if the proportion of workers exposed was small, the
increased disease rate in the total population could well be below the
threshold of clinical recognition. A further illustration is given
in Table 3-1. A population was exposed to both cigarette smoking and
arsenic trioxide, and experienced a three-fold increase in lung
cancer. This was not, in fact, noticed clinically. When the
situation was dissected in the light of knowledge of the effects of
cigarettes and arsenic on the human bronchial epithelium, the very
serious risks for some groups were revealed.

Occupational situations that increase the risk of common disease
by a factor of two or three can in fact be detected if a formal
epidemiologic analysis is done using a substantial number of
observations. For example, an increased risk of lung cancer among
welders has now been reported from studies of death certificates in
the U.S., Britain, and Canada (90). Ad hoc studies directed towards
the clarification of the etiology of a particular disease commonly do

Table 3-1. Relative Risks of Lung Cancer by Arsenic Trioxide
Exposure and Cigarette Smoking

Arsenic Category	Low	Medium	High	Very High	Total Group
Smoker	1.2	3.1	3.6	8.0	)
					) 3.1
Non-Smoker	1.0	0.9	2.9	6.2	)

Source: (92)
(The point can be illustrated from numerous studies, e.g., (93).)

this. Thus case-control studies of the occupational distribution of all the bladder cancers reported from a particular population may reveal that there was an excess of some jobs in the case group, indicating an increased risk. Similarly, if workers are observed for a long time, risks may be identified through the higher mortality of groups with particular exposures. Table 3-2 gives examples of hazards identified by these means.

The examples of the detection of previously unrecorded occupational hazards are all from the 1980's, and were collected by a brief and unsystematic search of the literature. It is clear that such occasions are common, but in the absence of data on the number of studies in total and of the number that gave no indication of occupational hazard, no estimate can be made of their prevalence. However, the number of positive findings is sufficiently large to suggest that many workers are unwittingly exposed to danger. Dubrow and Wegman (49), following an examination of a wide range of occupational studies concluded that after the effects of asbestos, the second priority should be research into the consistent excess of lung cancer found in motor vehicle drivers. The particular perspective of those taking care of patients gives them little opportunity for recognizing this type of relationship - an increase in a disease that is already common.

The epidemiologic methodology is neutral, and can on occasion provide evidence that a chemical under suspicion is really harmless to exposed workers - for example trichlorethylene (96, 97). Negative findings may be of great importance - for example, the demonstration that whatever the origin of the excess melanoma incidence at Livermore, it does not operate at the very similar facility of Los Alamos (98). This obviously narrows the search for the agent.

Contribution to Total Occupational Cancer

At the present time, there is an active debate about the numbers of cancers in human population resulting from occupational exposure, and their ratio to the total cancer incidence. The estimates that are at the low end of the range rely on excess risks reported from traditional methodologies (80, 112). Low level and currently unrecognized hazards may make an important contribution to the actual level of occupationally caused morbidity.

SOME STOCHASTIC ASPECTS OF OCCUPATIONAL SURVEILLANCE

In the ordinary course of medical practice considerable information is gathered and recorded about the illnesses of workers. If this information were systematically analyzed, and used to compare the experience of different groups in relation to the numbers exposed to different chemical agents, there is good reason to hope that human toxicity could be recognized more quickly than it is at present. Such

Table 3-2   Clinically Undetectable Increased Risks of Endemic Disease
            Found by Recent Epidemiologic Study*

Disease	Occupation	Relative Risk	Year
Cancers			
Nasal	Exposure to Lacquers & Paints	Large**	1983
Lung	Sugar Cane Farmers	2.4	1981
	Diesel Railroad Workers	1.4	1983
	Tin Miners	2.0	1981
	Painters	2.0	1983
Stomach	Coal Miners Who Smoke Cigarettes	3.1	1983
	Rubber Workers	1.8	1982
Large Bowel	Spectacle Lens Makers	3.2	1982
Digestive System	Benzotrichloride	4.0***	1983
Brain	Petro-Chemical Workers	2.1	1983
	Pesticide Applicators	2.0	1983
Testis	Farming	6.3	1984
Melanoma	Petro-Chemical Workers	2.2	1981
Lymphocytic Leukemia	Rubber Workers Exposed To Xylene	5.5	1983
Others			
Ischemic Heart Disease	Rubber Workers Exposed To Ethanol Or Phenol	1.8	1983

* Sources: (nasal, 99) (lung, 100, 103, 101) (stomach, 102, 104)
          (colon, 105) (digestive system, 66) (brain, 106, 107)
          (testis, 108, 109) (lymphocytic leukemia, 45) (IHD, 110)

** 12 observed against less than 1 expected
*** 5 cases observed against 1.24 expected - unlikely to be due to
chance, but too few for further subdivision.

a system would have to cover the complete population at risk, do this continuously, and have its data systematically analyzed by efficient statistical methods. Its task would be to identify increases in risk in the occupation above that reasonably to be expected at the time and place. The general need for surveillance systems, and their nature and formal structure has been discussed on a number of occasions, for example by Langmuir (113), Doll (114), Langmuir (115), Muir et al. (116), and Higginson (117).

Traditional surveillance systems deal with the experience of large, geographically defined populations. They deal with large numbers and long periods of time. The simple visual analysis of trends of adjusted rates that has sufficed to guide public policy for a hundred years (e.g., 118) is only now beginning to give way to methods that make better use of the data (for example, in influenza surveillance (119); and, as a beginning, in chronic disease (120, 121)).

Health Surveillance in Small Populations

Industrial problems can only be studied crudely in large populations – the death rate for carpenters is an aggregate of the experience of people doing the most diverse jobs and exposed to the widest array of toxins, occupational information given on a census form and on a death certificate may be very different, and so on. For both reliable data and sufficient detail, studies must be at the level of the company or individual plant. Further, a new toxic agent is likely to be introduced in a small number of firms at first. The only way to find its effects is to look at the individual work places. Both these factors ensure that any occupational study dealing with toxic agents that do not affect large numbers of workers in a gross and obvious way, must have their effects studied in small numbers of exposed subjects. Although the risk may be high, the numbers of cases must be small. The problem is illustrated by the following examples.

In 1976 two cases of choroidal melanoma were identified in the work force at a chemical plant in Belle, West Virginia. The disease is not common, and the population of workers was not large. Although the event could have occurred by chance, the hypothesis was thought sufficiently important that a substantial study, involving ophthalmologists, occupational hygienists, and a statistician, was mounted. A considerable degree of validation of the hypothesis was obtained when a third case treated elsewhere was identified in 1977, a further case was found in the company records, and a new case in occurred in 1978. The hypothesis of the generation of eye melanomas by something in this particular plant has thus been supported by the implied prediction that more would be found. The link is, of course, not absolute. Eye melanoma is an unpredictable disease that can remain undiagnosed for a long time. It is just possible that a similar intensity of investigation could uncover, under any circumstances, this number of cases previously unrelated to a work place (122, 123, 124).

Table 4-1 Observed and Expected* Numbers of Cases of Malignant
Melanoma of the Skin, Lawrence Livermore National Laboratory,
1967-1981.

Yr	´67	´68	´69	´70	´71	´72	´73	´74	´75	´76	´77	´78	´79	´80	´81	Total
OE	0	1	1	1	1	3	0	4	4	2	6	1	3	7	3	37
Ex																12.09

* On the basis of the melanoma rates for Alameda County (in which the
Laboratory is situated), adjusted for age, sex, and census tract of
residence of workers at the laboratory. Austin et al. (32), and
personal communication from Dan Moore, Ph.D.

There has been a major effort to establish whether the low
exposure to external radiation, and the unknown internal radiation,
was responsible for any ill effects in participants at the United
States´ atmospheric nuclear tests in the 1950´s (125, 126). The
statistically significant excess of leukemia was based on 10 cases,
compared with 4 expected.

Lack of numbers of cases has also made it difficult for the
investigators at Livermore to disentangle the causative agent,
particularly when it is considered that about one third of the cases
are not associated with occupational exposure (Table 4-1). Another
problem that has not yet been resolved, primarily due to lack of
numbers, is the relationship of the phenoxy herbicides to Hodgkin´s
disease (127).

Some Estimates of Power

Hence, as well as being concerned for the accuracy and
completeness of the data collected, an adequate health surveillance
system must be designed with attention to the statistical power that
is attainable with the numbers. If it is not going to be feasible to
detect smaller episodes than those that are currently recognized by
people in industry, there is no point doing anything more. There is
an extensive literature on the power of statistical tests, and some
studies on their use in surveillance systems. However, we have been
able to find little on the problem facing industry - surveillance
where a novel toxin can cause any one of a wide range of conditions.

To examine the point in a realistic way, we have calculated the
power of a health surveillance system to find various increased risks
in a plant with a population of employees of the same size and age and

sex composition as that at the Lawrence Livermore National Laboratory, and situated in a geographic area where the population experienced the same cancer rates as Alameda County. We have chosen to examine the position for malignant melanoma of the skin, and for lung cancer. These diseases, along with many others, would be on the list of diagnoses to be regularly and automatically scanned by the computer for deviations between the observed and the expected. The melanomas are of importance because we have evidence from Livermore of how the physicians, acting in a traditional way, were able to perform a surveillance role. Lung cancer has been chosen because of its high

Table 4-2. Numbers of employees by age and sex, incidence rate for malignant melanoma of skin and for lung cancer in the local population, and expected numbers of cases in the employee population. Hypothetical model

Age	Number of Employees	Incidence Rate of Melanoma*	Expected Number of Cases of Melanoma	Incidence Rate of Lung Cancer*	Expected Number of Cases of Lung Cancer
Males					
20-	702	5.2	0.036	0.45	0.00316
30-	1,277	11.0	0.140	6.35	0.08109
40-	1,416	17.0	0.240	47.40	0.67118
50-	1,157	17.0	0.200	143.40	1.65914
60-65	214	21.0	0.045	300.20	0.64240
Total	4,766		0.661		3.05697
Females					
20-	340	9.8	0.033	0.65	0.00221
30-	279	14.0	0.039	5.20	0.01450
40-	223	17.0	0.038	29.50	0.06579
50-	162	15.0	0.029	80.55	0.13049
60-65	30	19.0	0.006	124.70	0.03741
Total	1,034		0.145		0.25040
Total Persons	5,800		0.806		3.30611

*per 100,000

325

Table 4-3   Statistical Power by Length of Observation, Using Relative Risk (RR) or Excess Cases as the Criterion

Length of Observation	One Year				Five Years			
Disease	Melanoma		Lung Ca.		Melanoma		Lung Ca.	
Criterion	RR	Excess Cases	RR	Excess Cases	RR	Excess Cases*	RR	Excess Cases*
Power (%)								
50	5.5	4	2.5	5	2.5	1.3	1.6	2.0
80	9.8	8	3.8	9	3.5	2.2	2.0	3.3
90	12.6	10	4.6	12	4.1	2.7	2.2	4.0

* mean excess cases per year over the five year period.

incidence, and because a large number of chemical agents can produce it in people. The calculation of the expected numbers of melanomas and lung cancers to be newly diagnosed each year in the employee population is given in Table 4-2.

Increased risk may express itself multiplicatively, summarized by a relative risk greater than one, or additively, summarized by a risk difference greater than zero. Let the baseline probability of a disease (say melanoma) be p, and an occupational risk factor has raised this risk to Kp + G, where K is a number greater than or equal to 1, and G is a number between 0 and 1-p. K is the relative risk when G=0. G is the risk difference when K=1. We have available for surveillance a group of "N" employees at the target facility, 5,800 in the model. For comparison there are plants with "T*N " employees. The simplest comparison between two plants would calculate the proportion of people in each plant for a given year having a melanoma diagnosed, and comparing these two with a simple chi-square test. This, of course, assumes that the two plants were comparable for factors associated with the disease. Using a one-tailed test, and assuming normality, the power of this test is approximately the probability that a normal random variate will have a value higher than

$$Z= 1.645 - [(K-1)*p + G]*N**.5/[p*(K+1/T) +G]**.5$$

The probability of a value higher than Z, is the probability of rejecting the null hypothesis, or the power of the test in the situation described by the parameters N, p, K, D, G and T. The rest of this discussion describes power as a function of these parameters.

The results are summarized in Table 4-2. For a disease as common as lung cancer, comparing a plant of the given size of 5,800 workers with one similar one, and with a year of observation, a surveillance system would have an 80% chance of finding a relative risk of 3.8, that produced 9 cases extra to the 3 expected. This is an increased risk smaller than that usually found in cigarette smokers, and probably not detectable clinically. For a less common disease, such as melanoma, the power is less - one year's observations would require a 9.8-fold increase in risk to be detectable with 80% certainty.

The power of a surveillance system is sensitive to the number of cases, and if it is set up to examine rolling time periods longer than a year, its power increases greatly. For melanoma, with five years of data, a relative risk increased to 3.5 and producing 2.2 extra cases a year on average, would have been detected with 80% certainty by the system. Thus the purely mechanical operations of a surveillance system would do about as well as the actual physicians at Livermore. The medical department there was well staffed and operating under favorable conditions - close supervision of workers exposed to known toxic agents, stability of the work force, concentration of the work for the most part within a limited area. Many workers in large organizations are less well situated.

There are situations where the clinical approach offers almost no hope for the detection of a problem - for example, the exposure of workers in a single plant to a toxin so mild that it merely doubles their death rate from lung cancer. The surveillance system would only have a 29% chance of finding such a doubled rate with one year's experience. However, this chance would steadily rise, to reach 80% in 6 years. This is too long, but it is better than never recognizing the problem, which is likely without such a system. Further analyses confirmed that the power of the system increased slowly with increase in the size of the comparison population, but movement in this direction must produce problems of comparability. The higher the real relative risk, the greater the power of the system.

These preliminary studies thus suggest that a surveillance system could detect increased risks of plausible size in employee populations with a high degree of reliability. In recognizing increased risks of diseases with a substantial background level of incidence in the community, which is the area of greatest clinical difficulty, a well-designed health surveillance system provided with good diagnoses should be able to perform about as well as the physicians in most circumstances. It is possible to envisage situations where it could do a great deal better.

References

1. Pochin E. Risk and medical ethics. J Medical Ethics 1982;8: 180-84.

2. Anonymous. Leading work-related diseases and injuries - United States. (Center for Disease Control). MMWR 1983;32:24-32.

3. Attfield MD. Pneumoconiosis in coal miners: NIOSH research and surveillance. MMWR 1983;32:39SS-42SS.

4. Decoufle P, Blattner WA, Blair A. Mortality among chemical workers exposed to benzene and other agents. Environ Res 1983; 30:16-25.

5. Tsai SP, Wen CP, Weiss NS. Retrospective mortality and medical surveillance studies of workers in benzene areas of refineries. J Occup Med 1983;25(9):685-692.

6. Cherry N, Waldron HA. The prevalence of psychiatric morbidity in solvent workers in Britain. Int J Epi 1984;13(2):197-200.

7. Cooke WE. Pulmonary asbestosis. Br Med J 1927;II:1024-27.

8. Lynch KM, Smith WA. Pulmonary asbestosis III: carcinoma of lung in asbesto-silicosis. Am J Cancer 1935;24:56-64.

9. Wagner JC, Sleggs CA, Marchand P. Diffuse pleural mesothelioma and asbestos exposure in the north western Cape Province. Br J Ind Med 1960;17:260-71.

10. Ross R, Nichols P, Wright W, Lukes R, Dworsky R, et al. Asbestos exposure and lymphomas of the gastrointestinal tract and oral cavity. Lancet 1982;ii:1118-19.

11. Grubbe EH. The first X-ray burn. In: Grubbe EH (ed), X-Ray Treatment - Its Origin, Birth and Early History. Minneapolis: The Bruce Publishing Company, 1949, pp. 43-44.

12. Clapp CA. The pathogenesis of cataract. In: Clapp CA (ed.) Cataract its Etiology and Treatment. Philadelphia: Lea & Feibeger, 1934, pp. 68-85.

13. Frieben. Cancroid des rechten handruckens. Forschr Geb Rontgenstr 1902;6:106.

14. Lange K. Krebserkrankungen und geologische verhaltnisse im Erzgebirge. Ztschr f Krebsforsch 1935;42:306-10.

15. Lorenz E. Radioactivity and lung cancer; a critical review of lung cancer in the miners of Schneeberg and Joachimsthal. J Natl Cancer Inst 1944;5:1-15.

16. Creech Jr JL, Johnson MN. Angiosarcoma of liver in the manufacture of polyvinyl chloride. J Occup Med 1974;16:150-51.

17. Fielder RJ, Shillaker RO. Toxicity review 3 – carbon disulphide. London: Health and Safety Executive, 1981.

18. Chemical Abstract Services Registry passes 4-million mark; uses grow. CAS rep 1978;7:2.

19. Fishbein L. Potential Industrial Carcinogens and Mutagens, Publ. 560/5-77-005. U.S. EPA, Wa. D.C. 1977.

20. Maugh TH. Chemicals: How many are there? Science 1978;199:162.

21. Davis DL, Magee BH. Cancer and industrial chemical production. Science 1979;206:1356-1358.

22. Davis DL, Bridbord K, Schneiderman M. Cancer prevention: Assessing causes, exposures, and recent trends in mortality for U.S. males 1968-1978. Teratogenesis, Carcinogenesis, and Mutagenesis 1982;2:105-135.

23. Kerr PS. Recording occupational health data for future analysis. J Occup Med 1978;20(3):197-203.

24. Whorton D, Krauss RM, Marshall S, Milby TH. Infertility in male pesticide workers. Lancet 1977;ii:1259-61.

25. Weiss W. Chloromethyl ethers, cigarettes, cough and cancer. J Occup Med 1976;18:194-99.

26. Keogh JP, Pestronk A, Wertheimer D, Moreland R. An epidemic of urinary retention caused by dimethylaminopropionitrile. JAMA 1980;243:746-49.

27. MacBeth R. Malignant disease of the paranasal sinuses. J Laryngol 1965;79:592-612.

28. Figueroa WG, Raszkowshi R, Weiss W. Lung cancer in chloromethyl methyl ether workers. N Engl J Med 1973;288:1096-97.

29. Billmaier D, Yee HT, Allen N, Craft B, Williams N, et al. Peripheral neuropathy in a coated fabrics plant. J Occup Med 1974;16:665-71.

30. Cannon SB, Vaezey Jr JM, Jackson RS, Burse VW, Straub WE, et al. Epidemic Kepone poisoning in chemical workers. Am J Epidemiol 1978;107:529-37.

31. Smith DC, Prentice R, Thompson DJ, Herrmann WL. Association of exogenous estrogen and endometrial carcinoma. N Engl J Med 1975; 293:1164-67.

32. Austin DF, Snyder MA, Reynolds PJ, Biggs MW, Stubbs HA. Malignant melanoma among employees of Lawrence Livermore National Laboratory. Lancet 1981;712-16.

33. Viola PL, Bigotti A, Caputo A. Oncogenic response of rat skin, lungs, and bones to vinyl chloride. Cancer Research 1971;31:516-519.

34. Maltoni C, Lefemine G. Carcinogenicity bioassays of vinyl chloride 1. Research plan and early results. Env Research 1974; 7:387-405.

35. Tiller JR, Schilling RSF, Morris JN. Occupational toxic factor in mortality from coronary heart disease. Br Med J 1968;4: 407-11.

36. Ames B. Identifying environmental chemicals causing mutations and cancer. Science 1979;204:587-593.

37. International Agency for Research on Cancer (IARC) 1982. IARC monographs on the evaluation of the carcinogenic risk of chemicals to humans. IARC Monographs 1-29 and Suppl. 4.

38. Karstadt M, Bobal R, Selikoff IJ. A survey of the availability of epidemiologic data on humans exposed to animal carcinogens. In Quantification of Occupation Cancer (eds. Peto and Schneiderman) Banbury Report #9, Cold Spring Harbor Laboratory, 1981.

39. Mackenzie I. Breast cancer following multiple fluoroscopies. Brit J Cancer 1965;XIX(i):1-8.

40. Folley JH, Borges W, Yamawaki T. Incidence of leukemia in survivors of the atomic bomb in Hiroshima and Nagasaki, Japan. Am J Med 1952;13[?]:311-321.

41. Lewis EB. Leukemia and ionizing radiation. Science 1957;125: 965-72.

42. Milham S, Strong T. Human arsenic exposure in relation to a copper smelter. Environ Research 1974;7:176-182.

43. Kuratsune M, Tokudome S, Shirakusa T. Occupational lung cancer among copper smelters. Int J Cancer 1974;13:552-558.

44. Brinton JA, Blot WJ, Stone BJ, Fraumeni Jr JF. A death certificate analysis of nasal cancer among furniture workers in North Carolina. Cancer Res 1977;37:3473-74.

45. Arp EW, Wolf PH, Checkoway H. Lymphocytic leukemia and exposures to benzene and other solvents in the rubber industry. J Occup Med 1983;25(8):598-602.

46. Case RAM, Hosker ME. Tumour of the urinary bladder as an occupational disease in the rubber industry in England and Wales. Br J Prev Soc Med 1954;8:39-50.

47. Luboinski B, Marandas P. Cancer de l'ethmoide: etiologie professionnelle. Arch des Maladies Professionnelles, de Medicine du Travail et de Securite Sociale (Paris) 1975;36:477-87.

48. Siemiatycki J, Day NE, Fabry J, Cooper JA. Discovering carcinogens in the occupational environment: A novel epidemiologic approach. J Natl Cancer Inst 1981;66:217-25.

49. Dubrow R, Wegman DH. Setting priorities for occupational cancer research and control: Synthesis of the results of occupational disease surveillance studies. J Nat Cancer Inst 1983;71(6):1123-1142.

50. Lynge E, Andersen O, Kristensen TS. Lung cancer in Danish butchers. Lancet 1983;??[March]:527-528.

51. Milham SJ. Occupational mortality in Washington state 1950-1979. U.S. Dept. of Health and Human Services, National Institute for Occupational Safety and Health, Division of Surveillance, Hazard Evaluations and Field Studies, Cincinnati, Ohio, October 1983.

52. Menck HR, Henderson BE. Occupational differences in rates of lung cancer. J Occup Med 1976;18:797-801.

53. Mason TJ. Geographic patterns of cancer risk: a means for identifying possible occupational factors. Ann NY Acad Sci 1976; 271:370-76.

54. Stone BJ, Blot WJ, Fraumeni Jr JF. Geographic patterns of industry in the United States. An aid to the study of occupational disease. J Occup Med 1978;20:472-77.

55. Blot WJ, Fraumeni Jr JF. Arsenical air pollution and lung cancer. Lancet 1975;ii:142-44.

56. Cole P. Cancer and occupation: status and needs of epidemiologic research. Cancer 1977;39:1788-91.

57. Miller RW. Areawide chemical contamination. Lessons from case histories. JAMA 1981;245:1548-51.

58. Li FP. Clinical studies of cancer etiology. Cancer 1977;40:445-47.

59. Wright P. Untoward effects associated with practolol administration: Oculomucocutaneous syndrome. Br Med J 1975; (March 15):595-598.

60. Falk H. Epidemiological studies of vinyl chloride health effects in the United States. Proceedings of Royal Soc Med 1976;69(4): 303-306.

61. Herbst AL, Scully RE, Robboy SJ. Prenatal diethylstilbestrol exposure and human genital tract abnormalities. Natl Cancer Inst Monogr 1979;51:25-35.

62. Rehn L. Blasengeschwulste bei Fuchsin-Arbeitern. Arch Klin Chir 1895;50:588-600.

63. Wada S, Nishimoto Y, Miyanishi M, Kambe S. Mustard gas as a cause of respiratory neoplasia in man. Lancet 1968;I:1161-63.

64. Whorton MD. Dibromochloropropane health effects. In: Rom WN, (ed.), Environmental and Occupational Medicine. Boston: Little, Brown and Co., 1983, pp.573-77.

65. Sakabe H, Matsushita H, Koshi S. Cancer among benzoyl chloride manufacturing workers. Occupational Carcinogenesis. Annals of the New York Academy of Sciences 1976;271:67-70.

66. Sorahan T, Waterhouse JAH. A mortality study of workers in a factory manufacturing chlorinated toluenes. Ann Occup Hyg 1983; 27:173-82.

67. Norell S, Ahlbom A, Lipping H, Osterblom L. Oesophageal cancer and vulcanisation work. Lancet 1983;I:462-63.

68. Silverman DT, Hoover RN, Albert S, Graff KM. Occupation and cancer of the lower urinary tract in Detroit. J Natl Cancer Inst 1983;70:237-45.

69. Miller RW. The alert practitioner as a cancer etiologist. Cancer Bull 19??;29(6):183-185.

70. Lichtenstein S, Slovic P, Fischhoff B, Layman M, Combs B. Judged frequency of lethal events. J Exper Psychol Hum Learn Mem 1978; 4:551-78.

71. Nelkin D. Workers at risk. Science 1983;222(4620):?.

72. Najarian T, Colton T. Mortality from leukaemia and cancer in shipyard nuclear workers. Lancet 1978;i:1018-20.

73. Rinsky RA, Zumwalde RD, Waxweiler RJ, Murray WE, et al. Cancer mortality at a naval nuclear shipyard. Lancet 1981;i:231-36.

74. Lyon JL, Melville R, Klauber R, Gardner JW, Udall KS. Childhood leukemias associated with fallout from nuclear testing. New Engl J Med 1979;300:397-402.

75. Beck HL, Krey PW. Radiation exposures in Utah from Nevada nuclear tests. Science 1983;220:18-24.

76. Land CE, McKay FW, Machado SG. Childhood leukemia and fallout from the Nevada nuclear tests. Sci 1984;223:139-144.

77. Spitzer WO, Shenker SC, Hill GB. Cancer in a Montreal suburb: the investigation of a nonepidemic. Can Med Assoc J 1982;127:971-74.

78. Chiazze L, Silverman DT, Levin DL. The cancer mortality scare. JAMA 1976;236:2310-12.

79. Darby SC, Reissland JA. Low levels of ionizing radiation and cancer - are we underestimating the risk? J R Statistical Soc 1981;(Part 3):298-331.

80. Doll R, Peto R. The Causes of Cancer. Oxford: Oxford Univ. Press, 1981, p. 1245.

81. Taves DR. Fluoridation and cancer mortality. Origins of Human Cancer, Book A: Incidence of Cancer in Humans (eds. Hiatt, Watson, Winsten), (Cold Spring Harbor Conferences on Cell Proliferation, Vol. 4), Cold Spring Harbor Laboratory, 1977, pp.357-366.

82. Hoover RN. Fluoridated drinking water and the occurrence of cancer. J Natl Cancer Inst 1976;57(4):757-768.

83. Levy BS, Sigurdson E, Mandel J, Laudon E, Pearson J. Investigating possible effects of asbestos in city water: Surveillance of gastrointestinal cancer incidence in Duluth, Minnesota. Am J Epidemiol 1976;103:362-68.

84. Higgins IT. Mortality of reserve mining company employees in relation to taconite dust exposure. Amer J Epidemiol 1983; 118(5):710-719.

85. Doll R, Vessey MP, Beasler RWR, Buckley AR, Fear EC, et al. Mortality of gasworkers – final report of a prospective study. Br J Ind Med 1972;29:394-406.

86. Erickson JD. Mortality in selected cities with fluoridated and non-fluoridated water supplies. N Engl J Med 1978;298:1112-16.

87. Chilvers C. Cancer mortality by site and fluoridation of water supplies. J Epidemiol Comm Health 1982;36:237-42.

88. LaBarthe DR. Methodologic variation in case-control studies of reserpine and breast cancer. J Chron Dis 1979;32:95-104.

89. Winn DM, Blot WJ, Shy CM, Pickle LW, Toledo A, Fraumeni Jr JF. Snuff dipping and oral cancer among women in the Southern United States. N Engl J Med 1981;304:745-49.

90. Gallagher RP, Threlfall WJ. Cancer mortality in metal workers. Can Med Assoc J 1983;129:1191-1194.

91. Land CE, Boice JD, Shore RE. Breast cancer risk from low-dose exposures to ionizing radiation: Results of parallel analysis of three exposed populations of women. J Natl Cancer Inst 1980;65: 353-376.

92. Welch K, Higgins I, Oh M, Burchfiel C. Arsenic exposure, smoking, and respiratory cancer in copper smelter workers. Arch Environ Health 1982;37:325-335.

93. Liddell FDK, McDonald JC, Thomas DC. Methods of cohort analysis: appraisal by application to asbestos mining. J R Statist Soc A 1977;140(4):469-491.

94. Anonymous. Incidence of liver cancer and trichloroethylene manufacture: joint study by industry and a cancer registry. Br Med J 1983;286:846.

95. Schneiderman MA, Decoufle P, Brown CC. Thresholds for environmental cancer: biologic and statistical considerations. Ann NY Acad Science 1979;329:92-130.

96. Axelson O, Andersson K, Hogstedt C. A cohort study on trichloroethylene exposure and cancer mortality. J Occup Med 1978;20(3):194-196.

97. Paddle GM. A strategy for the identification of carcinogens in a large, complex chemical company. In: Peto R, Schneiderman M (eds) Banbury Report 9 – Quantification of Occupational Cancer. Cold Spring Harbor: Cold Spring Harbor Laboratory 1982, pp. 177-189.

98. Acquavella JF, Wilkinson GS, Tietjen GL. A melanoma case-control study at the Los Alamos National Laboratory. Health Physics 1983; 45(3):587-592.

99. Hernberg S, Collan Y, Degerth R. Nasal cancer and occupational exposures. Scand J Work Environ Health 1983;9:208-213.

100. Rothschild H, Mulvey JJ. An increased risk for lung cancer mortality associated with sugarcane farming. J Natl Cancer Inst 1982;68:755-60.

101. Howe GR, Fraser D, Lindsay J, Presnal B, Yu SZ. Cancer mortality (1965-77) in relation to diesel fume and coal exposure in a cohort of retired railway workers. J Natl Cancer Inst 1983;70: 1015-19.

102. Ames RG. Gastric cancer and coal mine dust exposure. A case-control study. Cancer 1983;52:1346-50.

103. Whorton MD, Schulman J, Larson SR. Feasibility of identifying high-risk occupations through tumor registries. J Occup Med 1983;25(9):657-660.

104. Parkes HG, Veys CA, Waterhouse JAH, Peters A. Cancer mortality in the British rubber industry. Br J Ind Med 1982;39:209-20.

105. Wang J-D, Wegman DH, Smith TJ. Cancer risks in the optical manufacturing industry. Br J Ind Med 1983;40:177-81.

106. Waxweiler RJ, Alexander V, Leffingwell SS, Haring M, Lloyd JW. Mortality from brain tumor and other causes in a cohort of petrochemical workers. J Natl Cancer Inst 1983;70:75.

107. Blair A, Grauman DJ, Lubin JH, Fraumeni Jr JF. Lung cancer and other causes of death among licensed pesticide applicators. J Natl Cancer Inst 1983;71:31-37.

108. Mills PK, Newell GR, Johnson DE. Testicular cancer associated with employment in agriculture and oil and natural gas extraction. Lancet 1984;1:207-210

109. Rushton L, Alderson MR. An epidemiological survey of eight oil refineries in Britain. Br J Ind Med 1981;38:225-34.

110. Wilcosky TC, Tyroler HA. Mortality from heart disease among workers exposed to solvents. J Occup Med 1983;25(12):879-885.

111. Higginson J. Proportion of cancers due to occupation. Prev Med 1980;9:180-88.

112. Milham S, Jr. Proportion of cancer due to occupation in Washington State. In: Peto R, Schneiderman M (eds), Banbury Report 9 - Quantification of Occupational Cancer. Cold Spring Harbor Laboratory, 1981, pp. 513-22.

113. Langmuir AD. The surveillance of communicable diseases of national importance. N Engl J Med 1963;268:182-92.

114. Doll R. Surveillance and monitoring. Intl J Epidemiol 1974; 3:305-14.

115. Langmuir AD. William Farr: Founder of modern concepts of surveillance. Int J Epidemiol 1976;5(1):13-18.

116. Muir CS, MacLennan R, Waterhouse JAH. Feasibility of monitoring populations to detect environmental carcinogens. INSERM 1976; 52:279-294.

117. Higginson J. The necessity for an international system of cancer surveillance and monitoring in selected environments. Rev Epidem et Sante Publ 1977;25:179-184.

118. Devesa SS, Silverman DT. Trends in incidence and mortality in the United States. J Environ Pathol Toxicol 1980;3:127-55.

119. Choi K, Thacker SB. Mortality during influenza epidemics in the United States, 1967-1978. Amer J Publ Health 1982;72(11):1280-1283.

120. Osmond C, Gardner MJ, Acheson ED. Trends in cancer mortality 1951-1980. Medical Research Council, Environmental Epidemiology Unit, Office of Population Censuses and Surveys, Her Majesty's Stationery Office, London, crown copyright 1983. (Series DH1, no. 11.)

121. Stevens RG, Moolgavkar SH. A cohort analysis of lung cancer and smoking in British males. Amer J Epidemiol 1984;119(4):624-641.

122. Albert DM, Puliafito CA, Fulton AB, Robinson NL, Zakov ZN, et al. Increased incidence of choroidal malignant melanoma occurring in a single population of chemical workers. Am J Ophthalmol 1980; 89:323-37.

123. Lee JAH. Increased incidence of choroidal malignant melanoma and the use of inappropriate statistical methods. Am J Ophthalmol 1980;90:272-73.

124. Albert DM, Smith AB, Leffingwell SS. Reply to editorial by JAH Lee on increased incidence of choroidal malignant melanoma and the use of inappropriate statistical methods. Am J Opthalmol 1980;90:273-74.

125. Caldwell GG, Kelley DB, Health Jr CW. Leukemia among participants in military maneuvers at a nuclear bomb test – a preliminary report. JAMA 1980;244:1575-78.

126. Caldwell GG, Kelley D, Zack M, Falk H, Heath Jr CW. Mortality and cancer frequency among military nuclear test (Smoky) participants, 1957 through 1979. JAMA 1983;250:620-24.

127. Coggon D, Acheson ED. Do phenoxy herbicides cause cancer in man? Lancet 1982;i:1057-59.

337

OCCUPATIONAL EXPOSURE TO IONIZING RADIATION

Jan Olof Snihs

National Institute of
Radiation Protection
Stockholm

INTRODUCTION

Occupational exposure comprises all the dose equivalents and intakes of radioactive nuclides incurred by a worker during periods of work.

This definition should in principle include all workers because of their permanent exposure to the natural radiation. However, from a regulatory point of view there are reasons for not including exposure to "normal" natural radiation, but only those components of natural radiation that result from man-made activities or that arise in special environments. There is no sharp dividing line, however, between levels of "normal" natural radiation and modified and enhanced natural radiation caused by human activities. Examples of the latter are aviation, mining and other underground work, use of some phosphate fertilizers etc. In aviation the aircraft crew is exposed to the increased cosmic radiation with height, in underground work the natural radiation is enhanced by uncovering uranium or thorium and/or increasing the concentration of the natural radionuclides in air by the underground work. When using phospate fertilizers with a higher than normal content of natural radionuclides the workers are exposed to enhanced external and internal irradiation.

Irrespective of the exact definition of occupational exposure, it is easily concluded that the number of workers exposed to ionizing radiation increases continually in the world. The exact number is difficult to determine because of the different routines used for recording occupational exposures and accounting workers as radiation workers. This difficulty is caused by different approaches to international recommendations on classification of workers and their registrations.

The relative number of radiation workers partly reflects the level of technical development and economic and social welfare of a country and in developed countries the number is at present of the order of 2 per 1 000 inhabitants and in developing countries of the order of 0.1 per 1 000 of population. The distribution of workers in different fields of occupation varies also but a major area of interest is always the medical field including doctors, nurses, laboratory personnel and dentists. Other fields are research institutions of universities and hospitals, industries where radiation is used as a tool in the industrial processes, radioisotope production etc. A field of increasing interest is the uranium fuel cycle. Even if there are national fluctuations in the economical and political interest in the nuclear field there is a general and global expansive trend of nuclear power. The installed world electrical generating capacity in 1983 was about 170 GW(e) with about 200 GW(e) under construction. In the year 2 000 an installed capacity of around 1 000 GW(e) is expected. At present about 10 % of the total electrical energy is produced by nuclear power and this is expected to increase to about 25 % by the year 2 000. The number of reactors in operation in 31 December 1982 was 298, and the number of workers involved was of the order of 100.000.

THE REGULATORY SYSTEM

The occupational exposure to ionizing radiation is regulated on the basis of international recommendations issued by ICRP. In order to understand and put the levels of exposure into perspective and possibly use the information for epidemiological purposes it is necessary to be familiar with the concepts and quantities used, the assumptions on the detrimental effects of radiation and the principles of the dose limitation system as recommended by ICRP. It is also necessary to be familiar with the monitoring and dose recording practice.

CONCEPTS AND QUANTITIES

The interaction of radiation with matter is described quantitatively by the energy deposited per unit mass. The energy deposition, the absorbed dose D, from all types of radiation is defined as

$$D = \frac{d\bar{\varepsilon}}{dm}$$

where $d\bar{\varepsilon}$ is the mean energy imparted by radiation in a volume element and dm is the mass of the volume element. The SI unit for absorbed dose is joule per kg and its special name is gray (Gy).

The quantity exposure has been used in the measurement of X- and gamma radiation. It is now used only as a quantity for reference standards. It is replaced by air kerma, K, defined by the relationship

$$K = \frac{dE_{tr}}{dm}$$

where dE_{tr} is the sum of the initial kinetic energies of all the charged ionizing particles liberated by uncharged ionizing particles in a material mass dm.

The biological effects do not depend solely on the energy deposition per unit mass, or absorbed dose, but also on the type of radiation. The correlation between dose and biological effect is also dependent on the type of biological effect and the distribution of the absorbed dose rate in time.

Effects of high absorbed doses that have a threshold below which they do not occur are called non-stochastic. For those effects for which there is no evidence of a threshold dose, such as cancer induction, it is known that if a group of people are irradiated then a proportion will show the effect, but there is no possibility of predicting which individuals will be affected. Therefore, an increase in the irradiation will only increase the probability for each individual that the effect will occur. These effects are called stochastic. For protection purposes it is assumed that the risk of stochastic effects from irradiation of a tissue is directly proportional to the absorbed dose in the tissue, although various other dose-response relationships have been observed.

With the assumption of a linear relationship between dose and its corresponding probability of effect the addition of doses implies corresponding addition of probabilities. In case of a non-linear relationship, e.g. a curvilinear, this will not be the case. For incremental doses, the incremental probability of a health effect corresponding to a small incremental dose will, for the curvilinear case, depend on the previous level of dose, whereas for the proportional case it is independent on other doses.

If the additional doses are not large in comparison with the pre-existing dose, the relevant portion of the curvilinear response can be approximated by a linear relationship. Small additional doses can then be treated independently of the pre-existing dose and of each other. This is the basis which underlies the use of risk factors to relate the incremental probability of a health effect to the incremental dose and these factors will be independent of the absolute level of dose.

To meet the need in radiation protection for a numerical relationship between the radiation exposure and its biological effects, the quantity <u>dose equivalent,</u> H, is used. H is defined by

$$H = DQN$$

where Q is the quality factor and N is the product of all other modifying factors specified by ICRP. For the present the ICRP has assigned a value of unity to N. Both Q and N are dimensionless. The SI unit of dose equivalent is the same as for absorbed dose, namely Jkg^{-1}, and has been given the special name sievert (Sv). The earlier unit for dose equivalent was rem (1 rem = 0.01 Jkg^{-1}).

The quality factor Q allows for the different effectiveness of different types of radiation and its value has been defined as a function of the <u>collision stopping power,</u> L_∞ in water at the point of interest. ICRP has specified the relationship at a number of values of L_∞ as shown in Table 1. Other values can be obtained by linear interpolation.

Table 1. Specified relationship between Q and L_∞

L_∞ in water (kev μm^{-1})	Q
$\leqq$ 3.5	1
7	2
23	5
53	10
$\geqq$ 175	20

ICRP has also recommended approximate values for all common types of ionizing radiation; these are given in Table 2.

It is important to know that the dose equivalent should not be used to assess the consequences of accidental exposures in man which may involve high doses causing severe non-stochastic effects. For that purpose, absorbed dose is the appropriate quantity after weighting for the <u>relative biological effectiveness</u> (RBE) of each type of radiation. It is defined as the ratio of the absorbed dose of a reference radiation to the absorbed dose of a test radiation to produce the same level of biological effect of the same extent and/or nature, other conditions being equal.

Table 2. Recommended permissible approximation of quality
factor for various types of radiation

Type of radiation	Approximate value of Q
X rays, gamma rays and electrons	1
Thermal neutrons	2.3
Neutrons, protons and singly charged particles of rest mass greater than one atomic mass unit of unknown energy	10
Alpha particles and multiply-charged particles (and particles of unknown charge) of unknown energy.	20

The probability of occurrence of a stochastic effect in an organ is assumed to be proportional to the dose equivalent in that particular organ. The proportionality factor differs for the various organs of the body. However, in assessing health detriment the total risk is usually required. If all the body is uniformly irradiated a single overall risk coefficient can be used. If the irradiation of different organs is non-uniform - as for instance in case of irradiation from many internally deposited radionuclides - a further quantity is necessary to represent the total risk.

ICRP has recommended a quantity for allowing for the different mortality risks associated with irradiation of different organs, together with a proportion of the hereditary effects. This quantity is defined by the sum:

$$\sum_T w_T H_T$$

where w_T is the weighting factor to represent the proportion of the stochastic risk resulting from irradiation of tissue T to the total risk when the whole body is irradiated uniformly and H_T is the mean dose equivalent in tissue T. This sum is called effective dose equivalent, H_E.

To assess the effective dose equivalent, the dose equivalent in each tissue from all sources is assessed and multiplied by the appropriate weighting factor and the resulting products are then summed. If all the tissues in the body were uniformly irradiated the result would be numerically equivalent to the wholebody dose equivalent.

The values of w_T recommended by ICRP are shown in Table 3; they are appropriate for protection for individuals of all ages and both sexes, i.e. for workers and members of the public. The value for gonads includes serious hereditary effects, as expressed in the first two generations.

Table 3. Weighting factors recommended by ICRP for calculation of effective dose equivalent

Organ or tissue	Weighting Factor w_T
Gonads	0.25
Breast	0.15
Red bone marrow	0.12
Lung	0.12
Thyroid	0.03
Bone surfaces	0.03
Remainder	0.30

In practice the "remainder" organs or tissues are taken to be the five not specifically listed in Table 3 that receive the highest dose equivalents;

The hands and forearms, the feet and ankles, the skin and the lens of the eye are not included in the "remainder", and these organs should therefore be excluded from the computation of effective dose equivalent.

The absorbed dose from external irradiation is delivered at the same time as the tissue is exposed to the radiation field. To take account of the time distribution of absorbed dose to internal organs caused by incorporated nuclides ICRP has defined the committed dose equivalent, which is the time integral of the dose equivalent rate in a particular organ following an intake of radioactive material into the body. The integration time is 50 years after intake, taken to correspond to a working lifetime. The formal definition of committed dose equivalent is:

$$H_{50} = \int_{t_0}^{t_0+50y} \dot{H}(t)dt$$

for a single intake of activity at time t_0 where $\dot{H}(t)$ is the relevant dose equivalent rate in an organ or tissue at time t.

With the assumption that the effect is directly proportional to dose equivalent it is sometimes useful to define a quantity to measure the total radiation exposure of a group of individuals. This quantity is called the collective dose equivalent, and is given by

$$S = \int_0^{\infty} H\ N(H)\ dH$$

where N(H) dH is the number of individuals receiving a dose equivalent between H and H + dH; or by

$$S = \sum_i \bar{H}_i\ N(\bar{H})_i$$

where N $(\bar{H})_i$ is the number of individuals in a population subgroup receiving an average dose equivalent of $\bar{H}_i$.

If the dose is expressed in terms of effective dose equivalents the resultant definitions give the collective effective dose equivalent, S_E.

In most practical situations the collective dose equivalent is obtained by summing doses received over a specified time period, often 1 year. However, the collective committed effective dose equivalent from intakes of radionuclides in that year includes the 50 year integration of dose equivalent rates in the relevant organs resulting from the intakes.

The per caput effective dose equivalent is the average of a range of actual dose equivalents to individuals. It is obtained by dividing the collective dose equivalent over a given time in a specified population by the number of individuals in the population at the time, or, more directly, by calculating the average absorbed dose rate, or intake of radionuclides, from the source, and hence the average dose equivalent or committed dose equivalent.

The integration of the per caput dose from a practice given as a function of time gives the dose equivalent commitment, H_c, defined by

$$H_c = \int_0^{\infty} \bar{H}(t)\ dt$$

where $\bar{H}(t)$ is the per caput dose equivalent rate as a function of time. If the upper time limit of integration is infinity the resultant quantity is the dose equivalent commitment; if the integration is terminated at a time T, then the resultant quantity is named the truncated or incomplete dose equivalent commitment.

If the practice continues at the same rate and all other relevant factors are constant it can be shown that the maximum future per caput dose equivalent rate per unit practice will, at equilibrium, be numerically equal to the dose equivalent commitment per unit practice. This provides a means for estimation of the maximum future annual per caput dose equivalent from a continued practice.

Similarly, if a practice continues at the same rate for T years, the maximum future per caput dose equivalent rate is equal to the truncated per caput dose equivalent commitment.

A source or practice will also give rise to a collective effective dose equivalent rate which varies with time. By integration the collective effective dose equivalent commitment is achieved.

$$S_{E.c} = \int_0^\infty \dot{S}_E(t) \ dt$$

The collective effective dose equivalent commitment is associated with the total health detriment caused by a given decision or a practice. It can therefore by used for justification or optimization studies.

ICRP SYSTEM OF DOSE LIMITATION

ICRP has recommended a system of dose limitation in terms of three components:

1. The justification of the practice

    No practice shall be adopted unless its introduction produces a positive net benefit.

2. The optimization of radiation protection

    All exposures shall be kept as low as reasonably achievable, economic and social factors being taken into account.

3. The dose limits for individuals

    The dose equivalent to individuals shall not exceed the limits recommended for the appropriate circumstances by ICRP.

Justification

The expression "positive net benefit" invokes the idea of cost-benefit analysis. However, the choice between practices will depend on many factors, only some of which will be associated with radiation protection. Therefore, more general decision-making methodologies would need to be applied to decisions on the justification of practices. In any case there is a need to ensure that the total detriment from a practice is appropriately small in relation to the expected benefit of the practice.

Optimization

Since any exposure to radiation is assumed to involve some degree of risk, all exposures should be kept as low as reasonably achievable, i.e. the protection should be optimized.

The optimization applies for doses below the dose limits and therefore non-stochastic effects are precluded. For the stochastic effects the mathematical expectation of the amount of harm in an exposed group of people is proportional to the collective effective dose equivalent.

The selection of a level of protection that meets the optimization requirements includes consideration of several factors. Several methods can be used for this decision-making, such as multicriteria methods, which compare by pairs the various options, aggravative methods which combine the values of the criteria in each option into a single value ranking the results from different options in order to select the best. The most normal aggregative methods are based on utility functions to quantify the criteria. An important method based on utility functions is the cost-benefit analysis which expresses the criteria in monetary terms.

The basis of cost-benefit procedures for radiation protection optimization is that an option is selected if the resulting net benefit exceeds that of the next best alternative and not otherwise. The net benefit can be expressed as $B = V - P - (X + Y)$, where B is the net benefit from the practice, V is the gross benefit, P is the production cost excluding the cost of protection, X is the cost of achieving the selected level of radiation protection and Y is the cost of the detriment. The optimization requirement means minimizing the sum of the cost of protection X and the cost of detriment Y.

The cost of protection and the detriment is dependent on the level of protection which can be characterized by a protection parameter, W. A protection parameter can be ventilation rate, thickness of lead etc. The objective of optimization is to find the "optimized" value W when $X(W) + Y(W)$ is minimum i.e.

347

$$\frac{dX(W)}{dW}\bigg|_{W_0} = - \frac{dY(W)}{dW}\bigg|_{W_0}$$

This procedure is called differential cost-benefit analysis. The level of exposure in the optimized situation as defined by this equation is such that a marginal increase in the cost of radiation protection is exactly balanced by a marginal reduction in the cost of detriment.

If X(W) and Y(W) have only discrete values, the optimized level is reached by a step-by-step improvement of the protection. The decision to go from one level of control, A, to a more costly one, B, would then be taken if

$$\left[\frac{X(W_A) - X(W_B)}{Y(W_A) - Y(W_B)}\right] < 1$$

In that case, optimization can be achieved through an iteration process, testing increasingly higher levels of radiation protection and stopping when the expression above no longer holds.

The optimization procedure necessitates expression of cost of protection and detriment in the same unit. Since the health detriment is proportional to the collective effective dose commitment S, it is also assumed that the cost of the health detriment also is proportional to that quantity so that

$$Y = \alpha \cdot S$$

where α is a dimensional constant expressing the cost assigned to the unit collective dose for radiation protection purposes. If other detriments such as anxiety are quantified and corresponding costs are taken into account, they should be added.

Thus the optimization may be expressed as

$$X(W) + \alpha \cdot S(W) = minimum$$

which at the optimum W corresponds to the expression

$$\frac{dX}{dW}\bigg|_{W_0} = - \alpha \frac{dS}{dW}\bigg|_{W_0}$$

or

$$\frac{dX}{dS}\bigg|_{S_0} = - \alpha$$

348

If the functions are discontinuous, the expression takes the
form

$$- \frac{X_B - X_A}{S_B - S_A} \leqq \alpha$$

where A and B stand for different levels of protection.

There are some limiting factors in the optimization. If the
optimization procedure leads to excessively high individual doses,
the maximum acceptable individual dose is the limiting condition.
If the optimization will be too expensive, available resources will
be limiting. In these cases, a cost-effectiveness analysis may be
appropriate, this is an analysis of how a given level of protection
can be achieved at the minimum cost or how the maximum protection
can be obtained at a given cost-level.

The cost of health detriment in monetary units is the cost the
society is willing to pay to avoid this detriment. This cost is
expressed as $\alpha \cdot S$. The value of $\alpha \cdot S$ is a controversial matter. The
collective dose multiplied by the risk factor gives the statistical
prediction of the number of cancers and hereditary effects in a
population as a result of the exposure. If a given value could be
assigned to each statistical death, the value of alpha could be
estimated by division of that value by the relevant risk factor.

Several attempts have been made to define a value for the
collective dose (expressed as man Sv) and the values have ranged
from \$ 1,000 manSv^{-1} to \$ 100,000 manSv^{-1}.

Dose limits

A limit is the value of a quantity which must not be exceeded.

The limits used in radiation protection are:

(1) <u>Primary dose equivalent limits</u>. The primary limits relate to
the dose equivalent, effective dose equivalent, committed dose
equivalent or committed effective dose equivalent, depending on the
exposure circumstances. These limits apply to an individual or, in
the case of exposure of the public, to the critical group, i.e. the
most exposed group.

(2) <u>Secondary limits</u> are needed when the primary dose limits cannot
be applied directly. In the case of external exposure, secondary
limits may be expressed in terms of the so-called dose equivalent
index. In the case of internal exposure, secondary limits may be
expressed in terms of annual limits on intake.

(3) <u>Derived limits</u> are related to the primary limits by a defined model such that if the derived limits are observed, it is likely that the primary limits would also be observed.

(4) <u>Authorized limits</u> are limits for any quantity specified by the competent authority or by the management of an installation (operational limits). These should generally be lower than the primary or derived limits.

Furthermore, <u>reference levels</u> are used in radiation protection. A reference level is the value of a quantity which is used to determine a particular course of action. It is not a limit. Examples of reference levels are:

(1) <u>Recording level</u> is a level of dose or intake above which the information is of sufficient interest from a radiation protection point of view to be worth recording and keeping.

(2) <u>Investigation level</u> is a level of dose or intake above which the results are considered sufficiently important to justify further investigations.

(3) <u>Intervention levels</u> are usually specified for use in abnormal situations. If the value of a quantity does not exceed or is not predicted to exceed the intervention level, then it is highly improbable that intervention will be warranted.

The limit for the annual effective dose equivalent for workers is 50 mSv. In addition, the annual dose equivalent limit for individual organs and tissues of workers is 500 mSv except in the case of the lens of the eye for which the limit is 150 mSv. For women of reproductive capacity any necessary exposure should be as uniformly distributed in time as is practicable. The purpose of this is the protection of the embryo before a pregnancy is known. When a woman is known to be pregnant she should work only in such working conditions where it is most unlikely that the annual exposures will exceed three-tenths of the dose equivalent limits.

The dose equivalent from external radiation is delivered at the same time as the radiation is received and the dose equivalent from external radiation received during a year can therefore be compared with the limit. However, the dose equivalent from an intake of radioactive materials may be spread over future years, and in this case it is the committed effective dose equivalent that must be compared with the limit.

For comparison of the committed effective dose equivalent from intakes with the dose equivalent limits, secondary limits for individual radionuclides giving the maximum intake in a year can be used. The secondary limits are known as <u>annual limits on intake</u>

(ALI); they correspond to the committed effective dose equivalent from an intake of a given radionuclide equal to the dose equivalent limit for workers. Keeping the intakes in each year less than the ALI ensures that the maximum annual dose equivalent from that radionuclide will always be less than the dose equivalent limit even if intake continues every year for 50 years.

When both external and internal exposures are received in a year, the annual dose limit will not be exceeded if the following condition is met:

$$\frac{H_E}{50 \ (mSv)} + \Sigma \frac{I_j}{I_{j,L}} \ \leqq \ 1$$

where H_E is the actual annual effective dose equivalent, I_j is the annual intake of radionuclide j and I_{jL} is the annual limit on intake for radionuclide j. Sometimes it is necessary to explicitly require that the condition

$$\frac{H_{sk}}{500 \ (mSv)} \ \leqq \ 1$$

shall also be met where H_{sk} is the shallow dose equivalent index ($\sim$ dose to the skin).

In some situations derived air concentrations (DAC) are of practical use. These are obtained by dividing the ALI by a standard volume of air inhaled in a working year of 2000 hours at a breathing rate of 1.2 m^3h^{-1}.

THE RISKS CORRELATED TO THE LIMITS

The objective of radiation protection is to prevent the non-stochastic effects and to limit the probability of stochastic effects to an acceptable level. That means that even if the dose is very small there is still a small probability of a detrimental health effect. This effect can be genetic and somatic. The average risk factor for hereditary effects, as expressed in the first two generations, is for radiation protection purposes given by ICRP to be about $4 \cdot 10^{-3}$ Sv^{-1}. The additional damage to later generations is of the same magnitude.

The somatic risks are distributed in time after each exposure. After the time of exposure the probability of a detrimental effect increases from approximately zero for a few years (= latent period) up to a maximum value and then declines to zero again. The cancers can be divided into leukemia and all other cancers because of their different latent periods. For leukemia the average annual risk is about $0.8 \cdot 10^{-4}$/year per Sv during 25 years which leads to a lifetime risk of mortality from leukemia of $2 \cdot 10^{-3}$ per Sv. For other cancers the shape of the risk curve is less certain but if the average annual risk is taken to be $2 \cdot 10^{-4}$ per Sv during 40 years this corresponds to a lifetime risk of $8 \cdot 10^{-3}$ per Sv. The total risk of leukemia and other cancers is therefore 10^{-2} per Sv.

If there is a continuous exposure of 10^{-2} Sv/year the annual risk will continuously increase to reach a level of 10^{-4}/year after several tens of years. The accumulated risk after 50 years of exposure will be 0.24 % eventually rising to 0.5 %.

The limit for the effective dose equivalent for workers is 50 mSv/year. A continuous exposure of 50 mSv/year during 50 years will accordingly result in an annual risk of $5 \cdot 10^{-4}$/year and a lifetime accumulated risk of 1-3 %.

In the ICRP recommendations it is said that a valid method for judging the acceptability of the level of risk in radiation work is to compare this risk with the risks in other occupations known to have a high standard of safety.

The risk for radiation workers and other workers can be compared in various ways. One way is to compare the average risks, another to compare the risk to maximum exposed groups. This is illustrated in Table 4.

Table 4. Comparison of risks

Causes	Average risk		Maximum risk	
	Radiation workers	Other workers	Radiation workers	Other workers
Accidents	A_1	A_2	A_3	A_4
Occupational diseases	0_1	0_2	0_3	0_4
Total	$T_1 = A_1 + 0_1$	$T_2 = A_2 + 0_2$	$T_3 \neq A_3 + 0_3$	$T_4 \neq A_4 + 0_4$

In a comparison between two occupations the average accident risks for radiation workers should be compared with average accident risk for workers in another occupation, i.e. A_1 and A_2 respectively. Similarly 0_1 should be compared with 0_2 and T_1 with T_2. In radiation work A_1 is small and 0_1 is well identified and quantifiable. In other work there is good statistical data on the accidental risks, A_2, but the knowledge of cause and effect relationship for

occupational diseases is very limited. The ideal comparison mentioned above can therefore hardly be carried out and in its publication 26 ICRP has therefore compared the risk of occupational
disease caused by radiation with the risk of fatal accidents in
other occupations. This risk comparison relates to O_1 and A_2.

Occupations recognized as having a high standard of safety are
those in which the average annual mortality risk due to occupational
hazards is less that 10^{-4}. In these occupations fatalities are
accompanied by a much larger number of less severe consequences
and in a comparison account should be taken of all components of
harm, both fatal and non-fatal effects.

In radiation work it is very unlikely that workers will get an
annual dose of 50 mSv, year after year. Because of optimization and
good radiation protection practice the actual average doses to
workers are less, and often much less. Considering, this it is concluded that the average risk in radiation work is comparable with
the average risk in other safe occupations. The actual exposures
in various occupations are presented and discussed below.

Another comparison of interest would be to compare the risk
profile of various occupations, i.e. to include a comparison of the
maximum risk groups, identified in Table 4 by A_3, O_3, T_3 and A_4,
O_4, T_4. The maximum total risk T_3 and T_4 is not the sum of the two
components because they probably do not represent the same individuals. In radiation work there is a great deal of information on the
dose distribution to workers and those groups which are regularly
more exposed than others are easily identified. In other work,
however, the corresponding information is very poor and often non-
existent and it is therefore difficult to make any comparison
between radiation workers and other workers on this basis. On the
other hand, comparisons can be made between different kinds of
radiation occupations.

ICRP´s comparison with average doses and risks has occasionally been misunderstood to mean a recommended limit of the average
dose to a worker over a working lifetime, in other words a recommendation of a limit for the lifetime dose. That was not the intention
of ICRP. It is also to be observed that if such a limit should be
introduced it would interfere with the rights of an individual to
follow the career of his choice. Statement of that meaning was
made by the Committee on Radiation Protection and Public Health,
NEA, OECD, in 1982.

TRAINING AND ADMINISTRATIVE CONTROL

The control of occupational exposure is maintained by optimization of the radiation protection in the design and the operation.
This also includes education and training of the workers in radia-

tion protection. The workers are thereby aware of the potential health hazards in their work and how these can be reduced by safe working methods and techniques. Even if the main safety should be built into the design, the importance of well educated and trained personnel should not be underestimated. Failures of the protection system can occasionally be caused by so-called "human factor", i.e. unplanned, irrational or undisciplined actions against everything learnt and regulated. This is minimized by applying good ergonomic principles in the planning of design and equipment. However, even when this has been done there are several examples of incidents or accidents caused by the human factor and some of them have led to very serious consequencies.

An education and training program could also, hopefully, increase the workers awareness of the limited reliability of all technical safety systems. Also here there are several examples of severe accidents when there has been a failure in a safety system, e.g. when a failure of the interlock system to a gamma radiography exposure room has not been observed by the worker.

Other methods to improve the radiation protection are more of an administrative nature. Examples are classification and marking of working areas with varying need for supervision and control, record-keeping of workplace monitoring and persondosimetry results to follow up the routine working conditions and special events or doses of interest etc. All these results would be used for improvements of the radiation protection by optimization procedures. Investigation levels are used to initiate special investigations. These can be triggered by measurements or predicted doses. For instance, there might be an investigation level for the expected collective dose caused by planned work. If the predicted collective dose is higher than the investigation level the employer must report and discuss the radiation protection problem with the responsible authority. Examples of such levels of the order of 0.1 manSv exist.

MANAGEMENT OF OVEREXPOSED WORKERS

ICRP´s recommended dose limits in publ. 26 do not apply to accidents and emergencies but only to those conditions where the source of exposure is under control. However, ICRP gives some recommendations and guidance on the planning of actions or countermeasures after an accident. These recommendations and guides only state general principles because of the individual nature of the decisions to be made for worker involved in the accident. Recently, the Committee on Radiation Protection and Public Health, NEA, OECD, made a study among member states on their regulations and/or experience of measures taken in case of over-exposure of workers. In their answers the following common elements could be identified.

354

(a) Notification

Provisions are made for the notification of the worker, immediate responsible person, employer, medical advisor, and responsible authority under specified conditions, when a suspected overexposure occurs.

(b) Assessment of dose and immediate medical attention

Immediate action is required to be taken to assess the dose incurred and communicate this imformation to the medical advisor.

(c) Investigation

A detailed investigation is required to identify and record the circumstances causing the overexposure and recommendations are made for corrective action if indicated, to ensure that recurrence of the circumstances causing the accident is unlikely. An important element in the corrective action is to ensure that information developed in the investigationis widely disseminated so that other activities can profit from the experience.

(d) Recording of exposures

Requirements are included for the recording of the dose by the employer, the medical advisor and, in some cases, a central state authority.

(e) Medical followup and future employment restrictions

Medical followup and future employment restrictions are handled on a case-by-case basis through consultations between the employer, worker, medical advisor and competent authority. In one case there would be generic requirements in regulations that following an overexposure the individual must not be assigned to tasks which are likely to result in the dose equivalent exceeding one percent of the annual limit during the remainder of the calendar year in which the exposure occurred.

MONITORING AND DOSE ASSESSMENTS

The radiation protection principles are in general applied by the following steps.

1. An annual individual limit (50 mSv) is established.

2. A derived limit corresponding to the annual individual limit is established. That could be a dose rate, a concentration of radionuclides in air or water, a level of contaminations of surfaces etc.

3. Optimization of the protection is carried out.

4. The optimized level of protection is expressed in terms of quality of design, conditions on operation, external dose rate, activity concentration in air etc. If these levels are expressed as limits they are called authorized limits.

5. An operational level might be established as a reference level for special actions.

Monitoring is carried out to check the compliance with given regulations. The results of monitoring are also sometimes directly or indirectly used for dose assessment. The monitoring includes measurements on air, water surfaces and man and concerns external and internal irradiation. The measurements are made continuously or occasionally on a regular or irregular basis. The results of the measurements are impaired by inaccuracies of varying significance. The external exposure of man is normally measured by a personal dosemeter. TLD and film dosemeters are used for external dosimetry. The film dosemeter has the advantage of preserving its information on dose and can be examined repeatedly afterwards. TLD is easier and more rapid to handle in an automatic system for dose measurements and dose data statistics in computers. In nuclear power plants, maintenance personnel work at several plants in a year and therefore it is essential to have a rapid and reliable system for continuous and automatic information on the accumulated dose.

Standards on quality assurance tests are given by the international standard organisation (ISO). They include guidance on how tests should be made and how the results should be understood. The uncertainties and errors in the results from dosemeter measurements depend on several factors associated with the standards and reference values used, reproduceability, linearity with dose, energy dependence. The overall uncertainty for a given practice with occupational exposure may be ± 50 % or more. If it is less than ± 20 % it is certainly to be considered very good.

The primary assessment of external exposures is in terms of effective dose equivalent or the dose equivalent to special parts of the body. In many cases the body can be considered to be rather homogenously irradiated and the assessments be made of the deep dose equivalent (depth 1 cm) and the skin dose equivalent (depth 0.007 cm). The deep dose equivalent assumed to be taken as the effective dose equivalent is measured by the dosemeter on the trunk of the body in the most exposed position. In case of exposure to soft x-rays the dosemeter is placed underneath the apron and often supplemented by a dosemeter on the collar or the head. These two dosemeters can be used to assess the effective dose equivalent and the dose equivalent to the eye. Special hand and finger dosemeters are used if those extremities are particularly exposed.

The measurement of skin dose in case of beta radiation is often uncertain because of inadequate dosemeters and difficulties in interpreting the significance of the results. The thickness of the sensitive layers of the skin varies on the body and for different persons.

If the external exposure of man is measured by fixed monitors in a room additional uncertainties are introduced, like the varying representativity of the measured result for the real exposure of man. The representativity depends on how the location of the source varies in relation to the monitor and how the worker is exposed in relation to the measured exposure. Because of these uncertainties fixed monitors are used only to supplement individual monitoring and as a warning device. They can be used alone in working places where the source is fixed and the normal exposure and potential risks of high exposures are small.

The internal exposure is mostly controlled by indirect measurements on the concentration of radionuclides in air, water or on surfaces. The compliance to given regulations is shown by comparison with derived limits associated with the primary limit (50 mSv/ year) or secondary limit like ALI or with the authorized limit as is required by the competent authority. For this purpose it is therefore not necessary to assess any dose caused by internal radiation. However, sometimes the assessment of the relationship between, for instance, an air concentration of a radionuclide and the corresponding intake in the body or dose is very difficult and unreliable. In these cases biological monitoring is made including external body measurements and measurements on excreta or exhaled air. By appropriate metabolic models the activity concentrations in relevant organs or tissues of the body can be assessed and, if the time of intake is known, also the amount of intake. However, the reliability of the result is dependent on the pattern of intake, whether the intake is multiple or single, the metabolic differences among various persons, the kind of nuclide etc. Some nuclides with long physical and biological halflives in the body, such as actinides, present difficult problems to measure in excreta (only a small part is released from the body) and to assess the annual intake (because some part of the body burden depends on earlier intake). Others like ^{3}H are easier to determine by biological monitoring. In many occupations the intakes of radionuclides are very small in comparison with ALI or any authorized limit and the corresponding effective dose equivalents are also very small compared to the external doses and are therefore neglected in the dose records.

The relative number of workers subject to monitoring in various occupations and working places is not consistent in relation to the actual and potential risk of exposures. ICRP considers that in cases where it is most unlikely that annual doses will exceed three-tenths of the dose limit, individual monitoring is not necessary. However, personal dosemeters are often used also in these occupations and in general monitoring is more common than ICRP considers to be justified. The reasons are of social and personnel-political character and are intended to confirm that the conditions are satisfactory.

These circumstances cause special problems in calculating average doses to workers, because an increased number of dosemeters to unirradiated workers will decrease the average.

Another problem is the differences in the procedures used for reporting dosemeter results less than the minimum detectable level. These results are reported as zero or the minimum level of detection or something in between. However, it is generally agreed that the recording level below which the dose is recorded as zero should not exceed one-twentieth of the annual limit pro-rata for the monitoring period.

A third problem is the differences in the procedures used for reporting missing dosemeter results. The recorded dose is either an estimated dose or a pro-rata proportion of the annual authorized limit. This can distort the records and make any assessment of average and collective doses uncertain.

PRESENTATION OF DOSE DISTRIBUTIONS

The results of monitoring expressed as an annual effective dose equivalent, a fraction of ALI or a derived limit, or as other quantities for the purpose of radiation protection, are periodically collected, assessed and presented. The purpose is to show the workers, management, authorities and the public whether given limits are complied with, the distribution of doses and the average as a measure of average individual risks, the collective dose as a measure of detriment, the changes and tendencies as compared with earlier years etc.

The individual doses can also be grouped in different types of work to illustrate the various degrees of radiation protection problems. These results might also indicate the fields in which the need for radiation protection improvement is greatest although this would eventually be decided on the basis of optimization.

The collective dose is a measure of the radiation detriment caused by the practice. It is of interest to follow the change of the collective dose to judge the justification of continued practice.

It might also be of interest to group the collective doses delivered at various individual doses, e.g. those from individual doses, less than 5 $mSva^{-1}$, those between 5 and 15 $mSva^{-1}$ and those delivered at doses exceeding 15 $mSva^{-1}$. The purpose of that is to study the relative contribution to the radiation detriment from various levels of individual risk.

It is also of interest to make comparative studies of the collective dose from various practices or work places and for that purpose it is sometimes preferable to normalize the occupational collective dose per unit of practice, e.g. per GW-year for nuclear power production, per film used for X-ray medical examination per year at hospitals. The normalized collective dose can also be used for comparison with the collective dose from exposure of the public, caused by the practice by its radioactive releases into the environment, by use of the produced radioactive material as a consumer product, by exposure of people as patients etc. Sometimes it occurs that the collective occupational dose per unit of practice is also used for expressing a level of ambition for the radiation protection of workers.

The annual dose distribution is often found to be log-normal, especially for doses much below the dose limit. A variable x is said to have a log-normal distribution if y = ln(x) has a normal distribution. A log-normal distribution can be identified by plotting the cumulative frequency on a probability axis against the logarithm of dose. By use of the log-probability plot technique, deficiences in the data (like missing data, data less than the limit of detection limit etc.) are compensated for by extrapolation.

AVAILABLE DATA ON OCCUPATIONAL EXPOSURES AND THEIR USE FOR EPIDEMIO-LOGICAL STUDIES

As described above there is a stringent and logical system of dose limitation for radiation workers with special quantities, formalistic and practical protection procedures, monitoring and methods for assessments and control. A lot of monitoring and dosimetric data are available. As has already been pointed out, the data are impaired by errors and uncertainties but neverthless, used as a part of the radiation protection system, serve their purpose to ensure good radiation protection practice. Whether the data can be used for epidemiological studies is much more uncertain. The information given here might help in that judgement.

Successful epidemiological studies on occupational radiation exposures are sparse. The reason for that is less due to bad epidemiology than to low radiation doses, which of course is a very satisfactory situation. Assuming that the average annual effective dose equivalent for workers is 5 mSv, the expected number of cancers in a group of 10^4 workers would be of the order of 1 per year at equilibrium. That number of cases would not make the epidemiology study easy.

However, there are special groups of workers with higher risks than others and they can be identified by the monitoring and dosimetry system. One such group, the uranium miners, has been examined by epidemiologists and correlations have been found between radon daughter exposure in mines and the excess rate of lung cancer. This correlation has also been found for non-uranium miners with high radon daughter exposures.

The United Nations Scientific Committee on Atomic Radiation (UNSCEAR) has recently given extensive information in its 1982 Report on occupational exposure for various occupations, countries and time. As expected, there are great variations in average doses and collective doses depending on varying standard of radiation protection, numbers of workers and facilities, reporting system, etc. Table 5 is a rough summary table indicating the orders of magnitude.

Table 5. Average individual doses and collective doses to workers in various occupations.

Occupation	Average dose (range) $mSv\ a^{-1}$	Collective dose
Nuclear		
Mining	10-20	1 manSv $(GW_{(e)}a)^{-1}$
Milling	2-4	0.1 _"_
Fuel manufacture	1-3	1 _"_
Reactors	3-10	10 _"_
Reprocessing	3-10	10 _"_
Research	1-5	5 _"_
Total		30 _"_
Medical	0.3-3	1 manSv per 10^6 population
Industrial radiography	1-3	} 0.5 _"_
Research	0.3-5	

Some comments on the table. The total collective occupational dose equivalent from nuclear power production can be estimated by multiplying by the total energy generated. In 1979 that was 70 $GW_{(e)}a$ which gives about 2000 manSv. This corresponds to 0.5 manSv per 10^6 population as a comparison with the other occupations.

In the nuclear field a general tendency of the occupational doses with time is that the average doses decrease, the collective doses increase and the normalized collective doses per $GW_{(e)}a$ are decreasing slightly. Groups with higher-than-average occupational radiological risks are uranium miners and health physicists and some maintenance workers at reactor plants.

In medicine, industry and research the average doses are generally low. In industrial radiography with radioisotopes, the potential risk of serious accidents is a significant risk factor.

REFERENCES

United Nations. Ionizing Radiation: Sources and Biological Effects. United Nations Scientific Committee on the Effects of Atomic Radiation 1982 report to the General Assembly, with annexes. United Nations sales publication No. E.82.IX.8. New York, 1982.

ICRP. ICRP Publication 26. Annals of the ICRP 1, #3, Pergamon Press, N.Y., 1977.

NON-OCCUPATIONAL EXPOSURE TO IONIZING RADIATION

Jan Olof Snihs

National Institute of
Radiation Protection
Stockholm

INTRODUCTION

Non-occupational exposure comprises all the dose equivalents
and intakes of radioactive nuclides incurred by people but not
associated with their work. It includes natural radiation, medical
exposure of patients, radiation from fallout caused by nuclear
weapon tests, releases from nuclear power installations etc. The
levels of exposure vary in time and place. Some part of non-occupational exposure is not controllable, e.g. cosmic radiation,
radiation from the ground etc.; some is controllable, e.g. medical
exposure and releases from nuclear power. Enhanced natural radiation exposure is partly controllable, e.g. enhanced radiation in
houses.

The non-occupational exposure is dominated by the contribution from natural and medical exposure. Normally there is no special benefit to balance the natural radiation, it is only a detrimental factor for people and society. Medical exposure, on the
other hand, is expected to be balanced by the benefit of the medical examination. A minor source of public exposure is the releases
from nuclear power. The corresponding detrimental effect is expected to be balanced by the benefit of the electrical energy produced by the nuclear installation.

The levels of and possible problems with public exposure and
how they are managed and regulated are discussed below.

CONCEPTS AND QUANTITIES

The same concepts, quantities and units are used in connection with public exposure as for occupational exposure. Any supplementary concepts etc will be explained when they are introduced in the following text.

ICRP SYSTEM OF DOSE LIMITATION

Justification and optimization

For the purpose of justification and optimization the collective dose equivalent commitment (here called collective dose) is estimated. Justification and optimization are source-related requirements and need consideration of both the occupational and public exposure. Their application for the protection of the public implies some practical and conceptual problems such as uncertainties, time distribution, small individual doses etc. They are discussed below.

The uncertainties in the assessment of the resultant collective dose should be minimized by using models and dose calculations which are as realistic as possible. This is important in the optimization procedure in order to avoid biased solutions rather than the truly optimized option. In the final judgement of the result of the optimization, the significance of the uncertainties should be taken into consideration.

In case of very long-lived nuclides released to the environment now and after a very long time, as for example from geological repositories for high level waste, there will be a very long term exposure.

The uncertainties of the dose assessment increase as the time of interest increases. In a time period of $10^3 - 10^4$ years the uncertainties increase mainly because of insufficient knowledge of people's diets and habits during these time periods. The dose-effect relationship is also uncertain in these long-term perspectives because of possible greatly improved medical treatment of radiation-induced diseases. However, these thoughts can never be more than speculative and do not justify less concern for future doses than doses occurring today. For time periods of more than 10^4 years environmental changes will also occur, new ice-ages, changed climate, geographical dislocations because of ground and seabottom movements etc. This will make the dose assessments even more uncertain.

In geological repositories the radioactive nuclides may be isolated for more than 10^4 years and after that appear in the biosphere during various lengths of time. If that time period is short in geological terms the environmental distributions may be assumed to be the same as now. However, if the release time to the biosphere from the repository is long in geological terms there are fundamental difficulties. It might be argued that all the uncertainties associated with future doses particularly those occurring after say 10^4 years should be reflected in the consideration of these doses in the discussion of various options and levels of radiation protection. Is it reasonable to use the same monetary effort to optimize the protection when the collective doses under discussion occur in the distant future as when they occur during the time for which the dose assessments are much more reliable?

There does not exist any rationale for selecting any special monetary value of a collective dose differing from the present value. Discounting techniques have been proposed for allocating future doses lower monetary values then present collective doses. This is, however, much debated.

The collective dose should include all doses irrespective of where they occur. In many cases releases to the environment of long-lived nuclides will give a much higher collective dose caused by global exposure than that caused by local exposure. Therefore, it would be quite inappropriate for the optimization and justification procedure to consider only the local contribution. If differential cost benefit technique is used the monetary value of the global collective dose (α-value) should be the same as that used for the local components and should not be lower than an internationally agreed value.

There are proposals to use <u>cut-off</u> for small doses, i.e. doses less than the cut-off are not considered in the calculation of collective doses. This could result in a substantial decrease in the magnitude of the assessed collective dose and thus the efforts to improve the radiation protection to the optimum could no longer be justified. The argument for cut-off may be that small doses correspond to such small risks that neither the individual nor society should take an interest and pay special attention to them. This argument would possibly apply if there were only one source in the world and if the judgement (made by the one country having the source) of the insignificance of small doses occuring in other countries is also accepted by these countries. Because neither of these assumptions is true, the argument is not applicable . The only relevant argument would be that small doses may have no biological effect. Because the natural background is of the order of 1 mSv a^{-1} the "small" doses considered must be of that order of magnitude.

Limits

ICRP´s recommended effective dose equivalent <u>limit</u> for members of the public is 5 mSv in a year. It applies to the mean dose equivalent in a so-called critical group. A critical group should be representative for those individuals in the population expected to receive the highest dose equivalent. The dose limit is based on considerations of other risks in the society that are regularly accepted. On this basis a risk in the range of 10^{-6} to 10^{-5} per year would probably be acceptable for any individual member of the public. With an assumed risk factor of about 10^{-2} Sv^{-1}, this acceptable risk would imply restriction of the lifetime dose to members of the public to 1 mSv per year of life-long exposure.

This limit should not be used for the purpose of planning the design and operation of a facility from the point of view of radiation protection. It is a constraint for the optimization and in practice the doses to the public are much smaller than the limit.

The limits suggested above refer to the stochastic effects. In order to prevent the induction of non-stochastic effects on individual organs an overriding annual dose equivalent limit of 50 mSv should apply.

The limits are individual-related and should include the contributions from all administratively controlled sources. That implies proper distribution of permissible contributions from the various sources. A practical approach is the use of "upper bounds" as constraints for the optimization of each source. The upper bound value for a given category of sources should be an appropriate apportionment of the individual dose limit, taking into account the expected contribution from other sources. The accumulation of doses caused by the release of long-lived nuclides should be considered. This is made by assessment of the dose commitment. If the dose commitment from one year of practice does not exceed the upper bound expressed as an annual dose limit for a particular source, the annual doses in the future caused by continued use of this source will never exceed the upper bound.

This method of limiting future individual doses is straightforward if the number of sources is constant. If this is not the case, the expected maximum future number of sources of the category of interest must be foreseen. If this number is correlated to the number of people using or getting benefit from the source the maximum future individual annual dose can be controlled by maximizing the resulting collective dose equivalent commitment per unit of practice. For nuclear power, in some countries, this is made by setting a limit on the collective dose equivalent commitment per installed electric power and year, i.e. in manSv $(MW \cdot a)^{-1}$.

Because a time-unlimited use of a source is usually unrealistic, for example because of limited resources, the collective dose in this case and for this purpose is assessed by integration over the time during which the source is assumed to be used. For nuclear power a time period of 100-500 years has been used. It must be stressed that this limited integration is made only to meet the purpose of this particular calculation, which is limitation of future individual doses. It does not imply an undervaluation or neglect of future doses. The upper bound for individual dose is set on the basis of apportionment and acceptability of risk. This is a matter of national responsibility but also assumes an international understanding of the global dispersion and consequences of certain releases of radioactive nuclides in air and water. Otherwise, national efforts to keep individual doses below established upper bounds and even below ICRP's recommended primary dose limits would be seriously jeopardized by contributions from foreign countries.

In radiation protection in general, when some doses are received with certainty, doses are compared with dose limits or upper bounds. The dose limits represent the beginning of an unacceptable probability of stochastic effects.

In the case when doses are not received with certainty, but with some small probability (p), the individual would be protected at the same level as in the previous case, if the total probability of stochastic harm does not exceed the probability (p_o) related to the dose limit (D_o). The total probability would be the product of the probability (p) of a given dose and the probability (s) of stochastic harm, given that dose. This probability (ps) will not exceed the probability at the dose limit, if the product of the dose (D) and its probability does not exceed the dose limit (i.e. $pD \leqslant D_o$). It should be understood however, that this product, which is formally the mathematical expectation of dose, represents a dose which may never occur and that the expectation value has a standard deviation which, at low probabilities is $1/\sqrt{p}$ times its own value. The whole argument is therefore based on a comparison of probabilities and not on an assessment of the expectation value. All doses that might occur must also be less than, say, 100 mSv in order not to introduce any non-linear relations which would invalidate the assumptions.

It is sometimes argued that the solution to a problem would not necessarily need to be good in the long-time perspective but it is left for future generations to solve the long-term problems. That would be their share of the bill for the inherited welfare. There are at least two objections to that. Firstly, there is no guarantee that the resources available in the future will be sufficient to solve the problems which arise. Secondly, the application of such a principle to all long-term problems would make the future burden of unsolved problems unacceptable, reducing the future margins for expenses and efforts of the future generations to solve their own problems and increase their own prosperity.

Therefore, the major effort should be directed to obtaining reasonable assurances today that the individual doses and corresponding quantity for level of protection in the future do not exceed acceptable values. The acceptable dose level should not exceed those accepted today.

As for occupational exposures, there are secondary and derived limits for the public. The secondary limit ALI need special comments. The values of ALI recommended in ICRP publ. 30 are for workers based on a Reference Man and there are many factors by which they would differ from those appropriate for members of the public. The relative values for infants of the committed dose equivalent in a number of tissues per unit of intake of several nuclides are more than 1 up to 1000 times greater than those for adult workers. The resulting ALI will accordingly be similarly less.

DOSE LIMITATION SYSTEM FOR NATURAL RADIATION

The dose limits recommended by ICRP do not apply to contributions from "normal" natural radiation. However, there are levels of natural radiation that should be controlled in the same way as for artificial sources. ICRP has recently published recommendations applicable to natural sources of radiation, publ. 39.

ICRP makes a distinction between existing and future sources. If the radiation from an existing source is considered to be too high, remedial action should be taken. The competent authority should specify action levels specific to the initiation of the remedial action being considered. ICRP does not consider it appropriate to recommend any general action level but recommends, for the specific case of radon in houses if the remedial action is fairly simple, an action level for equilibrium equivalent radon concentration in the region of 200 Bqm^{-3} (corresponding to an annual effective dose equivalent of 20 mSv).

Future sources can be subject to limitation and control during the planning and decision stages and their introduction should be justified and the protection optimized. However, ICRP´s recommended dose limits should not be applied. Instead, it is recommended that competent authorities set an upper bound of individual dose in the optimization assessments.

MEDICAL EXPOSURE

With the exception of the natural exposure, medical exposure represents the greatest contribution to the exposure of the public. Increased economical and social welfare in a society increases the medical exposures because of the increased number of medical examinations. But it would also simultaneously or eventually decrease the exposure per examination because of improved radiation protection practice.

ICRP´s system of dose limitation is also applicable to medical exposure except for the limits. Limits are set where benefits and detriments are not received by the same members of the population. In the case of medical examinations they are normally the same persons and ICRP´s limits are therefore not applicable. However, the examinations should be justified and the radiation protection should be optimized. The decision as to whether an examination is justified is the responsibility of the physician.

Some types of examinations require special attention since they may need special protection and dose limitation. Examples are periodic health checks where the justifications depends on the probability of achieving important information and the benefit of that information for the patient. The justification of mass screening and dose limitation should be based on consideration of the benefit to the individual and the whole population and the costs in terms of detriment, equipment and manpower. Another example is medical research which is not always beneficial to the exposed patient. The question of voluntariness and knowledge of the risks is essential and imperative. In these cases authorized limits might be set.

MONITORING AND DOSE ASSESSMENT

Exposure of the public is controlled by monitoring and modelling. Monitoring normally concerns the source but occasionally also the environment. Modelling is needed to assess the doses from contaminated water, air or food but sometimes also to assess doses caused by external radiation from contaminated ground or surfaces.

The objectives of regulative monitoring are one or several of the following:

- to assess doses to the critical group
- to demonstrate compliance with authorized limits
- to check the condition of the source
- to warn in case of unforeseen conditions
- to initiate special actions or countermeasures
- to provide data for information of the public
- to provide data for verification and improvements of models etc.

Besides the regulative monitoring, specific monitoring might occur for special investigations and research. The doses due to public exposure are assessed on the basis of monitoring and/or modelling.

Some examples are given below of methods for assessing the exposure of the public caused by various sources of radiation.

a) Releases from nuclear power reactors:

Releases are measured at the source, doses are assessed by use of environmental models for the dispersion in air and water and uptake in plants, vegetables and animals and by use of metabolic models and models of human behaviour in the environment, shielding effects etc. Some environmental monitoring and sampling are made to improve the assessment. Sometimes stationary monitoring equipment is used in the near environment to measure continuously the external doses and the concentration of airborne radionuclides released from the plant. The measurements are made with respect to the critical group. The collective doses are based only on source monitoring and modelling, even though the models themselves were originally based on measurements in the environment. The doses are assessed as (collective) effective dose equivalent commitment per year of practice or as annual effective dose equivalent.

b) Repositories for high level waste:

The releases are predicted and the resulting doses are assessed exclusively by the use of modelling.

c) Radon in houses:

Long-term measurements are made either by sampling in representative houses or by random grab sampling or using both methods. Factors influencing radon levels in houses such as the ventilation, building material, age of the building, radon releases from ground etc. are measured and analyzed for various houses to get quantitative relationships and the doses are assessed on the basis of statistical treatment of these results and on metabolic models for the correlation between radon daughter levels in air and radiation dose in the lung.

d) Consumer products.

The exposure of the public is estimated on the basis of primary measurements on the product, assumptions on its use, and possible misuse, and metabolic models.

e) Fallout

Measurements are made on the external radiation from deposited radionuclides on the ground, on the concentration of radionuclides in air and food and by whole-body measurements on people. The results of the measurements are extrapolated to the whole population by knowledge of the representativity of the grab sampling and measurements, and by metabolic modelling.

The examples given show that most of the dose assessments are based on modelling even though monitoring is also continuously performed to support and improve the models. The reliability of the assessed doses varies with the source and the exposure. The most reliable assessments are those of doses such as those due to external radiation from the cosmos and from the ground, internal radiation from ^{40}K, ^{3}H and noble gases and ^{137}Cs from fallout. Examples of less reliable assessments are those of doses from releases into rivers, actinides on the ground and radon in houses. Nevertheless, there are extensive data on the exposure of the public around the world and they are regularly reported by UNSCEAR.

AVAILABLE DATA ON PUBLIC EXPOSURE AND THEIR USE FOR EPIDEMIOLOGICAL STUDIES

The public exposure varies depending on the time, the place and the standard of living. Data are reported from all parts of the world and by weighting them with the number of people in various countries, weighted averages are obtained for the global mean annual dose. The collective doses are less dependent on the variations. A summary is given in Table 1 and it refers to the years around 1980.

Table 1. Annual average, individual doses and collective doses caused by exposure of the public

Source	Average annual effective dose equivalent mSv	Annual global collective dose equivalent manSv
"Normal" natural sources	2	$8 \cdot 10^6$
Coal power plants	$0.5 \cdot 10^{-3}$	2 000
Commercial aviation	–	2 000
Luminous timepieces	–	2 000
Smoke detectors	–	10
Fallout	10^{-2}	$3 \cdot 10^7$ commitment
Nuclear power	10^{-4}	500
Medical	(0.4)	$2 \cdot 10^6$

Some comments on the table:

a)   "Normal" natural sources. About half of the dose is caused
     by inhalation of radon daughters in indoor air. There are
     great variations in the radon daughter levels in houses
     depending on different ventilation rates, radium concentrations
     in building materials, radon emanation from the ground etc. In
     some countries the radon daughters in houses cause a great
     public health problem. For instance in Sweden the inhalation
     of radon daughters might cause 10-50 per cent of the lung
     cancers. Some of the houses have had very high radon daughter
     concentrations corresponding to an annual effective dose
     equivalent of the order of 1 Sv. The various country-average
     values of radon daughter concentration are generally higher
     in the temperate latitudes than in the tropical latitudes
     (by a factor of 4) due to the rate of ventilation and type
     of dwelling. The other components of the natural radiation
     are cosmic radiation, radiation from ground and buildings and
     internal radiation from incorporated radionuclides in the
     body, each of these components giving about 0.3 mSv per year.

b)   Coal power plants. Coal contains small amounts of natural
     radionuclides and to some extent they are dispersed in the air
     when coal is burnt. The pathways of exposure of the population
     are inhalation during passage of the plume, external exposure
     and inhalation and ingestion of radionuclides deposited on
     the ground.

c)   Commercial aviation. The cosmic radiation increases with the
     altitude. From 4 to 12 kilometers altitude the dose rate
     increases by a factor of 20. During occasional intense solar
     flares the dose rate may increase even more. In Table 1 the
     average dose is not given because the individual doses are
     from zero (those who do not fly) to the order of 1 mSv per
     year for aircraft personnel. Supersonic aircraft fly at
     higher altitudes (<20 km) than standard jet aircraft (<12 km)
     and the dose equivalent rate is therefore higher. But because
     the speed is higher, the flying time for a given trip is
     shorter and the total dose equivalent for a flight will be
     about the same.

d)   Luminous timepieces. ^{226}Ra, ^{3}H and ^{147}Pm are the radionuclides
     used for the illumination of clock and watch dails. The con-
     tent in watches varies but if the international standards
     are followed the annual effective dose equivalent from watches
     with ^{226}Ra is about 40 µSv, with ^{3}H about 0.3 µSv and with
     ^{147}Pm about 2 µSv. The doses are caused by external radia-
     tion, inhalation of tritium and external radiation respec-
     tively.

e)   Smoke detectors. The ones refferred to are so-called ioniza-
       tion chamber smoke detectors. Most of them contain about
       0.1 MBq^{241} AM and the exposure of the public is mainly caused
       by the external radiation from the detector. The annual collec-
       tive dose equivalent given in the table is an extrapolation
       from the value given for the United States (1-2 manSv per
       year).

f)   Fallout. The most intensive nuclear explosions in the atmos-
       phere occurred in the years 1954 to 1958 and 1961 to 1962.
       But testing in the atmosphere still occurs occasionally. The
       resulting fallout exposes people for a very long time al-
       though at low dose rates. It has been estimated that all the
       nuclear tests conducted up to 1980 have committed the world
       population to an additional exposure as large as that corres-
       ponding to about four years of natural radiation. The major
       part of the exposure from fallout is caused by 4 radionuclides,
       ^{14}C, ^{137}Cs, ^{95}Zr and ^{90}Sr.

g)   Nuclear power. Because of the very small releases from nuclear
       power production the resultant radiation doses have to be
       assessed merely on the basis of modelling. Furthermore, it is
       not practicable to assess doses caused by all individual sites
       but to assume hypothetical sites with characteristics repre-
       sentative of each stage of the fuel cycle namely, mining and
       milling, fuel fabrication, reactor operation, reprocessing and
       waste management, storage and disposal. Also, the environment
       has to be hypothetical with the characteristics of existing
       site environments. Most of the releases consist of relatively
       short-lived radionuclides and therefore they are only of local
       concern. Some radionuclides are long-lived and can contribute
       to a global irradiation of man. The average dose equivalent
       given in the table is estimated as an global average and in
       practice the individual doses fluctuate around that value
       depending on the distance from the nuclear installation. The
       annual dose equivalent rate for the most exposed individuals
       is generally less than 0.1 mSv a^{-1}.

       The doses given in Table 1 refer to an annual projected
       nuclear production of 80 GW(e)·a. This number is expected to
       increase in the future and consequently also the individual
       and collective doses. A way to predict the future doses is to
       assess the collective dose equivalent per GW(e)·a of electri-
       cal energy produced and multiply by the expected magnitude
       of nuclear power production in the future. That has been done
       by UNSCEAR in its 1982 report and with the assumption that
       there are no technical improvements and that current levels
       of discharge per GW(e)·a continue for 500 years, the expected
       doses at the year 2500 are calculated. The results are an
       annual collective effective dose equivalent of 250 000 manSv

from 10 000 GW(e)·a per year to 10^{10} people with an annual per caput dose of 25 μSva^{-1}.

h) Medical exposures. The medical exposure is the largest component to man-made irradiation of man. The frequency of diagnostic x-ray examinations vary between 300 and 900 examinations per thousand inhabitants per year in industrialized countries excluding mass surveys and dental examinations. Absorbed doses to various organs vary between 0.01 and 50 mGy per examination. The annual collective effective dose equivalent caused by diagnostic radiology in developed countries is of the order of 1 000 manSv per million population. In developing countries the corresponding number would be one order of magnitude less and a weighted value for the whole world population would be about 400 manSv per million population per year. Nuclear medicine examinations contribute insignificantly to the doses caused by x-ray diagnostic procedures, although its relative contribution may vary in different countries.

REFERENCES

United Nations. Ionizing Radiation: Sources and Biological Effects. United Nations Scientific Committee on the Effects of Atomic Radiation 1982 report to the General Assembly, with annexes. United Nations sales publication No. E.82.IX.8. New York, 1982.

ICRP. ICRP Publication 26. Annals of the ICRP 1, #3, Pergamon Press, N.Y., 1977.

RISK ASSESSMENT OF LOW DOSES OF RADIATION AND CHEMICALS

R. B. Setlow

Biology Department
Brookhaven National Laboratory
Upton, N.Y. 11973

INTRODUCTION

Any credible assessment of the effects of low doses of radiation or chemicals on humans is difficult for several reasons (Setlow, 1983): 1) human data are almost always statistically inadequate with a few possible exceptions such as cigarette smoking and asbestos exposure (Peto, this volume), 2) extrapolation from experimental data on animals to predictions for exposed humans often involves many poorly understood factors, such as pharmacokinetics (Hoel et. al., 1983), DNA repair, intrinsic cell sensitivities, etc., 3) most animal experiments use high doses so as to obtain significant effects with small numbers of animals but the responses to high doses may involve different effects and a very different pharmacokinetic than do low doses.

I shall exemplify some of the extrapolation difficulties in estimating mutagenic and carcinogenic effects by using DNA damage as the central theme. However, to analyze the extrapolation problem at the DNA level it is essential to know which DNA products of radiation or chemical exposure are bad and which are innocuous (Setlow, 1980). For example, methylating agents, such as MNNG or dimethylnitrosamine (DMN) methylate many different positions on the DNA chain. The major numerical product is N-7 deoxyguanosine, but this product seems to have negligible biological consequences compared to the relatively minor product O^6-methyldeoxyguanosine (m^6dGuo) (Pegg, 1984). The latter product tends to base pair with thymine as well as with cytosine, whereas the former does not. For ethylating agents, the situation is more complicated because a number of O-ethylation products, not only O^6-ethyldeoxyguanosine seem to be of carcinogenic importance (Singer, 1984).

A number of experimental tricks have been used to show that the photoproducts of major importance arising from ultraviolet radiation of wavelength less than 320 nm are cyclobutane pyrimidine dimers (Setlow and Setlow 1974). Ionizing radiation makes many alterations in DNA. In addition to single and double strand breaks there is some experimental evidence indicating that base damage is very important, but at least for cytotoxicity there is good evidence that double strand breaks are the important damages (Setlow and Setlow, 1972). It has been shown recently that Chinese hamster cells selected for cytotoxic sensitivity to ionizing radiation are deficient in the ability to repair double strand breaks (Kemp et al., 1984).

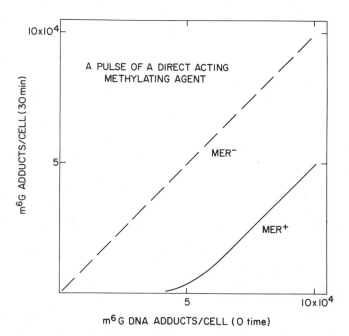

Fig. 1. Hypothetical curves to illustrate the effect of DNA repair on the amount of m^6dGuo as a function of dose for a rapid acting, direct methylating agent. The dose is represented on the abscissa as m^6dGuo at 0 time. The effect of repair is shown by the amount of m^6dGuo per cell at 30 minutes after treatment. Mer⁻ cells lack repair protein, Mer⁺ cells are assumed to contain approximately 50,000 acceptor sites per cell.

METHYLATING AGENTS

The repair of DNA damaged by methylating agents is well understood (Setlow, this volume). The most important product, m^6dGuo,
is repaired rapidly by a stoichiometric reaction that uses up the
repair protein. Hence low doses that yield few products may have
no biological effect, whereas larger ones would saturate the methyl
accepting protein and result in a linear increase in m^6dGuo with
dose (Fig. 1).

The exogenous and endogenous alkylating agents to which people
usually are exposed are not direct acting ones, as hypothesized in
Fig. 1, but are chemicals such as DMN that require metabolic activation to reactive intermediates before DNA products can be formed.
Since the liver is the seat of major concentration of activation -
detoxification systems, it is not surprising that the alkylation of
hemoglobin shows a curvilinear dose - response curve for DMN (Fig.
2). The chemical is activated and reacts or is detoxified in the
liver at low doses so that it does not get into the circulation,

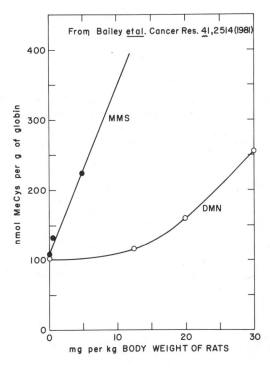

Fig. 2. The observed methylation of cysteine of globin as a function of dose for IP injection of methylmethanesulfonate
(MMS), a direct acting agent, and dimethylnitrosamine (DMN)
an indirect acting agent (Bailey et al., 1981).

Table 1. Mutation frequencies at seven specific loci in the offspring of male mice injected interperitoneally with ethylnitrosourea[a]

| | | Mutations per locus x 10^5 | |
Dose (mg/kg)	offspring	average	induced
0	531,500	0.75	0.0
100	24,900	43.6	43
10 x 10^b	20,000	6.4	6

a. Russell et. al., 1982b
b. 10 mg/kg once a week for 10 weeks

but at high doses the enzyme system is saturated and DMN escapes to
be activated and react in the blood. On the other hand, a direct
acting agent of long half life, such as methylmethanesulfonate
shows a linear dose response curve for the methylation of hemoglobin.

The two effects illustrated in Figs. 1 and 2 imply that extrapolation from high to low doses of alkylation can not be made by a
linear interpolation for either direct or indirect acting chemicals
and that the tissues affected may depend critically on the size of
the administered dose. Moreover, if all tissues were affected
equally the end result may still depend on the DNA repair level in
the tissue (Goth and Rajewsky, 1974).

An excellent example of some of the above concepts is the
induction of specific locus mutations in the offspring of male mice
treated, by IP injection, with the direct acting ethylating agent
ethylnitrosourea (ENU). The dose response curve for acute exposure
is nonlinear (Russell et. al. 1982a) and there is a large dose rate
of effect (Table 1) (Russell et. al. 1982b), consistent with the
idea that at high doses or dose rates DNA repair is saturated.

BACKGROUND DAMAGE

The background damage from the wear and tear of living is the
irreducible minimum against which to measure DNA damage from exogenous radiations or chemicals (Table 2). The rate of accumulation
of background damage is so high that it would amount to approximately 2×10^9 endogenous damages per cell per life time. Since
there are only approximately 10^{10} nucleotides per cell, one is

De Fabo, E.C., and Noonan, F.P., 1983, Mechanism of immune suppression by ultraviolet irradiation in vivo. I. Evidence for the existence of a unique photoreceptor in skin and its role in photoimmunology, J. Exper. Med., 157:84.

Goth, R., and Rajewsky, M.F., 1974, Persistence of O^6-ethylguanine in rat-brain DNA: Correlation with nervous system-specific carcinogenesis by ethylnitrosourea, Proc. Natl. Acad. Sci. USA, 71:639.

Hoel, D.G., Kaplan, N.L., and Anderson, M.W., 1983, Implication of nonlinear kinetics on risk estimation in carcinogenesis, Science, 219:1032.

Kemp, L.M., Sedgwick, S.G., and Jeggo, P.A., 1984, X-ray-sensitive mutants of Chinese hamster ovary cells defective in double-strand break rejoining, Mutat. Res., 132:189.

Morison, W.L., 1983, Effects of UV radiation on immune reaction in humans, in: "Photoimmunology," pp. 205-214, J.A. Parrish, M.L. Kripke, and W.L. Morison, eds., Plenum Press, New York.

Pegg, A.E., 1984, Methylation of the O^6 position of guanine in DNA is the most likely event in carcinogenesis by methylating agents, Cancer Invest., 2:223.

Russell, W.L., 1963, The effect of radiation dose rate and fractionation on mutation in mice, in: "Repair from Genetic Radiation Damage," pp. 205-217, F.H. Sobels, eds., Pergamon Press, Oxford.

Russell, W.L., Hunsicker, P.R., Raymer, G.D., Steele, M.H., Stelzner, K.F., and Thompson, H.M., 1982a, Dose-response curve for ethylnitrosourea-induced specific-locus mutations in mouse spermatogonia, Proc. Natl. Acad. Sci USA, 79:3589.

Russell, W.L., Hunsicker, P.R., Carpenter, D.A., Cornett, C.V., and Guinn, G.M., 1982b, Effect of dose fractionation on the ethylnitrosourea induction of specific-locus mutations in mouse spermatogonia, Proc. Natl. Acad. Sci. USA, 79:3592.

Setlow, R.B., 1980, Damages to DNA that result in transformation, Adv. Biol. Med. Phys., 17:99.

Setlow, R.B., 1983, Quantitative assessment of risks, in: "Short-Term Tests for Environmentally Induced Chronic Health Effects," pp. 1-10, A.D. Woodhead, ed., U.S. Environmental Protection Agency, Washington.

Setlow, R.B., 1985, Saturation of DNA repair, in: "Assessment of Risk from Low-Level Exposure to Radiation and Chemicals: A Critical Overview, " in press, A.D. Woodhead, C.J. Shellabarger, and V. Pond, eds., Plenum Press, New York.

Setlow, R.B., and Setlow, J.K., 1972, Effects of radiation on polynucleotides, Annu. Rev. Biophys. Bioengineer., 1:293.

Singer, B., 1984, Alkylation of the O^6 of guanine is only one of the many chemical events that initiate carcinogenesis, Cancer Invest., 2:233.

GENETIC EFFECTS OF RADIATION

William J. Schull

The Epidemiology Research Center
School of Public Health, UT Health Science Center
Houston, Texas

INTRODUCTION

Evaluation of the genetic risk of exposure to ionizing radiation rests on a variety of experiences. These include (1) exposure to diagnostic and therapeutic doses of X-ray and radioactive materials such as radium or cobalt, (2) occupationally incurred exposures, e.g., in uranium mining or the maintenance of nuclear reactors, (3) geographic areas with "high" natural or man-made background radiation levels, and (4) the atomic bombings of Hiroshima and Nagasaki. Exposure from these sources varies substantially, qualitatively and quantitatively. It may be acute or chronic, of a single quality or several, whole body or partial, prompted by illness and hence possibly confounded by health status, and so forth. So disparate is such exposure and the methods of ascertainment used that it is impossible to examine these data in any collective manner. Accordingly, for this and several other reasons, this presentation will emphasize the studies of the offspring of the A-bomb survivors conducted initially by the Atomic Bomb Casualty Commission (ABCC) and now the Radiation Effects Research Foundation (RERF). First, from these experiences has been gathered the largest body of data, exceeding that from all other studies collectively. Second, these data do not confound medical indications for the use of ionizing radiation with the effects of the latter. Third, the survivors themselves represent both sexes, and a variety of ages, socio-economic statuses, occupations and the like; they are a "general population." Fourth, although there remain uncertainties about the precise amount of radiation survivors may have received, their individual doses are better known than for most other groups. Finally, at one time or another many of the various mutational surveillance strategies that have been suggested, have been

employed; these include a search for changes in the frequency of
(a) certain population characteristics, for example, the
occurrence of major congenital defect and premature death; (b)
sentinel phenotypes; (c) chromosomal abnormalities; and (d)
biochemical variants of a structural or kinetic nature. Although
these alternatives are diverse, their aims are the same -- to
estimate the probability of mutation per unit exposure to ionizing
radiation and to ascertain the public health implications of an
increase in the mutations measured.

POPULATION CHARACTERISTICS

     Continuous genetic surveillance of the children born in
Hiroshima and Nagasaki subsequent to the atomic bombing began on a
substantial scale in 1948. As previously stated, a variety of
studies have ensued, the first utilized the post-war Japanese
rationing system as a case-finding mechanism. A provision of this
system entitled pregnant women, who registered their pregnancies
after the fifth lunar month, to access to supplementary
foodstuffs. As a consequence of the stringency of the postwar
economic circumstances, most women registered their pregnancies,
and through this means, it was possible to identify more than 95%
of all pregnancies in these cities persisting for at least 20
weeks of gestation; and upon the termination of each to examine
the outcome. These observations, made in the home generally, were
supported by an infant autopsy program and a second examination of
some 20 percent of surviving infants 8-10 months after their birth
at the clinical facilities of ABCC (see Neel and Schull, 1956, for
a fuller description of this study).

     The indicators of possible genetic effects obtainable from a
program of examination of newly born infants, such as that just
described, include sex, birth weight, viability at birth, presence
of gross malformation, occurrence of death during the first month
of life, and physical development at age 8-10 months -- all
confounded by a variety of extraneous factors. A comprehensive
analysis of the data accumulated through 1953 revealed marginal
findings on the sex-ratio and survival of liveborn infants, and
prompted a continuation of the collection of data on these latter
two variables. Eventually over 140,000 births were involved in
the sex-ratio study (Schull, Neel and Hashizume, 1966), but these
data now seem less relevant, or at least less readily incorporated
into an assessment of the mutagenic effects of ionizing radiation
in man. The simple theory of sex-linked inheritance on which
prediction of an effect of parental exposure on the sex ratio
rested seems no longer tenable; it is compromised by the
occurrence of X-chromosomal inactivation and sex chromosomal
abnormalities that can confuse simple anthroposcopic determination
of sex.

384

The study of survival which ensued, the F_1 Mortality Study (Kato and Schull, 1960; Neel, Kato and Schull, 1974), continues. It focuses on three age, city and sex-matched cohorts; the first involves all infants liveborn in the two cities between May 1946 and December 1958 one or both of whose parents were within two kilometers of the hypocenter at the time of the bombing; the second, an age, city and sex-matched cohort randomly drawn from the remaining births in the two cities during this same period, for which one parent was exposed at 2500 meters or beyond and the other similarly exposed or not exposed at all and finally, a second age, city and sex-matched cohort randomly drawn from the births in these cities in these years where neither parent was present at the time of the atomic bombing. Recently, these cohorts of children have been enlarged to include births occurring in the period from January 1959 through December 1980.

Before the findings of these two programs are examined, it is necessary to describe the estimates of dose that have been used. The so-called T65 dosimetry (Milton and Shohoji, 1968) has served as the basis for the dose-response analyses of data collected in Hiroshima and Nagasaki for the last decade and a half; it assigns to each survivor separate estimates of gamma and neutron exposures, and total kerma based upon the stated distance from 'ground zero' in Hiroshima or Nagasaki and the shielding which may have attenuated the "free-in-air" dose. The appropriateness of these estimates has been questioned (Kerr, 1981; Loewe and Mendelsohn, 1981; see also, RERF, 1983, 1984). It is maintained that the neutron exposures in Hiroshima and Nagasaki may have been only 15-23% those previously thought, and the energies involved "softer", less penetrating. These developments do not affect individual exposures in Nagasaki greatly, but their effect in Hiroshima is more substantial. A precise evaluation does not exist as yet, for at the moment individual exposure under the new dosimetry can only be estimated for those persons who were exposed in the open, a minority of the survivors within two kilometers. Overall, some reduction in estimated total kerma is likely in Nagasaki but an increase seems probable in Hiroshima, especially at distances of two kilometers or so. This could alter the slope of the regression relationship and hence the estimates of risk to be presented shortly.

Clinical Findings

In 1948 through 1953, as a part of the clinical program previously described, 76,617 pregnancy terminations were studied of which 6,535 are unsuitable for analysis, mostly because the requisite data are incomplete or the pregnancy was unregistered. The clinical findings identify those pregnancies that terminated in a child with a major congenital defect, who was stillborn or

385

died during the first week of life. Genetic theory predicts an increase in such terminations proportional to the radiation dose of the parents because of the induction of mutations with deleterious effects. However, some of these types of outcome are not independent of one another -- a severely malformed infant is more likely to be stillborn, or if born alive, to succumb shortly after birth than a child without conspicuous defect. The analytic and interpretive issues posed by these interrelationships are circumvented if all pregnancies terminating in a malformed infant or one stillborn or dying in the first month of life are viewed as 'similar events,' and the data on the 70,082 acceptable pregnancy terminations summarized under the rubric "untoward pregnancy outcome."

The distribution of "untoward outcome" by parental exposure when the cities and sexes are combined, and the results of an analysis which regresses the frequencies of these events on parental exposures and a variety of concomitant variables known to influence their occurrence have been described elsewhere (Schull, Otake and Neel, 1981a, b). The increase in frequency of an untoward outcome per Sievert (100 rem) of gonadal exposure, as measured by the regression coefficient, was 0.001824 (standard error = 0.003232). In this analysis, a period characterized by an infant and childhood mortality rate of about 7 percent (see Ministry of Welfare, 1957), if one assumes that approximately one in every 400 liveborn infants died before reaching maturity because of radiation-related mutation (point or chromosomal), the gametic doubling dose, based on the regression estimate above, becomes simply [0.0025/0.0000182]/2 or 0.69 Sv. The assumption of one in 400 is conservative; values as high as one in 200 are defensible.

Here we present a somewhat different analysis, a more pragmatic one. Untoward pregnancy outcome has been distributed by maternal age, paternal age and parity, arguably the three most important sources of extraneous variation. The observed frequencies of untoward pregnancies among all parents were used to define a series of "maternal age-paternal age-parity" specific probabilities of an untoward outcome. These values were used, in turn, to calculate the expected number of such pregnancies in five dose categories, namely, less than one, 1-9, 10-49, 50-99 and 100+ cGy, based upon the combined parental exposures. The difference between the observed and expected numbers in each category, the "excess cases," was then regressed on average dose -- an analysis similar to that commonly used with the mortality data generated by the Life Span Study of the Radiation Effects Research Foundation (see, e.g., Beebe, Kato and Land, 1978; Kato and Schull, 1982).

Before the results of this analysis are presented the assumptions inherent in what has been done must be made explicit.

First, even though the sample on which the "maternal age-paternal age-parity" specific probabilities are based is large, these values are necessarily estimates of the "true" risk and hence are not without their own sampling errors. These are ignored in the analysis. Second, to combine parental exposures, as we have done, tacitly assumes that the risk to the child is the same irrespective of the sex of the exposed parent if only one was exposed, or if both parents were, upon total exposure rather than how doses were distributed over the parents. This may not be justified. There are significant differences in gametogenesis in the two sexes, and furthermore, there is evidence that the oocytes of the mouse and squirrel monkey are uncommonly sensitive to ionizing radiation. A single traversal of the cell membrane by a photon of energy may be sufficient to kill the cell (Dobson et al., 1978). Although the BEIR and UNSCEAR Reports on the genetic effects of exposure to ionizing radiation assume this is also true for the human oocyte, and discount a maternal contribution to the genetic impact of exposure, it is not known whether the human oocyte is equally sensitive. Under the circumstances, it is more conservative to assume maternal exposure to have an effect equal to that of paternal exposure. Finally, there are other sources of extraneous variation for which we have not adjusted that could obscure a radiation effect or create a spurious one. Of these, variation in infant mortality with time, not explicable in terms of changes in parental ages and the like, may be the most important. However, as extensive as the experience within these cities is, it does not support still further subdivision.

Table 1. Excess untoward pregnancy terminations and their relative risks in different exposure categories, Hiroshima and Nagasaki combined, 1948-1954.

Exposure groups (cGy)	Number of Pregnancies	Number of untoward outcomes Observed	Expected	Relative Risk
< 1	57908	2746	2745.90	1.00
1 - 9	6974	306	336.86	0.91
10 - 49	2854	153	137.55	1.11
50 - 99	1221	67	59.05	1.13
100 +	1125	60	51.89	1.16

Table 1 sets out the sample sizes in the five dose categories, the observed and expected number of untoward pregnancy outcomes in each, and the relative risk. The observed frequency of untoward outcome was regressed on the mid-value of the dose interval, and the regression was fitted through an intercept of zero. The resulting regression coefficient is 63 untoward pregnancy outcomes per million pregnancies per cGy. To compare this value with the absolute risk of leukemia or cancers other than leukemia the genetic risk must be related to time. Since the cancer risks are on an annual basis, and since the genetic one represents the time from the atomic bombing to the average year of birth -- six years, as a first approximation -- the pregnancy risk per year per cGy is about 10. This differs less than a factor of two from the excess cancer incidence cases per million person year rad (see Wakabayashi et al., 1983; Kato et al., personal communication).

Mortality

Originally the F_1 mortality cohort involved 52,621 live, single births where the exposure of both parents was known (Kato and Schull, 1960; Kato, Schull, and Neel, 1966; Neel, Kato and Schull, 1974). To this group has been added 22,984 births in the years from January 1959 through December 1980 of which 11,196 are to parents of known exposure status. Most of the latter parents were too young at the time of their exposure to have had children in the years from 1946 through 1958. Their inclusion provides insight into possible time dependent repair mechanisms and age differences in sensitivity to mutation, similar to the differences that have been seen in absolute and relative risks of radiation-related malignancy (Kato and Schull, 1982).

Deaths within the cohort are ascertained through examination of the household censuses required by law (Naruge, 1956). A copy of the death schedule is obtained on every individual who has died since his or her koseki was last perused. Normally a five-year cycle intervenes between one scrutiny of the koseki and the next.

Among the 63,817 individuals whose parents' exposures are known, there have been 3,786 deaths (3,552 in the original cohort and 234 in the extension). Our remarks here are restricted to the original cohort, for two reasons. First, the bulk of the deaths recorded involve individuals in this portion of the data, and second, individual doses have not as yet been assigned to most of the parents in the extension. Although the distance from the epicenter is known, the shielding has not been evaluated. Through December 1971, 3,231 deaths occurred in the original cohort; 321 additional deaths (about 10% more) occurred in the years 1972-1980. The results of the analysis to which reference has been made and one which includes the years 1972-1980 are shown in Table 2. Two analyses are presented, one which does and one which does not take cognizance of concomitant variation which could influence the risk of death. The gametic doubling dose remains essentially unchanged with the addition of eight more years of experience. Concomitant variation affects the estimate somewhat, but not greatly when one considers its inherent error. At face value, the impact of parental exposure to one Sievert is only one-fifth to one-eighth that associated with a year's difference in the time of birth over these years.

Table 2. Increments or decrements in the frequency of death in the F_1 mortality cohort per Sievert of gonadal dose (T65 estimate), based on an assumed RBE of 5. The standard error of each regression coefficient is indicated in parentheses. [after Schull et al., 1982]

Variable	Years at risk of death	
	1946-1971[1]	1946-1980[2]
Concomitant sources of variation ignored		
Joint parental exposure	0.000927 (0.001140)	0.000513 (0.001165)
Gametic doubling dose	1.35 Sv	2.44 Sv
Concomitant sources of variation considered		
Joint parental exposure	0.001130 (0.001900)	0.000730 (0.001390)
Year of birth	-0.005880 (0.000307)	-0.006207 (0.000316)
Gametic doubling dose	1.10 Sv	1.71 Sv

[1] Data drawn from Neel, Kato and Schull (1974)

[2] Analysis of Schull et al. (1982)

Seventy-two of these 3,552 deaths were ascribed to malignancy. The most common site was leukemia (35 cases). No clear trend in the occurrence of these deaths exists. The frequency of deaths per 1000 individuals at risk varies from 0.36 (both parents exposed) to 1.18 (father only exposed). The statistical errors associated with these estimates are substantial. Ishimaru, Ichimaru and Mikami (1981) have examined the relationship of the incidence of leukemia in this cohort to parental exposure more exactly. They find no radiation-related excess. The relative risk of leukemia among the children of survivors, after adjustment for city and sex differences, was 0.8 (as contrasted, of course, with 1.0 among individuals whose parents collectively received less than one cGy of exposure). Cancer of the stomach was the next most frequent site (9 cases); again, there is no trend with exposure. This might seem an unusual number, given the ages of the cohort, but cancer of the stomach is the most common malignancy in Japan and the number encountered in the F_1 Study is consistent with published age-specific rates (Otake, 1979).

SENTINEL PHENOTYPES

It has been argued that one potentially useful mutational surveillance strategy involves the search for changes in the rate of occurrence of the isolated case (within the family) of certain phenotypes, so-called sentinel ones, which have a high probability of being due to dominant mutation (Mulvihill and Czeizel, 1983). Among these phenotypes are aniridia, chondrodystrophy, epiloia, neurofibromatosis, and retinoblastoma. Some of these are, or have been until recently, fatal tumors, and most are presumably readily diagnosable. Among surveys of sentinel phenotypes, we include those clinical (as contrasted with cytogenetical) surveys that have sought to establish changes in the "normal" frequencies of phenotypes such as Down's, Klinefelter's and Turner's syndromes.

Insofar as the phenotypes earlier enumerated are concerned, in the absence of continuing clinical examination of the F1, the only ones under constant scrutiny in Hiroshima and Nagasaki have been those associated with childhood malignancy -- leukemia, retinoblastoma, Wilms' tumor and the like. The Tumor Registries in these cities make possible the identification of these occurrences as well as malignancies among cancer prone diseases such as those associated with immunodeficiency or neurofibromatosis. In the years the Registries have existed only one case of retinoblastoma and two of Wilms' tumor have been encountered. These small numbers offer no persuasive evidence of a relationship between the occurrence of cancer and parental radiation.

Three separate studies of Down's syndrome and the syndromes associated with sex chromosomal aneuploidy have been made. First, no relationship between maternal radiation and Down's syndrome

could be demonstrated in the clinical study previously described
(see Schull and Neel, 1962, for details). Second, Slavin, Kamada
and Hamilton (1966) studied some 92 individuals with Down's
syndrome drawn largely from eight schools for mentally retarded
children, five in Hiroshima Prefecture and three in Nagasaki.
Twelve additional non-institutionalized cases were ascertained
through five large hospitals in Hiroshima. Of these 92 cases, in
nine instances one or both parents were exposed and the child
conceived subsequently. Seven of these cases were simple trisomy
21, one was trisomy with a D/D translocation and the final case
involved mosaicism. Among these nine cases only two had exposures
of greater than one cGy -- one mother received 8 and another 16.
These estimates are the T65 "free-in-air" doses. Although
appropriate denominators for these cases are not clear, even the
case numbers themselves are not compelling.

Finally, a buccal smear survey was conducted in April-May
1963 on 8192 students in Hiroshima scheduled for dental screening
examinations at two junior and five senior high schools in
Hiroshima (Omori et al, 1965). Most of these students (all save
921) were born between April 1946 and March 1949. Of the smears
obtained on these 8192 students, 7141 (4481 males, 2660 females)
were deemed acceptable for analysis. No abnormalities were seen
among the 2660 females, but three cases of Klinefelter's syndrome
were seen among the 4481 males. None of the latter three were
conceived by parents exposed to the atomic bombing. Clearly, these
studies do not lend themselves, singly or collectively to doubling
dose estimation so sparse are the data.

CHROMOSOMAL ABNORMALITIES

Although studies of radiation related chromosomal damage
among the survivors began as early as 1949, reliable information
had to await the development in the late 1950s of the use of
leukocyte cultures with phytohemagglutinin and the other
technological steps now in vogue. An investigation of the
children of exposed parents was initiated in 1968, the subjects
being drawn from the cohorts established for the F_1 Mortality
Study. Awa and his colleagues (1981) have described this
undertaking and summarized the cytogenetic findings through 1980.
Since the youngest children in the study were 13 and the oldest 37
at the time of their examination, the survey will not yield
adequate data on the frequency of cytogenetic abnormalities
associated with increased mortality rates, such as unbalanced
autosomal structural rearrangements or autosomal trisomies.
However, the data on sex chromosomal abnormalities and balanced
autosomal structural rearrangements should, however, be relatively
unbiased even now. Data have not as yet been published on the
frequency of sister-chromatid exchanges and the like although such
observations are being made.

Awa and his coworkers find the frequency of sex-chromosome aneuploids in the children of parents exposed beyond 2499 meters to be 13/5058 or 0.00257. They have seen 3 XYY males, 6 XXY, 2 XXX females and 2 others. The frequency in the children of parents exposed within 2000 meters, with an average combined exposure of 0.87 Sv, is 16/5762 or 0.00278. There were 3 XYY, 2 XXY, 2 XXX, 1 XXq- and 1 X/XXX. These figures, though not statistically significantly different, can be taken at face value to generate zygotic and gametic doubling doses. The former is 10.71 Sv and the latter 5.35.

BIOCHEMICAL VARIANTS

Electrophoretic techniques for the identification of abnormal protein molecules created a new means to assess the genetic effects of A-bomb exposure. This approach, like the cytogenetic one, is free of many of the ambiguities inherent in the study of population characteristics or sentinel phenotypes. Accordingly, after a pilot study, a full-scale investigation employing this technique was undertaken in Hiroshima and Nagasaki in 1976. The subjects have been drawn from the cohorts of children born to exposed parents identified for the mortality study previously described. The same blood sample serves the needs of both. Each child is examined for rare electrophoretic variants of 28 proteins of the blood plasma and erythrocyte, and since 1979, a subset of the children is further studied for deficiency variants of eleven of the erythrocyte enzymes.

A rare electrophoretic variant is defined as one with a phenotype frequency of less than 2% in the population and an "enzyme deficiency" or "low activity" variant as one which results in an enzyme level three standard deviations below the mean (or less than 66% of normal activity). When either a structural or activity variant is encountered, its occurrence is first verified and then blood samples from both parents are examined for the presence of a similar variant. If the variant is not also found in one or both parents, and a discrepancy between putative and biological parentage is improbable, it presumably represents a mutation. Some eleven different red cell antigenic systems and the HLA phenotypes are used to explore discrepancies between the child and his or her putative parents.

Satoh and her colleagues (1982, unpublished) have estimated that they have information on the equivalent of 642,004 locus tests on 13,052 children born to parents whose average combined gonadal dose is approximately 0.59 Sv. Three probable mutations were described -- one, a slow migrating variant of glutamate pyruvate transaminase, another a slow migrating variant of phosphoglucomutase-2, and finally one involving nucleophosphorylase. Three probable mutations have also been seen in the equivalent of 478,803 locus tests on 10,609 children whose parents, one or both, were exposed beyond 2400 meters, that is, received less than one cSv. These variants involve the haptoglobin, 6-phosphogluconate dehydrogenase and adenosine deaminase systems. The two estimates of the rate of mutation are 0.47 and 0.63 x 10^{-5}, respectively. These numbers will undoubtedly increase still further for the family studies necessary to establish a probable mutation proceed slowly.

More recently, Satoh and her colleagues (1983, unpublished) have reported the results of the first 44,010 determinations, distributed over 11 enzymes, to assess the impact of parental exposure on the frequency of "deficiency variants." One probable mutation has been found, giving a mutation rate of 2.27 x 10^{-5}. Patently, neither these data nor those on structural variants are sufficiently extensive to warrant strong inferences.

ESTIMATES OF RISK

Conventionally, two parameters have been used to characterize the risk of radiation-related mutation. These are the probability of a mutation at a specific locus per unit of exposure, and the so-called "doubling dose." The latter is that dose at which the ratio of the spontaneous mutation rate to the slope of the dose response curve is precisely two. Each has its use and its advocates. Experimentalists favor the first for it reflects the nature of the data they collect and the issues they confront. Population biologists, however, favor the doubling dose. This is especially true of human population geneticists for no estimates of specific locus rates of induced mutation exist save the limited biochemical data previously described.

While there may be a mutability common to all DNA, as a public health issue, only those mutational events that are potentially transmissible are important and these clearly depend upon the biology of the organism involved. One out of every two or three human conceptuses, for example, is aborted spontaneously (see Abramson, 1971, for a review of the literature). If abortion is a random event, one would expect transmitted mutations to number only a third of those that actually occur. However, if mutations are generally deleterious, as the evidence supports, abortions are likely to be non-random, and the number 'recoverable' even lower. Human populations may purge some portion of newly arisen mutations, and thus lessen their public health impact. Be this as it may, we have three estimates of the doubling dose, on untoward pregnancy outcome, F_1 mortality and sex chromosome aneuploids, respectively. As we have seen, they differ. The preferred estimate would seem to be some function of the three. The best function, perhaps, is the weighted average of the individual estimates where the weights are the inverses of the variances of the several estimates; this, in effect, places the greatest credence in the estimate with the smallest sampling error.

As rough approximations to the three standard deviations of the doubling dose estimates we obtain 0.93, 3.88 and 24.26 Sv for untoward pregnancy outcome, F_1 mortality, and sex chromosome aneuploids. The coefficient of variation is especially large in the latter case, for the doubling dose lies well outside the dose interval covered by the observations. The weighted average of the estimates is 1.4 Sv with a standard deviation of 1.6 Sv. The true variance must actually be somewhat larger, for the doubling dose estimates for untoward pregnancy outcome and F_1 mortality are not wholly independent (neonatal deaths contribute to both estimates).

Earlier, we described an analysis that yields an estimate of the risk of an untoward pregnancy outcome with exposure. The estimate itself proved to be 63 per million pregancy-rad. In terms of impact, this suggests, first, that out of a million pregnancies terminating under the circumstances that prevailed in these years (when 47,500 pregnancies would have naturally ended untowardly within the first year of life), exposure to one cGy would have increased this number by some 63 cases. The relative risk would have increased to 1.001! Second, as we have earlier noted, this pregnancy risk is about twice that of cancer among the survivors (Kato and Schull, 1982; Wakabayashi, Kato, Ikeda and Schull, 1983). If at least a half of the pregnancy risk is attributable to radiation-related mutations, a conservative estimate presumably, then the genetic and cancer risks would be approximately equal.

The approximate nature of this estimate cannot be overly emphasized. First, it is based on the use of the mid-interval dose as representative of the values within an interval. In fact, the average dose, at least in those categories below 100 cGy, is somewhat less. However, this should lead to an underestimation of the dose-response relationship. Second, it treats all pregnancies as independent of one another; however many mothers registered on more than one occasion. To the extent, then, that successive outcomes to the same woman are correlated, the sampling error of this estimate is even larger than has been estimated. Third, of necessity we have ignored temporal trends in stillbirth and neonatal death rates. But these, particularly the latter, have fallen with time, and so too has the birth rate. Thus, relatively more children were born to exposed parents in the years when socio-economic circumstances contributed more to pregnancy wastage.

Measures of mortality and congenital malformation have
immediate meaning to the public; whereas the occurrence of a new
mutant form of glutamate pyruvate transaminase, for example, does
not. But to the geneticist, events of the latter kind have a
precision of measurement of the frequency of mutation not to be
found in changes in the frequencies of variables where the role
of genetic factors are uncertain. Similarly, mortality
surveillance, such as the one in Hiroshima and Nagasaki, is
inexpensive, but the biochemical studies are not. Undoubtedly
technological developments will, with time narrow these cost
differences and undoubtedly contribute new endpoints to measure.
Indeed, even now, the feasibility of such techniques as two-
dimensional electrophoresis, DNA sequencing, and the use of
restriction fragments to assess polymorphism are being explored.
These alternatives, unquestionably more elegant than those used in
the past to assess mutagenesis in this population, must still
confront the issue of their relevance to the concerns of the
public, and these focus on the health and well-being of their
children.

ACKNOWLEDGMENTS

The observations here described stem from a study conducted
originally by the Atomic Bomb Casualty Commission (ABCC) in
cooperation with the Japanese National Institute of Health of the
Ministry of Health and Welfare (JNIH), and presently pursued by
the successor to ABCC, the Radiation Effects Research Foundation
(RERF). The ABCC was a research agency of the U. S. National
Academy of Sciences-National Research Council and was supported by
Contract AT-49-1-GEN-72 of the U. S. Atomic Energy Commission.
The study is presently funded by the Japanese Ministry of Health
and Welfare and by the National Academy of Sciences-National
Research Council with support from Contract Ex-76-C-28-3161 from
the Department of Energy.

REFERENCES

Abramson, F. D., 1971, "Spontaneous fetal death in man: A methodological and analytical evaluation," Ph. D. Dissertation, University of Michigan, Ann Arbor, Michigan.

Awa, A., Honda, T., Neriishi, S., Hamilton, H. B., 1981, Cytogenetic study of the children of A-bomb survivors--An interim report, Jap. J. Hum. Genet., 26:130.

Beebe, G. W., Kato, H. and Land, C. E., 1978, Life Span Study Report 6. Mortality experience of atomic bomb survivors, 1950-74. Radiat. Res., 75:138.

Dobson, R. L., Koehler, C. G., Felton, J. S., Kwan, T. C., Wuebbles, B. J. and Jones, D. C. C., 1978 Vulnerability of female germ cells in developing mice and monkeys to tritium, gamma rays, and polycyclic aromatic hydrocarbons, in, "Developmental Toxicology of Energy-related Pollutants," D. D. Mahlem, M. R. Sikov, P. L. Hackett, F. D. Andrew, eds, Technical Information Center, U. S. Department of Energy, Washington, D. C.

Ishimaru, T., Ichimaru, M. and Mikami, M., 1981, Leukemia incidence among individuals exposed in utero, children of atomic bomb survivors, and their controls, Hiroshima and Nagasaki, 1945-1979. Radiation Effects Research Foundation Technical Report 11-81.

Kato, H. and Schull, W. J., 1960, Joint JNIH-ABCC life-span study of children born to atomic bomb survivors, research plan. Atomic Bomb Casualty Commission Technical Report 4-60.

Kato, H. and Schull, W. J., 1982, Studies of the mortality of A-bomb survivors. 7. Mortality, 1950-1978: Part I. Cancer mortality. Radiat. Res., 90:395.

Kato, H., Schull, W. J., Neel, J. V., 1966, A cohort-type study of survival in the children of parents exposed to atomic bombings, Am. J. Hum. Genet., 18:339.

Kerr, G. D., 1979, Organ dose estimates for the Japanese atomic bomb survivors. Health Phys., 37:487.

Kerr, G. D., 1981, Review of the dosimetry for the atomic bomb survivors, in, " Proceedings of the Fourth Symposium on Neutron Dosimetry, Gesellschaft fur Strahlen-und Umweltforschung, Munich-

Neuherberg, June 1-5, 1981", Vol. 1, pp 501-513, Office for Official Publications of the European Communities, Luxemburg.

Kerr, G. D. and Salomon, D. K., 1976, The epicenter of Nagasaki weapon: A reanalysis of available data with recommended values, Oak Ridge National Laboratory ORNL-TM-5139.

Loewe, W. E. and Mendelsohn, E., 1981, Neutron and gamma doses at Hiroshima and Nagasaki. Lawrence Livermore Laboratory Publ UCRL-86595.

Milton, R. C. and Shohoji, T., 1968, Tentative 1965 radiation dose estimation for atomic bomb survivors, Hiroshima-Nagasaki. Atomic Bomb Casualty Commission Technical Report 1-68.

Ministry of Welfare, 1957, "Vital Statistics 1955, Japan," Volumes 1 and 2, Division of Health and Welfare Statistics, Ministry of Welfare, Tokyo.

Mulvihill, J. J. and Czeizel, A., 1983, Perspectives in mutation epidemiology, 6. A 1983 view of sentinel phenotypes. Mutation Res., 123:345-361.

Naruge, T., 1956, "Koseki no Jitsumu to sono Riron [The Koseki: Theory and Practice]," Nihon Kajo-Shuppan, Tokyo.

Neel, J. V. and Schull, W. J., 1956, "The effect of exposure to the atomic bombs on pregnancy termination in Hiroshima and Nagasaki," NAS-NRC Publ. No. 461, Washington, D. C.

Neel, J. V., Kato, H. and Schull, W. J., 1974, Mortality in the children of atomic bomb survivors and controls, Genetics, 76:311.

Omori, Y., Morrow, L. B., Ishimaru, T., Johnson, K. G., Maeda, T., Shibukawa, T. and Tabaki, K., 1965, A buccal smear survey for sex chromatin aberration in high school students, Hiroshima. Atomic Bomb Casualty Commission Technical Report 11-65.

Otake, M., 1979, Patterns in cancer mortality in the United States and Japan. Radiation Effects Technical Report 13-79.

RERF (Radiation Effects Research Foundation), 1983, "First US-Japan Joint Workshop for Reassessment of Atomic Bomb Radiation Dosimetry in Hiroshima and Nagasaki," Radiation Effects Research Foundation, Hiroshima, Japan.

RERF, 1984, "Second US-Japan Joint Workshop for Reassessment of Atomic Bomb Radiation Dosimetry in Hiroshima and Nagasaki, with Special Reference to Shielding and Organ Doses," Radiation Effects Research Foundation, Hiroshima, Japan.

Satoh, C., Awa, A. A., Neel, J. V., Schull, W. J., Kato, H., Hamilton, H. B., Otake, M., Goriki, K., 1982, Genetic effects of atomic bombs, in, "The Unfolding Genome," Part A., B. Bonne-Tamir, ed, Alan R. Liss Inc., New York.

Satoh, C., Neel, J. V., Yamashita, A., Goriki, K., Fujita, M., Hamilton, H. B., 1983, The frequency among Japanese of heterozygotes for deficiency variants of 11 enzymes, Am. J. Hum. Genet., 35:656.

Schull, W. J., Neel, J. V. and Hashizume, A., 1966, Some further observations on the sex ratio among infants born to survivors of the atomic bombings of Hiroshima and Nagasaki. Am. J. Hum. Genet., 18:328-338.

Schull, W. J. and Neel, J. V., 1962, Letter-to-Editor: Maternal radiation and mongolism, Lancet, ii:537.

Schull, W. J., Neel, J. V., Otake, M., Awa, A., Satoh, C., and Hamilton, H. B., 1982, Hiroshima and Nagasaki: Three and a half decades of genetic screening, in, "Environmental Mutagens and Carcinogens," T. Sugimura, S. Kondo, and H. Takebe, eds, University of Tokyo Press, Tokyo.

Schull, W. J., Otake, M. and Neel, J. V., 1981, Genetic effects of the atomic bombs: A reappraisal. Science 213:1220-1227.

Schull, W. J., Otake, M. and Neel, J. V. 1981 In: Hook, E. (Ed) Human Mutation: Biological and Population Aspects.

Slavin, R. E., Kamada, N. and Hamilton H. B., 1966, A cytogenetic study of 92 cases of Down's syndrome, Hiroshima-Nagasaki. Atomic Bomb Casualty Commission Technical Report 2-66.

Wakabayashi, T., Kato, H., Ikeda, T., and Schull, W. J., 1983, Studies of the mortality of A-bomb survivors, Report 7. Part III. Incidence of cancer in 1959-1978, based on the Tumor Registry, Nagasaki. Radiat. Res., 93:112-146.

ON THE EFFECTS OF EXPOSURE TO RADON DAUGHTERS IN METAL MINES AND IN HOMES

Olav Axelson

Department of Occupational Medicine
University Hospital
S-581 85 Linköping, Sweden

INTRODUCTION

Mining is a hazardous trade because of accidents and occupational illnesses. Already in the 16th century, both Paracelsus and Agricola reported that lung disorders were frequently occurring among the miners in central Europe. In our time it has been suggested that these early observations might have had to do with lung cancer (Hueper, 1966), although other conditions like silicosis and tuberculosis presumably were prevalent as well. In 1879, however, a malignant lung disease was clearly identified (Härting and Hesse, 1879) among the miners at Schneeberg in Germany and this cancer hazard was further reported on by Arnstein in 1913. A similarly high lung cancer mortality was somewhat later found also in Joachimsthal or Jachymov in Czechoslovakia (Löwy, 1929; Pirchan and Sikl, 1932). For quite some time, these miners were referred to as providing a rather unique example of occupational lung cancer, due to "radium emanation", or radon, in the mine atmosphere (Ludewig and Lorenser, 1924). The percentage of deaths from lung cancer out of all deaths was high and around 40 %, as reported for the period 1875-1912, i.e. 276 out of 665 miner deaths were due to this single cause.

MINING AND LUNG CANCER

In the context of uranium mining in the US around 1950, the potential lung cancer hazard became a matter of concern and even controversy as to the actual risks involved (Hueper, 1966). However, at this time, also an important step forward was taken by the development a new exposure concept, the working level (WL), one unit

of which means any combination of short-lived radon daughters in
one litre of air, that finally would result in an ultimate emission
of 1.3 x 10^5 MeV of potential alpha energy. Then, by taking in
the time aspect, the final measure of exposure, the "working level
month" (WLM), was obtained, one month refering to an exposure time
of 170 hours in this context. This development was essential because it permitted later dose-response evaluations of lung cancer
among the uranium miners, first provided in the studies presented
in the late 60s and early 70s (Wagoner et al., 1965; Archer and
Lundin, 1969; Lundin et al., 1971).

However, reports on an increased lung cancer mortality also
in non-uranium miners began to appear, e.g. concerning British
hematite miners (Faulds and Stuart, 1956), US copper miners (Wagoner
et al., 1963), French iron ore miners (Rousell et al., 1964),
African gold miners (Osburn, 1969) and Canadian fluorspar miners
(DeVilliers and Windish, 1964) and there was some further updating
on the Czechoslovakian miners at Jachymov (Horacek, 1969). Most
of these populations had apparent exposure to radon and radon
daughters, but arsenic exposure might perhaps have played the greater role for the lung cancer hazard among the African goldminers.

Several more reports on lung cancer among non-uranium miners
have followed in the 70s and 80s, e.g. a further report on the
Cumberland iron miners (Boyd et al., 1970) along with similar observations on Swedish zinc-lead miners (Axelson et al., 1971;
Axelson and Sundell, 1978) as well as iron miners (Jörgensen, 1973;
Renard, 1974; Edling, 1982; Radford and Renard, 1984), all of the
respective mines with moderate levels of radon daughters, i.e.,
roughly up to about one working level. The reports on the epidemics
of lung cancer among uranium miners have also continued from the
US (Archer et al., 1973), Canada (Hewitt, 1979) and Czechoslovakia
(Sevc et al., 1976; Kunz et al., 1978; Kunz et al., 1979). It is
noteworthy in this context, that no clear excess of lung cancer
has been reported from coal and salt mines, known to be low in
radon and daughters (Waxweiler et al., 1973). Consequently, the
epidemiologic evidence is quite convincing that radon daughter
exposure is the causal agent behind the presumably world-wide lung
cancer hazard among miners, not only in uranium mines but also
in metal mines, whenever radon occurs in the work environment.

Some Features of Miners' Lung Cancer

Quite some interest has been devoted to the specific character of lung cancer in minders, especially with regard to the influence of smoking, but also to the histological characteristics.
Hence, when one of the early reports on US uranium miners and their
smoking habits was published in 1969 (Lundin et al., 1969), there
were 60 cases versus 15 expected among the smokers but also 2 versus

0,5 expected among the nonsmokers. Therefore, it seemed as if a multiplicative risk might have been at hand for radon daughter exposure and smoking. Furthermore, there was a very considerable relative excess of small cell undifferentiated cancers, i.e. oat cell cancers and related types. However, later on, also epidermoid cancers and finally even the less smoking-dependent adenocarcinomas have been found to appear in excess (Lundin et al., 1971; Saccomanno, 1980; Saccomanno et al., 1981), but in general, there tends to be some predominance of the small cell undifferentiated forms.

This originally observed pattern of a strong dependence of miners' lung cancer on a combination of radon daughter exposure and smoking has not been consistent in later studies of other miners, although it still seems to prevail among the US uranium miners (Whittemore and McMillan, 1983). Some of the other studies show merely additive effects (Edling, 1982; Radford and Renard, 1984), and even a relative protection from smoking has been observed, in a formal sense at least (Axelson and Sundell, 1978; Dahlgren, 1979). Taking the confidence interval for this protection into account, however, these latter reports might very well be consistent with an additive model. It has been suggested though, that also some rather complex mechanisms might be involved and explain the seemingly curious findings, namely an actual reduction of the dose of the shortranging alpha-radiation by mucous, as more abundantly occurring in the respiratory tract of smokers; these aspects will be further dealt with and have also been discussed elsewhere (Axelson, 1984).

The somewhat inconsistent results of the various studies referred to might also have an alternative or an additional, but quite simple explanation, namely that these studies are viewing populations at different phases in the development of the lung cancer risk, i.e., those populations following a multiplicative model being young, those showing additive effects being intermediate in age and those with protection representing old, "mature" populations where the smokers already have passed through their maximum of lung cancer risk (Archer, 1984). This idea implies that the development of lung cancer would go faster among the smoking than among the non-smoking miners, an assumption for which there is some epidemiologic support (Archer, 1973; Axelson and Sundell, 1978; Edling, 1982; Archer, 1984), although again not particularly consistent throughout all relevant studies, one of them even without indication of such a difference in induction-latency time between smokers and nonsmokers (Radford and Renard, 1984). Furthermore, the differences found in induction-latency times are not fully convincing either, as they are ranging from about only 3 years (Edling, 1982) up to about 12 years (Axelson and Sundell, 1978), all estimates being based on relatively few individuals.

RADON IN HOMES - A LUNG CANCER HAZARD?

Energy saving, through reduced ventilation either in heating or cooling air, has focussed interest on increased indoor radon concentrations and the subsequent possibility of a lung cancer hazard. Measurements of radon in homes began in Sweden in the mid-50s (Hultqvist, 1956), indicating differences between wooden houses, brick houses and concrete houses. This information offered a natural basis for testing the possibility that lung cancer in the general population could be causally related to exposure to indoor radon and daughters (Axelson et al., 1979). Thus, cases of lung cancer and referents (controls) of non-cancer deaths were drawn from a rural population, i.e. from a stable population without appreciable influence from industrial risk factors, and these subjects were categorized with regard to the type of house they had lived in. The lowest exposure category referred to wooden houses without a basement and the highest to stone houses with a basement. The result of this study was a significantly increasing trend for the lung cancer risk over exposure categories, the risk being about five-fold for persons in the high exposure category, i.e. stone houses with a basement, as compared to those in the lowest category. However, the study approach was somewhat crude without allowance for smoking, nor for possible and probable emanation of radon from the ground into the houses, as by now known to be most important for indoor radon concentrations according to information that has been obtained mainly during and after this first study. Hence, areas with alum shale deposits have been found to leak out radon, as also many of the Swedish granites and deposits of granite gravel (Åkerblom and Wilson, 1982).

Because of this further information about the contribution from the ground to indoor levels of radon, another study (Edling et al., 1984) was taken up on the island of Oeland in the Baltic. A rather narrow strip of alum shale is located along the western side of the island, except in the north. This particular geological structure provided for a unique possibility to account for radon contribution from the ground, especially as the limestone ground of the rest of the island has a low radioactivity. Again the study population was rural, which helped the elimination of various interfering exposures in the urban environment, and only long term residents, 30 years or more in the same houses, were enrolled in the study. Furthermore, measurements could be made in 86 % of the houses, owners permitting, and smoking habits were also obtained except for one case out of 23 and for 24 out of 202 referents. Again a significant result appeared and indicated an effect of radon and daughters in homes with regard to lung cancer, although the size of the study is regrettably small. Table 1 provides some information from this study, although the original data have been reduced with regard to age stratification; for details the reader

Table 1. Distribution of cases of lung cancer (International Classification of Disease, code 162) and referents (all subjects having lived at the same address for >30 years) into exposure categories based on measurements with alpha sensitive film (modified from Edling et al., 1984).

Gender and smoking	Case/ Ref	Exposure level, Bq/m^3 as equilibrium eqvivalent radon*			
		<50	50-149	>150	>50
Males					
Smokers	C	4	4	1	5
	R	15	7	2	9
Nonsmokers	C	2	1	2	3
	R	40	15	2	17
Females					
Smokers	C	0	0	0	0
	R	5	1	0	1
Nonsmokers	C	2	3	0	3
	R	42	27	3	30
Crude rate ratio		1.0	2.4	4.9	2.8
Stand. mortality ratio		1.0	2.2	4.8	2.6
Mantel-Haenszel rate ratio					
- point estimate		1.0	2.3	5.1	2.7
- 90 % conf. interv.			0.9-5.8	1.4-18.5	1.1-6.4
Mantel-extension $\chi^2 = 4.73$					

Note: The various rate ratios were calculated also with allowance for three age categories, 40-69, 70-79 and 80+.

* Divide by 3700 to obtain working levels (WL)

is referred to the published report on this study (Edling et al., 1984).

There are also a few other studies on the possible import of radon in homes on lung cancer morbidity, both of the correlation type, as from Canada (Letourneau, 1983), Sweden (Edling et al., 1982) and US (Hess et al., 1982), and of a case-referent design, as from US (Simpson and Comstock, 1983) and Sweden (Pershagen et al., 1984). All of these studies are somewhat indicative of a relationship except for the Canadian correlation study and the case-referent study from the US. It is noteworthy though, that there are suggestive trends in this latter non-positive case-referent study and a more relevant classification of exposure than applied might even have lead to another result. With regard to the Canadian correlation study, it might be recalled, that immigration movements would tend to dilute any existing effects, and Canadian asbestos production could be another factor with obscuring influence. However, as a summary view, it seems reasonable to suggest by now that there probably is an impact of radon in homes with regard to lung cancer, a conclusion which might also be looked upon as unavoidable with regard to the generally held idea of a more or less linear, non-threshold relationship of exposure to ionizing radiation and risk of cancer.

SMOKING AND RADON DAUGHTER EXPOSURE

The possible influence of smoking on the induction-latency period for lung cancer among miners has already been discussed, and it seems as if non-smokers might be about as affected as the smokers in the long run, i.e. in the upper ages. It is also of interest here, that Navajo Indians in uranium mining have shown an at least 14-fold (lower 95 % confidence bond) increase in risk for lung cancer (Samet et al.,1984). These Indians were non-smokers and low grade smokers, again indicating that smoking is by no means any pre-requisite for lung cancer to develop in the context of radon daughter exposure. The high relative risk is to some extent presumably reflecting the fact that the reference population also consists of non-smokers and low grade smokers, having a very low lung cancer incidence. Similarly, the iron miners in another recent study (Radford and Renard, 1984) showed a rate ratio of 2.9 for smokers and 10.0 for non-smokers, whereas the excess deaths were 21.8 cases per 10^6 person-years for the smokers and 16.3 cases per 10^6 person-years for the non-smokers.

However, with regard to the house studies, it seems as if especially the smokers are those who develop lung cancer in the presence of radon daughter exposure (Edling et al., 1984; Pershagen et al., 1984), although the present results are based on small numbers and therefore have to be looked upon as preliminary. Nevertheless, these findings seem to be in contradiction with some of the observations on miners, but this is not necessary the case. Hence, it has been found that radon daughters, as electrically charged when created, tend to attach to air-born particles, increasing the indoor radon daughter concentrations in the presence of cigarette smoke (Bergman and Axelson, 1983; Bergman et al., 1984). The implication is simply that smokers get a relatively higher exposure through their own passive smoke and an explanation might also be obtained for the relatively high lung cancer risk, that has been observed among truely passive smokers (cf. Bergman and Axelson, 1983; Axelson, 1984 for further discussion and references).

A further aspect on this issue could be that miners, who work in contaminated air, where the air pollution particles, as carrying radon daughters, are about equally inhaled by smokers and non-smokers. In addition, especially the smokers tend to get bronchitis, (Sluis-Cremer et al., 1967; Jörgensen and Swensson, 1970), which theoretically should offer some protection against the shortranging alpha-radiation and could account for the merely additive or even protective effects seen in miners as already mentioned (cf. also Axelson and Sundell, 1978).No visible such effect should be expected for the general population, however, because of a much lower prevalence of bronchitis in comparison to miners. A phenomenon supporting this reasoning has been observed in smoking beagle dogs, exposed to uranium ore dust and radon daughters. Hence, 9 respiratory cancers developed among 19 non-smoking dogs, whereas only 2 were seen among 19 of the smokers (Cross et al., 1982). The smoking seems to have preceeded each daily radon daughter exposure in this case, i.e. mucous stimulation by the cigarette smoke could very well have offered some protection to the subsequent radon daughter exposure. It is of some interest in this context also, however, that there is a rather early epidemiologic observation suggesting protection from bronchitis against lung cancer among coal miners (Ashley, 1967) and also some other observations have gone in the same direction (cf. Axelson, 1984 for further details). So, considering the seemingly complex pattern of interaction between radon daughter exposure and smoking, one might perhaps suggest, that radon daughter exposure acts merely as an initiator and that smoking to the greater extent would be a promotor of radiation-induced cancers, but also that smoking through mucous stimulation sometimes might reduce the initiating capacity of radon daughter exposure. Animal experiments do also suggest that alpha-radiation acts as an initiator and that subsequent irritation of the respiratory epithelium (Little and Kennedy, 1979) as well as smoking promote the development of cancer (Chameaud et al., 1982).

QUANTITATIVE ASPECTS

From time to time, attempts have been made to obtain quantitative risk estimates for radon daughter exposure through the combination of information from different miner studies. The early risk estimates were relatively low in terms of excess lung cancers per WLM and 10^6 person-years at observation, e.g. 1.8 for US uranium miners, 2.6 for the Joachimsthal and Schneeberg miners and 5.6 for the British haematite miners as given without any age standard or age range (Lundin et al, 1971; Archer, 1971). More recent evaluations tend to give higher estimates, however, i.e., overall figures more close to 20 excess cases per WLM and 10^6 person-years, still without any age limitations, but increasing to about 30 or more, with restriction of the ages of 50 and above (BEIR III, 1980; Axelson, 1983; Edling, 1983).

Quite recently, also Radford and Renard (1984) have provided quantified data both from their own study and from other investigations as suggesting the risk to be in the range of 6-21 excess cases per WLM and 10^6 person-years. They failed to appreciate the importance of age standardization or at least age restriction, however, as revealed by their comment to the comparison with the seemingly higher risk estimates from another study of Swedish iron miners (Edling and Axelson, 1983). As a matter of fact, their estimation of the cumulative incidence over lifetime, taken as 1 excess case per WLM and 1000 men (and alternatively suggested to be slightly less), is quite close to but actually above the figures that can be derived from two other Swedish mining populations (Axelson and Sundell, 1978; Edling and Axelson, 1982). Hence, the utilization of the age-restricted estimates from these latter populations (Edling, 1983; Edling and Axelson, 1983) leads to calculated cumulative lifetime estimates of 0.7 to 0.9 excess cases per WLM and 1000 men (up to the age of 75), dependent on which of the alternatively given estimates of exposure that is utilized.

It is pertinent in this context to also consider the corresponding estimates obtained from studies of the general population with regard to radon daughter exposure in homes. Again for ages of 50 and above one obtains figures in the range of 24 to 32 excess cases per WLM and 10^6 person-years, as derived from one of the Swedish studies (Axelson et al, 1979; Axelson, 1983), and from the other (Edling et al., 1984) one gets a corresponding range of 12-18, i.e. the lifetime excess would be about 0.3 to 0.8 per 1000 individuals and WLM. Hence, there is by no means any ground for a belief that the more recently obtained risk estimates from miners would overpredict the lung cancer morbidity in the general population, although such ideas are around in the literature (cf. Cohen, 1982; Harley, 1984), basically orginating from overestimates of the probable exposure in the past.

EPILOGUE

The relatively extensive experiences from studies on lung cancer among miners in various countries along with the findings in animal experiments, seem to suggest that radon daughter exposure is quite an effective initiator of lung cancer and that the influence from smoking might be mainly that of promoting a radiation-induced malignancy. At the same time, the role of bronchitis and its relation to smoking is somewhat confusing in this context, but increased mucous secretion might interfere with the induction of lung cancer, through sometimes hindering the short-ranging alpha-radiation to reach the basal cells of the epithelium.

The results of the presently rather limited number of studies on lung cancer and radon daughter exposure in homes seem to point towards the existence of an effect also in the general population. The quantitative risk estimates obtainable from miners and from "house studies" are presently quite consistent, but with the general population rather providing slightly lower estimates than the miners, although the data are quite scanty.

REFERENCES

Åkerblom, G., and Wilson, C., 1982, Radon - geological aspects
    of an environmental problem. Report No 30, Geological Survey
    of Sweden, Uppsala, (PO Box 670, S-75128 Uppsala, Sweden).
Archer, V. E., and Lundin, F. E., 1967, Radiogenic lung cancer
    in man: exposure-effect relationship, Environ. Res., 1:370.
Archer, V. E., 1971, Lung cancer among populations having lung
    irradiation, Lancet, 2:1261.
Archer, V. E., Wagoner, J. K., and Lundin, F. E., 1973, Lung cancer
    among uranium miners in the United States, Health Phys.,
    25:351.
Archer, V. E., 1984, Enhancement of lung cancer by cigarette smoking
    in uranium and other miners, in: "Proceedings from symposium
    on tumor promotion and enhancement in the etiology of human
    and experimental respiratory tract carcinogenesis," M. Mass,
    ed., Raven Press, to be published.
Arnstein, A., 1913, Uber den sogenannten "Schneeberger Lungenkrebs",
    Ver. Dtsch. Ges. Path., 16:332.
Ashley, D. J. B., 1967, The distribution of lung cancer and bronch-
    itis in England and Wales, Br. J. Cancer, 21:243.
Axelson, O., 1983, Experiences and concerns on lung cancer and
    radon daughter exposure in mines and dwellings in Sweden,
    Z. Erkrank. Atm.-Org., 161:232.
Axelson, O., 1984, Room for a role for radon in lung cancer causa-
    tion, Medical Hypotheses, 13:51.

Axelson, O., Edling, C., and Kling, H., 1979, Lung cancer and re-
    sidency - A case-referent study on the possible impact of
    exposure to radon and its daughters in dwellings, Scand.
    J. Work Environ. Health, 5:10.
Axelson, O., Josefsson, H., Rehn, M., and Sundell, L., 1971, Svensk
    pilotstudie över lungcancer hos gruvarbetare (Swedish pilot
    study on lung cancer among miners), Läkartidningen, 68:5687.
Axelson, O., and Sundell, L., 1978, Mining, lung cancer and smoking,
    Scand. J. Work Environ. Health, 4:46.
Bean, J. A., Isacson, P., Hahne, R. M. A., and Kohler, J., 1982,
    Drinking water and cancer incidence in Iowa. II. Radioactivity
    in drinking water, Am. J. Epidemiol., 116:924.
BEIR III, Committee on the biological effects of ionizing radia-
    tion:, 1980, "The effects on populations of exposure
    to low levels of ionizing radiation," National Academy of
    Sciences, Washington DC.
Bergman, H., and Axelson, O., 1983, Passive smoking and indoor
    radon daughter concentrations, Lancet, II:1308.
Bergman, H., Edling, C., and Axelson, O., 1984, Indoor radon daugh-
    ter concentrations and passive smoking. Proceedings from
    The 3rd international conference on indoor air quality and
    climate, Stockholm Aug 20-24, vol 2.
Chameaud, J., Perraud, R., Chretien, J., Masse, R., and Lafuma,
    J., 1982,Lung carcinogenesis during in vivo cigarette smoking
    and radon daughter exposure in rats, Recent Results Cancer
    Res., 82:11.
Cohen, B. L., 1982, Failures and critique of the BEIR III lung
    cancer risk estimates, Health Phys., 42:267.
Cross, F. T., Palmer R. F., Filipy, R. E., Dagle, G. E., and Stuart
    B. O., 1982, Carcinogenic effects of radon daughters, uranium
    ore dust and cigarette smoke in beagle dogs, Health Phys.,
    42:33.
Dahlgren, E., 1979, Lungcancer, hjärt-kärlsjukdom och rökning hos
    en grupp gruvarbetare (Lung cancer, cardiovascular disease
    and smoking in a group of miners), Läkartidningen, 76:4811.
Edling, C., 1982, Lung cancer and smoking in a group of iron ore
    miners. Am. J. Ind. Med., 3:191.
Edling, C., 1983, "Lung cancer and radon daughter exposure in mines
    and dwellings." Linköping University Medical Dissertations
    No. 157, Linköping.
Edling, C., and Axelson, O., 1983, Quantitative aspects of radon
    daughter exposure and lung cancer in underground miners.
    Br. J. Ind. Med., 40:182.
Edling, C., Comba, P., Axelson, O., and Flodin, U., 1982, Effects
    of low-dose radiation - a correlation study. Scand. J. Work
    Environ. Health, Suppl., 1:59.
Edling, C., Kling, H., and Axelson, O., 1984, Radon in homes -
    A possible cause of lung cancer, Scand. J. Work Environ.
    Health, 10:25.

Faulds, F. S., and Stewart, M. J., 1956, Carcinoma of the lung
in haematite miners. J. Pathol., 72:353.

Härting, F. H., and Hesse, W ., 1879, Der Lungenkrebs, die Bergkrankheit in den Schneeberger Gruben, Vjschr. Ned. Gerich.
K., 30:296, 31:102, 31:313.

Hess, C. T., Norton, S. A., Brutsaert, W. F., Casparius, R. E.,
Coombs, E. G., and Hess, A. L., 1980, Radon-222, in potable
water supplies of New England, New England Water Works
Association, 94:113.

Hewitt, B., 1979, Biostatistical studies on Canadian uranium miners.
Conference/workshop on lung cancer epidemiology and indust-
rial applications of sputum cytology, Colorado School of
Mines Press.

Horacek, J., 1969, Der Joachimsthaler Lungenkrebs nach dem zweiten
Weltkrieg (Bericht uber 55 Fälle). Z Krebsforsch., 72:52.

Hueper, W. C., 1966, "Occupational and environmental cancers of
the respiratory system", Springer-Verlag, Berlin.

Hultqvist, B., 1956, Studies on naturally occuring ionizing radiations, with special reference to radiation doses in Swedish
houses of various types. Kungl. svenska vetenskapasakademiens
handlingar, 4:e serien, Band 6, Nr.3, Almqvist
& Wiksell Boktryckeri AB, Stockholm.

Jörgensen, H.S., 1973 A study of mortality from lung cancer among
miners in Kiruna 1950-1970, Work Environ. Health, 10:126.

Jörgensen, H. S., and Swensson, A., 1970, Undersökning av arbetare
i gruva med dieseldrift, särskilt med hänsyn till lungfunk-
tion, luftvägssymptom och rökvanor (Investigation of workers
in a mine with diesel drift, especially regarding lung function, respiratory symptoms and smoking habits), AI rapport
No 16, Arbetarskyddsverket, Stockholm, (English summary).

Kunz, E., Sevc, J., and Placek, V., 1978, Lung cancer in uranium
miners. Health Phys., 35:579.

Kunz, E., Sevc, J., Placek, V., and Horacek, J., 1979, Lung cancer
in men in relation to different time distribution of radiation exposure. Health Phys., 36:699.

Létourneau, E. G., Mao, Y., McGregor, R. G., Semenciw, R., Smith,
M. H., and Wigle, D. T.,1983, Lung cancer mortality and
indoor radon concentrations in 18 Canadian cities. Proceeding
of the sixteenth midyear topical meeting of the Health
Physics Society on Epidemiology applied to health physics.
Albuquerque, N M Jan 9-13.

Little, J. B., and Kennedy, A. R., 1979, Evaluation of alpha radiation-induced respiratory carcinogenesis in syrian hamsters:
Total dose and dose-rate, Prog. Exp. Tumor Res., 24:356.

Ludewig, P., and Lorenser, E., 1924, Untersuchung der Grubenluft
in den Schneeberger Gruben auf den Gehalt and Radiumemana-
tion, Strahlenterapie, 17:428.

Lundin, Jr., F. E., Lloyd, J. W., Smidt, E. M., Archer, V. E., and Holaday, D. A., 1969, Mortality of uranium miners in relation to radiation exposure, hardrock mining and cigarette smoking - 1950 through September 1967. Health Phys., 16:571.

Lundin, Jr., F. E., Wagoner, J. K., and Archer, V. E., 1971, Radon daughter exposure and respiratory cancer. Quantitative and temporal aspects. NIOSH-NIEHS joint monograph No.1, Springfield, VA.

Löwy, J., 1929, Uber die Joachimsthaler Bergkrankheit; vorläufige Mitteilung, Med. Klin. 25:141.

Osburn, H. S., 1969, Lung cancer in a mining district in Rhodesia. S. Afr. Med. J., 43:1307.

Pershagen, G., Damber, L., and Falk, R., 1984, Exposure to radon in dwellings and lung cancer: A pilot study. Proceedings from The 3rd international conference on indoor air quality and climate, Stockholm Aug. 20-24, vol 2.

Pirchan, A., and Sikl, H., 1932, Cancer of the lung in the miners of Jachymov. Am. J. Cancer, 16:681.

Radford, E. P., Renard, K. G. St. C., 1984, Lung cancer in Swedish iron miners exposed to low doses of radon daughters, N. Engl.J. Med., 310:1485.

Renard, K. G. St. C., 1974, Respiratory cancer mortality in an iron ore mine in northern Sweden. Ambio, 2:67.

Roussel, J., Pernot, C., Shoumacher, P., Pernot, M., and Kessler, Y., 1964, Considération statistique sur le cancer bronchique des mineurs de fer du bassin de Lorraine, J. Radiol. Electr. 45:541.

Saccommano, G., 1980, Lung pathology and exposure to radon daughters, in: Rom, W. N., Archer, V.E., Health implications of new energy technologies, 29-35, Ann. Arbor. Science Publishers Inc., Ann Arbor.

Saccomanno, G., Archer V. E., Auerbach, O., Kuschner, M., Egger, M., Wood, S., Mick, R., 1981, Age factor in histological type of lung cancer among uranium miners, a preliminary report. International conference on radiation hazards in mining, Golden Colorado, Oct 4-9, 1981. Society of Mining Engineers of American Inst of Mining, Metallurgical and Petroleum Engineers Inc, New York,1981.

Samet, J. M., Kutvirt, D. M., Waxweiler, R. J., and Key, C. R., 1984, Uranium mining and lung cancer in Navajo men. N. Engl. J. Med. 310:1481.

Sevc, J., Kunz, E., Plasek, V., 1976, Lung cancer in uranium miners and longterm exposure to radon daughter products, Health Phys., 30:433.

Simpson, S.G., Comstock, C. W., 1983, Lung cancer and housing characteristics, Arch. Environ. Health, 38:248.

Sluis-Cremer, G. K., Walthers, L. G., Sichel, H. F., 1967, Chronic bronchitis in miners and non-miners: An epidemiological survey of a community in the goldmining area in Transvaal, Br.J. Ind. Med., 24:1.

DeVilliers, A. J., and Windish, J. P., 1964, Lung cancer in a fluorspar mining community. I. Radiation, dust and mortality
experience, Br. J. Ind. Med. 21:94.

Wagoner, J. K., Archer, V. E., Lundin, Jr. F. E., Holaday, D. A.,
and Lloyd, J. W., 1965, Radiation as a cause of lung cancer
among uranium miners, N. Engl. J. Med., 273:181.

Wagoner, J. K., Miller, R. W., Lundin, Jr. F. E., Fraumeni, J.
F., and Haij, N. E., 1963, Unusual mortality among a group
of underground metal miners. N. Engl. J. Med., 269:281.

Waxweiler, R. J., Wagoner, J. K., Archer, V. E., 1973, Mortality
of potash workers, J. Occup. Med., 15:486.

ATOMIC BOMB SURVIVORS: EPIDEMIOLOGY AND DOSE ESTIMATION

Seymour Jablon

National Research Council
2101 Constitution Avenue, N. W.
Washington, D. C. 20418, U. S. A.

INTRODUCTION

Within the space of three days, in August 1945, fission bombs were exploded at altitudes of five to six hundred meters above, first Hiroshima and then Nagasaki. The explosive yields were approximately 15 and 22 kilotons. We do not, to this day, know just how many people were in the cities at the time of the bombings, nor just how many died, either immediately or in the first few weeks after the bombings from the effects of blast, burns and radiation. The best estimates appear to be that the two cities contained just over 600,000 persons at the time of the bombings, and that the number of deaths, both immediately and during the following three months, was about 200,000.[1] Because the explosions were air bursts there was relatively little fallout, and what there was was concentrated in areas some kilometers outside the cities themselves. Neutron-induced residual radiation of any consequence was limited to the areas within a few hundred meters of the hypocenters, where destruction from blast was almost complete, and the residual radiation decayed to very low levels within a few days. The survivors, therefore, were subjected to acute doses of radiation, mostly gamma rays, received in just a few seconds.

The two cities were devastated; Japan, at the end of the war, was prostrate; the tasks of keeping people alive, feeding them, and reconstructing houses and businesses almost entirely consumed the energies of the inhabitants and the authorities, both Japanese and those of the occupation forces. Nevertheless, in the Fall of 1945 a Joint Commission of American and Japanese scientists undertook studies of the acute effects of the bombings upon the populations.[2] These studies led to a decision by the U. S. Government to sponsor long-term studies of the irradiated survivors. The Atomic Bomb Casualty Commission (ABCC) was formed as a field agency of the National Academy of Sciences, with funding supplied by the Atomic Energy Commission, and began work with an investigation of hematological disorders in 1947. In 1975, following negotiations between the governments of Japan and the United States, the ABCC was succeeded by a new, binationally supported organi- zation, called the Radiation Effects Research Foundation, or RERF. This change ended an uncomfortable and anomalous situation in which U. S. scientists managed a study, in Japan, of Japanese citizens, who had been injured by the United States.

METHODS

In 1950 the Government of Japan took a National Census and, at the request of the ABCC, used a supplemental schedule on which every inhabitant of Japan was asked "Were you in Nagasaki City or Hiroshima City at the time of the atomic bomb?". In the entire country, 284,000 persons replied affirmatively, and the schedules for all of the inhabitants of Hiroshima and Nagasaki who so replied were turned over to ABCC. There were 195,000 persons to be investigated by field interview to learn whether they had, in fact, been in one of the cities (10 percent were not), their exact location at the time of bombing and other necessary baseline data. No dosimetry information was available in 1955 when the studies were designed and the samples of persons to be studied were, perforce, based upon distance from the hypocenters. At a later date, collaboration with the Oak Ridge National Laboratory and the Japanese National Institute of Radiological Sciences did produce and attempt to validate experimentally dosimetry systems, the most recent version dating from 1965 and called the T-65 system.

In the T-65 system, data required for kerma dose estimates included not only the exact location of the survivor at the moment of detonation of the bomb, but details concerning possible shielding, as being in a house or factory building or, in some instances, in the open. For persons in houses, it was necessary to find out exactly where in the house. This information was obtained by field interviewers who were armed with pre-strike aerial photographs so that the survivor could find his house or other location. Some have expressed doubt concerning the survivors' ability to recall the circumstances accurately, several years later. The bombings, however, were very noticeable events. It turns out that survivors who were

414

sitting in their living rooms when suddenly the roof fell in retained vivid memories of the associated circumstances. For those who were in houses - more than 60 percent of the survivors - drawings were made in horizontal and vertical plan of their exact situations to permit application of the T-65 formulas.

In both cities, dose estimates were prepared for about 80,000 survivors - more than 30,000 being of less than one-half rad. Detailed shielding studies were, for logistic reasons, done only for 20,000 survivors, those who were exposed at the closest distances and for whom the dose estimates were more than 10 rads in most cases. For survivors at the greater distances where air doses were not large, average building transmission factors were used. For fewer than 2,400 survivors it was impossible to create an estimate because the needed data were unobtainable.

Unfortunately, within the past three years review of the problem has disclosed that the 1965 dosimetry is probably incorrect in some respects[3] and an intense effort is now under way to replace that system with a more modern and, we hope, more accurate one. That effort will not come to fruition, however, for another year or so. In the meantime, we are forced to depend upon the T-65 system, while recognizing probable inaccuracies. The most significant change in the dosimetry will be, in all likelihood, a reduction in the estimated neutron component to so low a level as to make doubtful the possibility of estimating neutron RBE's in this experience.

The ABCC-RERF program is fairly complex, but an attempt has been made to link different studies together by the use of a principal, large sample in which smaller samples for special studies are embedded (Figure 1). Studies are concerned on the one hand with somatic effects and on the other with genetic. The largest study on the somatic side is the so-called Life Span Study, in which 110,000 persons - both survivors and a not-in-city unexposed control group - are traced for mortality. Transcripts of death certificates are obtained and dates and causes of death, as shown by the certificates, are coded. The Autopsy Pathology program, which represented an attempt to obtain autopsies for deaths among survivors still resident in the two cities, covered some 70,000 persons, all included in the Life Span Study. Although the autopsy procurement program did not succeed in obtaining autopsies on even half of the deaths, many thousand of autopsies were done, and form the basis, at the very least, for careful and detailed

evaluation of the accuracy of various causes of death as
reported on death certificates. A still smaller subgroup of
20,000 persons constitutes the sample for the Adult Health
Study or AHS, a program which involves biennial physical
examinations and which has been marked by an examination rate
of about 80 percent. Information concerning such non-fatal
cancers as some breast cancers and, notably, thyroid cancer,
has resulted from the AHS. The program has also investigated
the possible radiation links of cardiovascular and other
diseases. Cytological specimens from members of the AHS sample
form the basis for investigations of radiation-induced chromosomal aberrations among the survivors. Finally, a small group
of less than 3,000 subjects who were in utero at the time of
the bombings are the subjects for studies of the effects of
radiation on the fetus.

Other sources of information concerning cancers include
Tumor Registries in the two cities, which were inaugurated in
1959, and Tissue Registries which include biopsy specimens.
These registries, like the Leukemia Registry, aim at the
complete enumeration of all cancers which are diagnosed in the
two cities. The names of the persons registered can then be
matched to the list of persons included in the study sample
and, in this way, it has become possible to study cancer
incidence, not merely mortality, in relation to the estimated
radiation dose received.

Incidence data are subject, however, to one severe
deficiency: No matter how complete the Registries may be with
respect to persons who are still resident in the cities, no
practicable method has been devised to learn of cancer
diagnoses which are made elsewhere. Since many of the younger
survivors have emigrated from the cities in search of employment or following marriage, the incidence data are subject to
bias which is of uncertain magnitude, but which is surely
age-related.

The data concerning cancer mortality have, of course, a
different deficiency. There is little or no problem concerning
their completeness; the excellent Japanese vital statistics
reporting and family registration systems make it relatively
easy and inexpensive to obtain a death certificate transcript
for every death that occurs among the members enrolled in the
Life Span Study. A difficulty, of course, beyond the problem
of inaccurate certification on death certificates is that one
can learn only about fatal cancers. This means that most of
the thyroid cancers and half of the breast cancers - both of
which are important radiogenic cancers - will be missed. Even

416

for cancers which have high fatality rates, variation among persons in survival time from onset to death will tend to obscure patterns of time dependence, that is, latency periods.

In any case, recognizing their different deficiences, both incidence and mortality data are obtained and, in some instances, the deficiencies of one method of ascertainment may be compensated by the virtues of the other.

Another arm of the program investigates genetic effects. Thirty years ago, when the program was young, there was as much concern, or more, about genetic effects of radiation as there was about somatic effects and the earliest large study at ABCC was, in fact, a search for genetic effects in children born in the first few years after the bombings.[4] Later, the sample of children was expanded somewhat to a little over 50,000 and a continuing study of mortality was instituted. More recently it has been possible to use deeper and more sensitive probes, and a study of genetic effects at the biochemical level has been in operation for several years. Here the idea is to detect mutations by identifying variant red cell proteins in a sub-group of about 34,000 children. Cytologic studies, seeking evidence of damage at the chromosomal level - chromosomal aberrations - are being pursued in a smaller group of about 19,000 children. Despite the intense effort which has gone into the studies of genetic effects, to this date no definite evidence of an increased mutation rate has yet been found.[5]

Techniques for investigating genetic material are evolving very rapidly at this time. Laboratory methods at RERF are constantly being improved and made more sensitive and, in an attempt to prepare for technology which is only a few years down the road, there is being started a program for storing white cells so that they will be available when the methodology is ripe for examining DNA itself. There is reason to hope that it will yet be possible to measure the specific locus mutation rate per rad in the children of the survivors despite our inability thus far to do more than to estimate an upper limit for that number.

Dosimetry

It has been necessary to reconstruct the dosimetry applicable to the survivors, not an easy task. Following some early, relatively crude attempts in 1965 the so-called T-65 system was devised by a group from Oak Ridge National Laboratory and put into place. This system, described by Auxier[6] involved estimates of the yields of the two weapons,

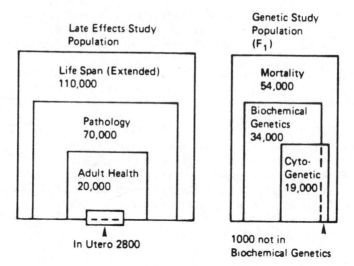

Figure 1: The Unified Population Studies at RERF Hiroshima and Nagasaki

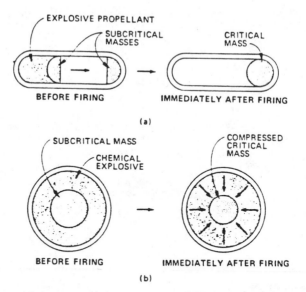

Figure 2: Schematics illustrating the principles of (a) Little Boy, a gun-assembly nuclear device, and (b) Fat Man, an implosion-type nuclear device (Glasstone and Dolan, 1977).

the prompt and delayed radiations which emanated from the
fissioning weapons and the subsequently rising fireballs,
radiation transport to the location of survivors, attenuation
by terrain and structures and, finally, attenuation by
overlying tissue of the radiation dose which actually affected
critical organs such as the bone marrow. Development of the
T-65 system required experimentation at the Nevada test site to
measure attenuation through air of neutron flux and gamma rays,
and to observe the consequences of interactions with building
materials. For this latter purpose replicas of Japanese
residential structures were built.

Actual application of the T-65 system to produce separate
estimates of gamma ray and neutron doses (kerma) for individual
survivors required field interviews of nearly 29,000 survivors
(or surrogate informants, to learn exact location at the time
of the bombings (ATB), the nature of the house or other
shielding structure if any, and the location within that
structure.[7] Milton and Shohoji have provided a detailed
description of the procedures involved in calculating the
estimated doses.[7]

After the introduction of the T-65 system all ABCC analyses
were based on dose estimates which were calculated according to
that system. Neutron doses were thought to be very small in
Nagasaki, but were appreciable in Hiroshima, while in both
cities many survivors had quite large gamma radiation
doses (Table 1). The fact that the ratio of neutron to gamma
doses was very different in the two cities promised the ability
to calculate the RBE - Relative Biological Effectiveness - of
neutrons compared with gamma rays by, in effect, contrasting
the two cities, and many such analyses were made, obtaining
values of the RBE which ranged from about 5 to about 25,
depending upon the biological endpoint (e.g., epilation or
leukemia) and on the dose response model employed.

It is convenient to consider separately two different
aspects of the dosimetry problem. It is first necessary to
determine the radiation field in open air at a distance from
the epicenter - the point in space at which the detonation
occurs. This involves the generation of radiation by the
exploding device and, subsequently, by the fireball, and the
radiation transport through the intervening distance, to the
place of interest. The second aspect consists of further
transporting the radiation through building materials to a
survivor, taking account of disturbances in the field which
result from the building and, possibly, adjacent buildings.

Table 1

The Life Span Study - Estimated T-65 Radiation Doses

Total dose (rad kerma)	Hiroshima			Nagasaki		
	Number	Mean Dose		Number	Mean Dose	
		Gamma	Neutrons		Gamma	Neutrons
400+	510	380	144	377	518	11.2
300-399	369	254	92	270	338	6.0
200-299	659	186	57	722	240	3.8
100-199	1,740	108	30	1,388	145	1.9
50-99	2,783	56.6	13.7	1,442	70.7	0.5
10-49	10,911	17.5	4.5	4,031	21.2	0.0
1-9	15,933	2.6	0.7	7,140	3.6	0.0
0	27,577	0	0	4,004	0	0
Unknown	1,429	-	-	957	-	-
Total	61,911	-	-	20,331	-	-

(Kato & Schull, 1982)

This produces the estimate of free-in-air kerma to the shielded survivor. Finally, it is necessary to examine the transport and attenuation within the human body itself to produce, at last, the dose to an organ of interest, such as the lung or the breast. This must be done for the gamma rays and for the neutrons emitted by the device.

To understand the problems it is necessary to consider just what happens when a fission bomb explodes, at the instant of detonation and during the first few seconds thereafter.

It is well known that a fission bomb consists of the means for creating a compact "critical mass" of either uranium 235 or plutonium 239, one whose ratio of mass to surface area is sufficiently large that more neutrons are born by fission than are lost through the surface, in each fission generation. Figure 2, after Glasstone & Dolan[8], shows schematically the gun-assembly device used in Little Boy in Hiroshima and the implosion device used in the Fat Man at Nagasaki. Parenthetically, the Little Boy was unique, so the characteristics of such a weapon have all to be derived theoretically and from observations of effects in Hiroshima, whereas many implosion devices, similar to Fat Man, were exploded in well-instrumented tests in Nevada.

At the instant of criticality, the fissioning mass is
emitting an enormous number of high energy neutrons and gamma
rays. This is part of the so-called prompt radiation. When
the neutrons escaped from the critical mass they encountered,
in Little Boy, about six inches of steel and other heavy
metals. Passage through this steel casing degraded the energy
of the neutrons, resulting in a much softer spectrum which
emerged from the still-unexploded bomb than a so-called
"fission spectrum." What is being discussed here is what
happens in the first micro-second after the critical mass has
been formed and before it destroys itself by exploding.

The Fat Man critical mass was, on the other hand,
surrounded by an enormous quantity of high explosive debris,
rich in hydrogen, in consequence of which neutrons passing
through lost energy through elastic scattering encounters with
hydrogen nuclei.

The situation is further complicated by the fact that
neutrons engage in different kinds of interactions with
ordinary matter. High energy neutrons lose energy in elastic
collisions, especially with hydrogen; while low energy neutrons
can be captured by nuclei, especially of nitrogen, creating an
excited nucleus which then decays, emitting a high energy gamma
ray.

Putting all this together, in Nagasaki, in the Fat Man
device, the large mass of "high explosive debris" which
surrounded the fissioning critical mass first degraded the
energy of the fission neutrons, then captured most of the
resulting low energy neutrons, and the device became an intense
source of gamma rays. In Hiroshima, on the other hand, the
neutrons which emanated from the Little Boy device had lost
energy during the passage through the steel casing, lost
further energy by elastic collisions with hydrogen present as
moisture in the humid air, and were then captured by
atmospheric nitrogen, resulting in the generation of gamma rays
in a large air mass surrounding the weapon.

Subsequently, the two devices exploded, quenching the chain
reactions, and producing fireballs which then rose. The
fireballs contained all of the debris of the weapons, which now
included a large store of unstable isotopes which had been
created by the intense neutron bombardment as well as fission
products. Most of these had very short half-lives and decayed
quickly, emitting gamma rays as they did so. The gamma ray
output of the devices was about equally divided between the
prompt gammas, emitted by the bomb and created by neutron

interactions with air, building materials and so on, and the delayed gammas, which emanated from the fireball during the first 5 to 10 seconds after the detonations.

In brief, for the prompt radiations:

1. Neutrons escaped from the weapon. Their number and energy levels were modified by the passage through the bomb casing and explosive debris.

2. Gamma rays produced in the bomb radiated out.

3. Gamma rays were produced at a distance from the epicenter by neutron capture reactions in air. This process is dependent upon the rate at which neutrons lose energy by elastic collisions with atmospheric hydrogen.

4. When gamma rays encountered building materials, or overlying tissues, they were attenuated.

5. When neutrons encountered materials, they lost energy through elastic collisions, and entered into capture reactions, with emission of gamma rays.

By contrast, the delayed radiation, almost all gamma rays, but including some neutrons, presents a much simpler problem. The radiation intensity is governed by time after detonation and the rate of rise of the fireball, but these are reasonably well understood.

Changes in the air dose curves as between those which underlie the T-65 system and the new estimates arise from new and, presumably, better estimates of the neutron leakage from the bombs during the instant of criticality and, as important, their energy spectrum; and from revision of the variation in neutron energy spectrum with increasing distance from the hypocenters resulting from water vapor present in the atmosphere. It should be emphasized that it was impossible, in the early 1960's, to make the kinds of theoretical calculations that are possible today. Instead, measurements were made at the Nevada test site. But the sources used for the measurements were not duplicates of the two bombs – and the radiations, therefore, had different energy spectra. Moreover, the neutrons behaved differently in the dry desert air in Nevada than they did in the moist August air in Hiroshima and Nagasaki, and the net result is as shown in Figure 3, taken from the paper by Kerr, Pace and Scott.[9] The neutron kerma in Hiroshima is reduced by a factor of about 10, while the

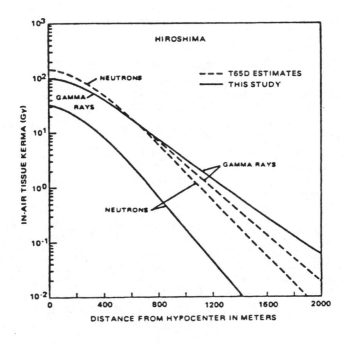

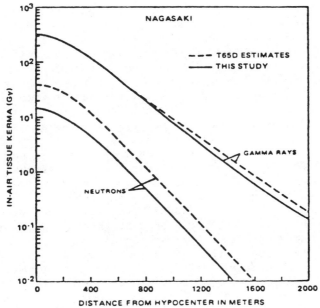

Figure 3: Air Dose Curves

gamma kerma has been increased beyond about 700 meters from the hypocenter. At 2,000 meters the gamma kerma free-in-air is increased by a factor of about 3. In Nagasaki the neutron kerma estimate has been lowered by a factor of about 2, while the estimate for gamma rays is little changed.

At this point, we have estimates of the gamma ray and neutron kerma free-in-air, to a survivor exposed in the open - a survivor who was neither in a building nor standing quite near to one. The majority of the survivors in the studies, however, were in Japanese houses of typical light construction. The T-65 system included a so-called nine parameter formula which had the purpose of translating the free-in-air kerma outside of the building to that at the location of the survivor within the building. An elaborate experimental system was used to develop the formula. Models of Japanese houses were built at the Nevada test site and were irradiated experimentally, with dosimeters outside and at several points inside the houses. Measurements were made during several bomb tests and also by use of the Health Physics Research Reactor as a neutron source and a cobalt 60 source for gamma rays. Estimates of the parameters in the nine parameter formula were made using a step-wise regression procedure.

Unfortunately, it turned out that much of the gamma radiation measured inside the houses resulted from neutron interactions with the building materials themselves, so the so-called shielded values for gamma radiation were seriously mis-estimated. Transmission factors under the nine parameter formula averaged, for gamma rays, about .90 in Hiroshima and .81 in Nagasaki; the neutron transmission factors were between .30 and .35. Marcum has estimated that, under the dosimetry system now being derived, the gamma ray transmission factors will average only .55 in Hiroshima and .50 in Nagasaki.[10] Combining these estimates with the ORNL estimates of the air-dose curves (Table 2), one can estimate the average mean dose in rems under a possible new dosimetry and compare that mean dose with the corresponding value for T-65D. The T-65 mean dose exceeds the new estimates by a factor that varies from about 1.6 to 2.2, depending on what value is used for the neutron RBE. The estimated ratio tells us that using the new dosimetry in relation to the cancer mortality data through 1978, the excess cancer mortality risk per rem will change by a factor in the neighborhood of two from the risk calculated using the T-65D dosimetry.

Table 2
RERF Life Span Study 1950–1978
Preliminary Estimate of Changes in Dose

	T–65D	Pace–Marcum
Mean Dose, Rems		
RBE 1	45.7	28.4
RBE 5	71.1	32.7
Ratio, T–65D to Pace–Marcum		
RBE 1	1.61	
RBE 5	2.17	

RESULTS

The only cause of death which has been elevated in irradiated survivors during the follow-up period is cancer (Table 3).[11] The relative risk of death from cancer was more than doubled in those with doses estimated at more than 400 rads. Although, superficially, it appears that mortality from causes other than cancer is slightly elevated in the highest dose groups, if the small number of deaths ascribed to diseases of the blood and blood-forming organs are excluded, the apparent effect virtually disappears. Pathology studies have shown that a small number of deaths really due to leukemia were certified as aplastic or other anemia. These errors occurred primarily in the early years, before it became generally known that leukemia rates were considerably increased among the survivors.

The relative risk of death from cancer is highest in exposed children and is a declining function of age at exposure (Figure 4). For leukemia, because of random noise in the system – there are not very many deaths from leukemia – the relative risks, although quite high, show no clear pattern of variation with age at exposure. The absolute risks, however, for both solid cancers and for leukemia are regularly increasing functions of age at exposure, except for the very youngest survivors, for whom the absolute leukemia risks are large. To some extent this picture may be incomplete and therefore deceptive. The data include deaths through 1978, or 33 years of follow-up after the bombings. Those who were aged 50 or more in 1945 had virtually completed their mortality experience 33 years later; however, those below 10 in 1945 were of average age only 38 in 1978, with most of their cancer experience yet to come. Since excess cancer rates are still increasing among the younger survivors it is entirely possible that the relationship between age at exposure and absolute cancer risks may become flatter with a increasing length of follow-up. The excess leukemia experience, however, appears to be virtually complete and the two leukemia curves can hardly change very much.

It is evident that the time trends for leukemia and for the solid tumors are very different (Figure 5). The relative risks for most of the solid tumors had risen by 1960 and did not change much thereafter. If relative risks merely remain constant as time passes, then the absolute risks must increase, since the average age of the population is constantly increasing and, with increasing age the natural, baseline cancer rates are also increasing - and very rapidly. In fact, the estimates of absolute risk per rad increased considerably in 1975-78. Since the BEIR 1980 risk estimates[12] were derived from data through 1974 only, it seems very possible that any future BEIR report, for which data through 1982 will be available, will derive somewhat larger risk estimates. If the absolute and relative risk estimates for a specific age group are compared, it seems clear that the large increase in absolute risk in 1975-78 is not parallelled by a corresponding increase in the relative risk (Figure 6).

It is important, however, not to lose sight of the fact that although we may be in some doubt as to the exact magnitude of the radiation risk, in absolute terms it is not large. Kato and Schull have extrapolated that, among all 283,000 A-bomb survivors in Japan, with a mean dose of around 16 rads, thus far a little more than 500 excess, radiation-induced cancer deaths have occurred, out of a total of nearly 68,000 deaths from all causes. The increase amounts to something under one percent. The chance that an average American will die someday in an automobile accident is about three times as large as the probability that an average A-bomb survivor will die from a radiation-induced cancer.

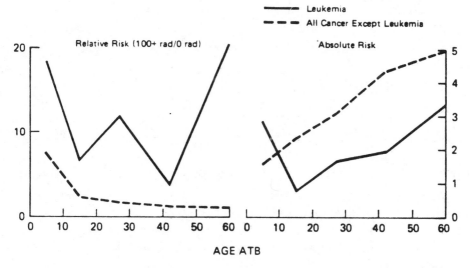

Figure 4:   Relative and Absolute Risk by Age ATB, 1950-78

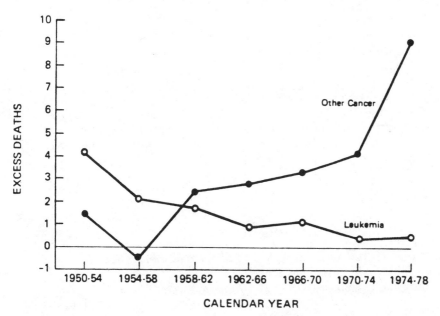

Figure 5:   Excess Deaths/Million Person-Year Rad Over Time Leukemia
and other Cancer

Table 3

'Mortality, 1950–1978

Relative Risks

Disease	0	1-9	10-49	50-99	100-199	200-299	300-399	400+	Trend statistics
				Radiation Dose (rads)					
Cancer	1	1.00	1.08	1.08	1.27	1.74	1.67	2.11	P$<$.001
Non-cancer	1	0.98	1.00	0.99	0.95	1.09	1.30	1.09	P$>$.10
	*(1	0.98	0.97	0.94	0.94	0.90	1.04	1.06)	P$>$.10)

*Excludes diseases of blood and blood-forming organs.

(Kato and Schull, 1982)

What is the implication of all this for radiological protection? Using A-bomb survivor data through 1974, the BEIR Committee, on the basis of a relative risk model, estimated that one million persons exposed to one rad of low LET radiation annually, from age 20 through 65, would generate about 5,500 extra deaths from leukemia and other cancer, compared with over 170,000 naturally occurring cancer deaths.[7] This is about a one-half of one percent increase in cancer.

It need hardly be added that these estimates are based on the notion that we know how to extrapolate radiation risks from exposures of 100 rads or more down to one rad. Before the T-65 dosimetry system was challenged, the data on exchange aberrations in chromosomes among survivors appeared to lend support to the idea that radiation effects that depend upon single hits might well follow a quadratic or second degree dose-effect relationship for low LET radiation as was seen in Nagasaki (Figure 7). The doses in Nagasaki were almost entirely from gamma rays. In Hiroshima, it was thought that

428

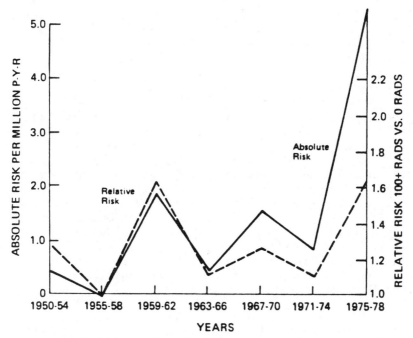

Figure 6: Absolute and Relative Risks of Death From Malignant Neoplasms Except Leukemia - Ages 35-49 at Exposure, 1950-1978

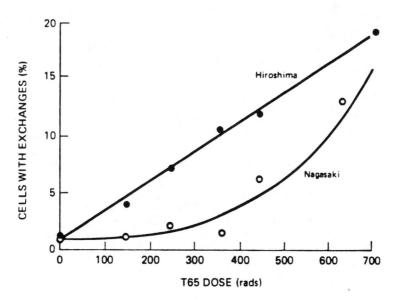

Figure 7: Chromosome Aberrations in the Adult Health Study by Exposure and City

the straight line relationship seen reflected high LET, neutron
effects. This was a very pretty and satisfying theory but in
the new dosimetry system which is now being created it appears
that the neutron dose in Hiroshima will be very markedly
reduced, and taking all changes together, the curves for the
two cities will probably resemble each other.

Finally to return to the subject of genetic effects, there
is little to say. As of September 1983 more than 600,000
electrophoretic tests had been made on more than 22,000
children, 55 percent of whom had at least one parent who was
exposed within 2,000 meters; the remaining 45 percent were
controls. Three mutations had been identified in each group so
that the mutation rates were indistinguishable. It is evident
that the ability to measure the specific mutation rate per rad
will depend upon examination of a vastly increased number of
genes. Since the number of children available cannot be
expanded, the hope lies in a several-fold expansion in the
number of genes which can be tested in each child. There is
hope that such an expansion can be realized by application of

REFERENCES

1. Committee for the Compilation of Materials on Damage Caused
    by the Atomic Bombs in Hiroshima and Nagasaki, ed.,
    "Hiroshima and Nagasaki," Basic Books, New York, (1981).
2. A. W. Oughterson and S. Warren, eds., "Medical Effects of
    the Atomic Bomb in Japan," McGraw-Hill, New York, (1956).
3. W. E. Loewe and E. Mendelsohn, Neutron and Gamma-Ray Doses
    at Hiroshima and Nagasaki, Nuclear Science and
    Engineering 81:325-350 (1982).
4. J. V. Neel and W. J. Schull, "The Effect of Exposure to the
    Atomic Bombs Pregnancy Termination in Hiroshima and
    Nagasaki," National Academy of Sciences, Publication
    461, Washington, D. C. (1956).
5. W. J. Schull, M. Otake and J. V. Neel, Genetic Effects of
    the Atomic Bomb: Reappraisal, Science 213:1220-1227
    (September 1981).
6. Auxier, J. A., "Ichiban: Radiation Dosimetry for the
    Survivors of the Bombings of Hiroshima and Nagasaki,"
    Energy Research and Development Administration,
    Technical Information Center, Oak Ridge, Tennessee
    (1977).

7. R. C. Milton, and T. Shohoji, Tentative 1965 Radiation Dose Estimation for Atomic Bomb Survivors, Hiroshima and Nagasaki, in: "Atomic Bomb Casualty Commission Techincal Report No. 1-68," Atomic Bomb Casualty Commission (1968).

8. S. Glasstone, and D. J. Dolan, "The Effects of Nuclear Weapons," U. S. Department of Defense and the Energy Research and Development Administration, U. S. Government Printing Office, Washington, D. C. (1977).

9. G. D. Kerr, J. V. Pace, III, and W. H. Scott, Jr., Tissue Kerma vs. Distance Relationships for Initial Nuclear Radiation from the Atomic Bombs, Hiroshima & Nagasaki, in: "U. S.-Japan Workshop for Reassessment of Atomic Bomb Radiation Dosimetry in Hiroshima and Nagasaki," D. J. Thompson, ed., Radiation Effects Research Foundation, Hiroshima, Japan (1983).

10. W. A. Woolson, J. Marcum, W. H. Scott, and V. E. Staggs, Building Transmission Factors In Revision, in: "Reevaluations of Dosimetric Factors, Hiroshima and Nagasaki," V. P. Bond and J. W. Thiessen, eds., U. S. Department of Energy, Technical Information Center Oak Ridge, Tennesse (1982).

11. H. Kato and W. J. Schull, Studies of the Mortality of A-bomb Survivors. 7. Mortality, 1950-1978: Part I. Cancer Mortality, Radiat. Res. 90:395-432 (1982).

12. Committee on the Biological Effects of Ionizing Radiation, "The Effects on Populations of Exposure to Low Levels of Ionizing Radiation: 1980," National Academy Press, Washington, D. C. (1980).

EPIDEMIOLOGY OF MICROWAVE RADIATION EFFECTS IN HUMANS

Charlotte Silverman

Food and Drug Administration
Center for Devices and Radiological Health
Rockville, Maryland 20857

INTRODUCTION

Microwave radiation is a form of nonionizing electromagnetic radiation of very low photon energies. Formerly part of the radiofrequency portion of the electromagnetic spectrum, it has been arbitrarily separated out and lies between infrared radiation and the radiofrequencies. Microwave radiation is generally defined as that portion of the electromagnetic spectrum between frequencies of 300 megahertz (MHz) and 300 gigahertz (GHz) associated with wavelengths between one meter and one millimeter (WHO, 1981) (Fig. 1). Microwaves have been subdivided into frequency bands designated loosely as extremely high frequency (EHF) or millimeter waves, super high frequency (SHF) or centimeter waves, and ultrahigh frequency (UHF) or decimeter waves. In addition there are letter designations (such as S,K,X,P) for special frequency bands which are used for radar (radio detecting and ranging), and there are industrial, scientific and medical (ISM) bands which have been assigned for specific applications, according to international agreements.

Microwave radiation occurs naturally but the natural background intensity is low. It is man-made sources developed since the 1940s that account for increasing and widespread exposure both of occupational groups and the general population. The extent of occupational exposure to microwave radiation sources is not known; one estimate put the number of workers potentially exposed to microwave and to radiofrequency sources at approximately 21 million in the United States in 1977, (Moss et al., 1977). With respect to general population exposure, a 1979 report listed nine million broadcasting transmitters, hundreds of thousands of microwave communications towers, tens of thousands of radar antennas

433

and almost 30 million CB radios in the United States (Glaser et al., 1979). The numerous uses of this form of radiant energy are shown in Table 1 and include, among others, radar, satellite communications, radionavigation, radio and television broad-

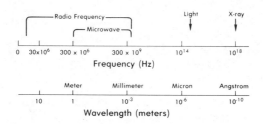

Fig. 1. Electromagnetic Spectrum

casting, and uses which are based on the heating properties of microwaves, such as microwave ovens, medical diathermy, hyper-thermia therapy, and heating and drying in innumerable industrial processes.

Exposure to microwave fields is generally described in terms of power density (intensity) under specified conditions and expressed in watts per square meter or milliwatts or microwatts per square centimeter (W/m^2, mW/cm^2, $uWcm^2$). Ranges of power density in relation to health effects have been a subject of controversy for over a quarter century because of differing views of low level and nonthermal effects. Occupational exposure limits in various countries range from 10 mW/cm^2 down to .01 mW/cm^2. Three arbitrary ranges of power densities for operational purposes were proposed at an international symposium (Czerski et al., 1974): (1) high, the range above 10 mW/cm^2 in which distinct thermal effects predominate, (2) low, the range below 1 mW/cm^2 in which thermal effects are improbable, and (3) an intermediate range in which weak but noticeable thermal effects occur as well as other unspecified effects. The specific absorption rate (SAR) has been introduced as a measure of the rate of energy absorption and is expressed as watts per kilogram (W/kg) (NCRP, 1981). Very complex energy distributions can occur in the external exposure field and in the biologic systems being exposed, and energy deposition can be markedly nonuniform. Clues to the hazards of microwave radiation have come mainly from accidental over-exposures, experimental laboratory research, and industrial hygiene surveys and surveillance programs.

Table 1. Radiofrequency Bands (Microwave)

Frequency	Wavelength	Band Designation	Typical Uses
30-300 GHz	10-1 mm	Extremely high frequency (EHF)	Satellite communications, radar, microwave relay, radionavigation, amateur radio
3-30 GHz	10-1 cm	Super high frequency (SHF)	Satellite communications, radar, amateur, microwave relay, airborne weather radar, ISM
0.3-3 GHz	100-10 cm	Ultra high frequency (UHF)	Microwave point to point, amateur, taxi, police, fire radar, citizens band, radio-navigation, UHF-TV, microwave ovens, medical diathermy, ISM
30-300 MHz	10-1 m	Very high frequency (VHF)	Police, fire, amateur FM, VHF-TV, industrial RF equipment, diathermy, emergency medical radio, air traffic control

MORTALITY STUDIES

Two cohort studies conducted during the past decade have investigated the mortality and morbidity experience of persons exposed during earlier years. Robinette et al., (1977, 1980) studied U.S. naval enlisted men occupationally exposed to radar during the Korean War period 1950-1954. The study was designed to make use of occupational differences in levels of exposure and of medical information recorded during military service and subsequently in the veteran period.

The study population was drawn from the thousands of enlisted men trained in the use and maintenance of radar equipment in technical schools maintained by the Navy since World War II. The 40,000 men selected for this study graduated during the period 1950 through 1954. Wartime service ensured virtually complete ascertainment of deaths, and exposure in the 1950s provided a period of over 20 years for long-term effects to develop. Measurements made by the Navy offered a guide for selecting the most highly exposed occupations. Occupational groups were classified as probably maximally exposed (those repairing radar equipment), and probably minimally exposed exposed (those operating radar equipment) (Table 2). The high exposure cohort of 20,000 was made up of electronics technicians, fire control (gunfire) technicians, and aviation electronics technicians. The groups in the low exposure cohort, who also numbered about 20,000, were classified as radioman, radarman, and aviation electrician's mate. The mean age in 1952 of the low exposure men was 20.7 and the average age of the high exposure group was 22.1 years.

Table 2. Exposure group and Occupational classification

Exposure group and Occupational classification	No.
Low exposure	
Radioman (RM)	9,253
Radarman (RD)	10,116
Aviation Electrician's Mate(AE)	1,412
Total	20,781
High exposure	
Electronics Technician(ET)	13,078
Fire Control Technician (FT)	3,298
Aviation Electronics Technician(AT)	3,733
Total	20,109

Table from Robinette et al. 1980

It was estimated from shipboard monitoring that radiomen and radar operators (the low exposure group) were generally exposed to less than 1 mW/cm^2 and that gunfire control and electronics technicians (the high exposure group) were exposed to higher but unspecifiable levels during their duties. It was not possible to assign exposure doses to any individuals in this study. An effort was made to develop an index of potential exposure for a sample of the high exposure group. This index called the Hazard Number required review of individual men's records and consisted of the sum of the power ratings of all gunfire control and search radars aboard the craft to which the technicians were assigned, multiplied by the number of months assignment.

436

Four health indexes were studied, largely through the use of automated record systems: mortality by cause of death, hospitalization during military service, later hospitalization in Veterans Administration (VA) facilities and VA disability compensation. Followup information was derived from search and linkage of Navy and VA records. Mortality information was retrievable for more than 95 percent of the Korean war veterans. Certified causes of death were obtained from copies of the death certificates.

The men in this study had a favorable mortality experience compared to the U.S. white male population of the same ages. This was to be expected because the men were screened before entering the service and again before acceptance in the technical training schools. Comparisons between the total low and high exposure groups revealed no difference in mortality from all diseases

Table 3. Number of Deaths from Disease and Mortality Ratios by Exposure Class (1950-1974)

Causes of death		Low exposure	High exposure
All diseases	No.	325	310
	MR+	1.04	0.96
Malignant neoplasms	No.	87	96
	MR	0.96	1.04
Digestive organs	No.	14	20
	MR	0.85	1.14
Respiratory tract	No.	16	24
	MR	0.85	1.14
Lymphatic and hematopoietic system	No.	20	26
	MR	0.83	1.18
Other malignant neoplasms	No.	37	26
	MR	1.19	0.82
Disease circulatory system	No.	167	151
	MR	1.07	0.93
Other disease	No.	71	63
	MR	1.08	0.92

+Mortality ratio standardized for year of bith; the combined low and high exposure groups taken as standard.
Data from Robinette et al. (1980)

Table 4. Mortality from Malignant Neoplasms of Lymphatic and Hematopoietic System

Cause of death	No. of deaths	
	Low exposure	High exposure
Lymphosarcoma and reticulum cell sarcoma	4	6
Hodgkin's disease	7	5
Other lymphoid neoplasms	1	1
Lymphatic leukemia	2	2
Myeloid leukemia	3	6
Monocytic leukemia	1	3
Other and unspecified leukemia	2	3
Total	20	26

From Robinette et al. 1980

combined (Table 3). Malignant neoplasms of the digestive organs, respiratory tract and lymphatic and hematopoietic system were found to be elevated in the total high exposure group compared with the low exposure group but none of the increases was statistically significant. Types of malignant neoplasms of the lymphatic and hematopoietic system in the two exposure groups are shown in Table 4; there are no differences between the groups. The study had a 90 percent chance of detecting 50 percent excess mortality at a significance level of $P = .05$ for comparisons between the total low and high exposure groups.

When comparisons were made within the high exposure group, across Hazard Number categories, respiratory tract cancer was significantly higher in those with the higher Hazard Number and the test for trend in mortality ratios with increasing Hazard Number produced a single significant result for all diseases combined. These may be fortuitous since occasional significant differences may be expected when numerous statistical comparisons are made; there were no supportive data and no smoking histories. Differential health risks attributable to occupational exposure to radar in the Navy 20 years earlier were not apparent with respect to mortality, an endpoint for which there was virtually complete information for the total study group. It should be noted, however, that the study subjects were very young when exposed, in their early 20s, and even a 20 year followup period may not be sufficient to detect long-term mortality effects.

The second cohort study concerns the mortality and morbidity experience of American Embassy personnel in Moscow. The long-term microwave irradiation of the American Embassy building in Moscow from 1953 to 1976 led to a two-year study of possible adverse health effects (Lilienfeld et al., 1978). Health histories of the U.S. foreign service staff and other personnel in Moscow and their dependents were compared with those of U.S. employees at eight other non-irradiated eastern European embassies or consulates during the same time period. The microwave irradiation of the Moscow embassy varied in intensity, direction and frequency during the 23 year period. Frequencies ranged from 0.6 to 9.5 GHz (U.S. Senate, 1979). Measured average power densities outside the building for several time periods ranged from 5 to 18 uW/cm^2. Tests for microwave radiation at all the eastern European comparison posts were reported as showing only background levels of 1 uW/cm^2.

A major effort was required to construct a basic list of all personnel who had served in any of the selected posts at any time during the 23 year study period and to identify their dependents who might have been with them during their tours of duty at any study post. The customary tour of duty was 2-4 years. The final identified total study population consisted of 4,388 employees and 8,283 dependents. Ninety-five percent of the employees were traced. Numbers and sex of employees who were traced and age categories of their dependents who were in residence are shown in Table 5.

Information on illnesses, physical conditions, and symptoms were sought from two major sources: (1) employment medical records, which were fairly extensive because of examination requirements for foreign duty, and (2) a self-administered health history questionnaire. Questionnaire responses were validated for

Table 5. U.S. Foreign Service Study

No. Traced and in Residence	Moscow Post	Comparison Post
Employees		
Male	1309	1710
Female	410	750
Total	1719	2460
Dependents		
Adults	436	787
Children	792	1285
Total	1228	2072

From Lilienfeld et al., 1978

a stratified sample by review of hospital, physician, and clinic records. Many sources were used to ascertain mortality status and the information was quite complete because of the high tracing success. It was not possible, however, to obtain death certificates for approximately one-third of the employees because of time constraints on the study and other sources of information were used to determine specific causes of death.

Standardized mortality ratios for various subgroups were calculated for each cause of death, by age, calendar period and sex. Similar procedures were used to develop summary indexes of morbidity. The observed mortality rates were lower than expected in both male and female employees, based on U.S. mortality rates, a reflection of much selection and the "healthy worker effect." The male employees had a more favorable experience than female employees. In both sexes, cancer was the predominant cause of death but the Moscow and comparison groups did not differ appreciably in overall and specific mortality. The population was relatively young, however, and it may have been too early to detect long-time mortality effects. About one-third of the employees were followed for 15-20 years and over half for longer then 10 years. There were approximately 50,000 person-years of observation for the total employee group. Among dependent children and adults, there were no differences between the Moscow and comparison groups. Problems of ascertainment of exposure could not be overcome in this study. Variation of field intensities within the building could not be determined, nor could records be located which indicated where employees had lived or worked; reliance had to be put on questionnaire responses and recollections to estimate an individual's potential for exposure. It should also be noted that exposure for 22 years was at the level of 5 uW/cm^2, an extremely low level even by Russian standards. The highest exposure level (18 uW/cm^2) was recorded for only 6 months in 1975-76; thus, the group exposed to the more intense fields had the shortest period of observation in the study (Table 6). Excess risk ratios which could be detected with a power of 80 percent at a significance level of .05 varied widely from 1.3 to 4 and above, depending on person-years of observation for various mortality or morbidity event ratios. There was no convincing evidence to implicate microwave radiation in the mortality experience of the Moscow employees.

Table 6. Microwave Exposure Levels at the U.S. Embassy in Moscow

Time Period	Exposed Area of Chancery	Power Density and Exposure Duration
1953 to May 1975	West Facade	Max of 5 μW/cm^2 9 h/day
June 1975 to Feb. 1976	South and East Facade	18 μW/cm^2 18h/day
Since Feb. 7, 1976	South and East Facade	Fractions of a μW/cm^2 18 h/day

Data from Lilienfeld et al. 1978

MORBIDITY STUDIES

General

Studies of microwave health effects have been made since the 1940s. The majority are occupational surveys and medical surveillance programs carried out to assess health hazards for persons exposed in industrial and military settings. Some selected studies of general health status are summarized in Table 7. An early American study (Barron et al., 1955, Barron and Baraff, 1958) reported findings from a physical examination program at an airframe manufacturing plant of 226 radar workers and 88 employees without industrial radar exposure. Some workers were re-examined periodically for a few years; duration of exposure ranged up to 13 years. Considerable effort was put into estimating exposures from the various radar frequencies but exposure times and power densities for individuals could not be estimated. No significant changes were found in physical status, clinical laboratory findings, eye pathology or fertility studies. Blood count changes in the first of the two studies were not subsequently validated. Methods of selection of the exposed and nonexposed were not stated and the small nonexposed group was considerably older than the radar workers.

Table 7. Selected Studies of Microwave Effects

Reference	Intensity (mW/cm^2)	Exposure (Years)	Effects
Barron et al. (1958, 1955)	4	0-13	No significant change in health status
Czerski et al., Siekierzynski et al. (1974)	<0.2-6.0	1-10	No differences in diagnosis between 2 exposure groups
Djordjevic et al. (1979)	<5	5-10	No clinical differences; more complaints in exposed
Lilienfeld et al. (1978)	.005-.018	2-4	No effect on illness patterns or cause of death
Robinette et al. (1980)	1-100	2-4	No effect on hospitalized morbidity or mortality

In Yugoslavia in 1979, Djordjevic et al. reported on clinical evaluations of 322 radar workers with a 5-10 year history of occupational exposure to microwaves and a control group of 220 nonexposed. The radar workers were 25-40 years of age and the controls were said to be matched for age, character of work regimen and socioeconomic status. The workers were exposed to pulsed microwaves within a wide range of intensities but generally at levels less than 5 mW/cm^2. Ten diagnoses were used in the comparative clinical evaluations (neurocirculatory asthenia, upper respiratory infection, neurosis, chronic rheumatoid disease, gastritis, duodenal ulcer, hypertension, cardiomyopathy, chronic bronchitis and ocular lens opacities). There were no statistically significant differences between the exposed and control group.

In the study of U.S. naval personnel described in the mortality section (Robinette et al., 1980), the cohorts of over 40,000 men were also followed for three morbidity endpoints: in-service hospitalization, VA hospitalization and disability compensation. Hospitalized illness during military service (around the period of exposure) was an endpoint for which there was virtually complete information for the total study group. Admission rates to Navy hospitals were computed by diagnostic class and by exposure category. Of the 18 comparisons between the total low and high exposure groups, two were statistically significant: the low exposure group had larger admission rates for mental disease and for accidents, poisonings and violence. For no disease class was the admission rate of the high exposure group significantly larger than that for the low exposure group and for some the rates were smaller. The differences in hospital admission rates could have resulted from differences in the occupational rosters relating to age and time of entry into service. There were no differential health risks that could be attributed to occupational exposure to radar with respect to hospitalization around the years of exposure. Later admissions to the VA hospital system revealed some significant difference between the low and high exposure group but the use of the VA hospital system was limited to less than 15 percent of the study subjects. With regard to service-connected disabilities, only actual compensation awards were available for analysis. A single difference was statistically significant for mental conditions, which occurred at a higher rate in the low exposure group than in the high exposure group. Claims rather than awards for service-connected disabilities would have greater relevance for differential morbidity but information on disallowed claims was not available for analysis.

In the study of American Embassy personnel in Moscow
(Lilienfeld et al., 1978), extensive analyses were performed on
information from employment medical records and a self administered health history questionnaire. Questionnaire responses,
which were received from about half of the personnel, were
validated for a stratified sample. Exhaustive comparative
analyses were made of all symptoms, conditions and diseases.
There were no essential differences in health experience between
the Moscow group and employees in the comparison eastern European
posts. The Moscow group had somewhat higher frequencies of most
of the common health conditions reported and males had a threefold
greater risk of acquiring protozoal infections. The size of the
study population and the period of observation were not sufficient
to detect excess risks less than twofold for many of the medical
conditions including all malignant neoplasms. For specific types
of neoplasms which occurred with low frequency, only a 5-10 fold
excess could be detected. There was no convincing evidence of a
microwave effect at the time of analysis.

Neural, Cardiovascular, Functional Effects

Nervous system and behavioral changes in experimental animals
following low level exposures have been reported for many years
from eastern Europe (Petrov, 1970; Baranski and Czerski,1976).
Until the 1970s virtually all of the numerous industrial health
surveillance programs and occupational surveys in the USSR and
eastern European countries reported functional disturbances of the
central nervous and cardiovascular systems among microwave workers
(Gordon, 1966; Sadchikova, 1974; Silverman, 1973). Exposures were
mainly low level (microwatts up to a few milliwatts/cm^2) and long
term.

Functional disturbances have been described as a typical kind
of radiowave or microwave sickness, the asthenic or neurasthenic
syndrome. Symptoms and signs include headache, fatigue, irritability, loss of appetite, sleepiness (or insomnia), sweating,
thyroid gland enlargement, difficulties in concentration or
memory, depression, emotional instability, loss of libido and
impotence. This clinical syndrome is reported to be generally
reversible if exposure is discontinued. Another frequently
described manifestation is a set of labile functional cardiovascular changes including bradycardia (or occasional tachy-
cardia), arterial hypertension (or hypotension) and changes in
cardiac conduction. This form of neurocirculatory asthenia is
also attributed to nervous system influence. More serious but
less frequent neurologic or neuropsychiatric disturbances have
occasionally been described as a diencephalic syndrome. Some
nervous system effects reported in studies before 1970 are shown
in Table 8.

Table 8. Nervous System Effects in Some Studies of Microwave
Workers Before 1970

Country	Number Exposed	Number Nonexposed	Sympt. signs	Neurol. exam.	EEG change
Czech.	72	0	+	+	+
Poland	149	0	+	+	+
U.S.S.R.	525	100	+	+	*
	66	34	+	*	*
	65	0	+	+	+
	26	0	-	-	+
	110	0	+	-	*

* not tested
Data from Silverman, 1973.

More recently, two industrial hygiene studies in eastern
Europe have failed to find microwave-related functional health
effects. In Poland (Czerski et al, I 1974; Sierkierzynski et al,
II 1974), 841 men occupationally exposed to pulse-modulated
microwave radiation of radar frequencies with exposure up to 10
years or more were studied. An unexposed control population could
not be found and the study group was subdivided into two groups
according to level of exposure. One group of 507 men was exposed
to mean power densities greater than 0.2 mW/cm^2, with short term
exposures estimated up to 6 mW/cm^2. The other group of 334 men
was exposed to levels less than 0.2 mW/cm^2. The results of
medical examinations were compared with respect to four health
status categories: no functional disturbance, neurotic syndrome,
digestive tract functional disturbances, and cardiocirculatory
disturbances with abnormal ECG findings. The two groups of men,
who were in the 20-45 year age group, were similar in health
status, and no association of symptoms with exposure level or
duration of occupational exposure could be demonstrated. It was
noted, however, that functional disturbances were found in about
60 percent of all individuals examined and in about 30 percent the
symptoms were severe enough to require removal from microwave
exposure under prevailing occupational standards. This was stated
to be an unusually high prevalence of functional disturbances.

In Yugoslavia (Djordjevic et al., 1979), the frequency of objective complaints related to the central nervous and cardiovascular systems was determined in a group of 322 workers in radar stations and a comparison group of 220. This was part of a comprehensive investigation of health status that included clinical examinations and laboratory tests. The radar workers, who had been exposed for periods of 5 to 10 years to pulsed microwaves of all radar frequencies and to intensities generally less than 5mW/cm^2, were matched with the nonexposed workers on age (25 to 40 years of age), some working conditions, and social and living conditions. Clinical, hematologic, biochemical and ophthalmologic findings were similar in both groups. Of the six complaints studied (headache, fatigue, irritability, sleep disturbance, impaired libido and memory impairment), three were found more frequently in radar workers. Headache, fatigue and irritability occurred in about 15% of the nonexposed workers but in 28% of the radar workers. The excess of subjective complaints in radar workers was ascribed to unfavorable environmental conditions of work in the radar stations such as high noise level, poor lighting, the necessity of paying attention to the radar screen and inadequate ventilation. This appears to contradict the authors initial statements that the working environments of the two groups were similar in all respects.

An American study of possible behavioral and physiologic effects of microwave radiation involved three small groups of U.S. Navy crewmen from a carrier ship: flight-deck crew who were expected to have the highest levels of exposure, hangar-deck crew with expected low level exposures and look-out crew with no expected exposure (U.S. Senate, 1977). No differences among the three groups were found, either in dockside or seagoing tests, with respect to task performance, psychologic tests or biologic effects.

The only American epidemiologic study to date of some of these symptoms and conditions is the cohort study of U.S. Embassy employees in Moscow and eastern European capitals (Lilienfeld et al., 1978). Although much symptomatology was found in the study subjects, no differences between them and the comparison groups were attributable to microwave exposure at the intensities measured outside the Moscow Embassy building, nor were there any differences between groups of dependent children or adults. These levels, however, were subtantially lower than the exposures reported in the eastern European occupational studies and the exposure periods were shorter. It is not possible at this time to characterize the functional changes and clinical effects which may be associated with exposure to microwaves.

Ocular Effects

The potential of microwave radiation to induce cataracts and minor lens defects has been the basis for much microwave research, particularly in the United States. Some experimental animals, notably the rabbit, develop cataracts under controlled laboratory conditions following a single high intensity exposure of 100-150 mW/cm^2 for 60 to 100 minutes (Cleary, 1980). There does not appear to be a cumulative effect of repeated exposures unless each exposure is high enough to be injurious to the lens. Human cataracts appear also to be a probable high threshold effect. In man, more than 50 clinical cases of alleged microwave-induced cataract have been reported, generally related to occupational exposures of high intensity. Most of these have been reported by a single ophthalmologist (Zaret, 1974) who contends that the posterior subcapsular type of cataract is characteristic of microwave radiation. In the opinion of most observers, however, microwave cataracts are not distinguishable from other cataracts.

Although there has been much interest in the cataractogenic effect of microwaves, only a minimal effort has been made to investigate cataracts as such, as distinct from minor lens changes which have been studied in numerous surveys as possible precursors of cataracts. The only case-control study of cataracts was reported in 1965 by Cleary et al. They used medical records from Veterans Administration hospitals and personnel records from the US Army and Air Force to study veterans of World War II and the Korean War. Cases were white males under the age of 55 who were treated for cataracts between 1950 and 1962. The diagnostic indexes of all Veterans Administration hospitals were screened to select a sample of 2946 men; a control sample was obtained from the same sources by selecting men with adjacent hospital numbers. Men over age 55 were excluded in order to minimize dilution of the sample with senile cataracts, and all cataract diagnoses that could be ascribed to a non-microwave factor were also eliminated from the sampling plan (that is, all congenital, traumatic, diabetic and other specified types). The study was designed to detect a twofold increase in relative risk, with a probability of 0.80 at an 0.05 level of significance. The military records of each veteran were abstracted to determine military occupational specialties, which were used to categorize members of the cataract and control groups as radar and nonradar workers. Relative risks are shown in Table 9; no excess risk of developing cataracts was detected among radar workers. The maximum time period after exposure was about 20 years but many of the men had far shorter post-exposure times. The exclusion of men over 55 leaves unanswered the question of excess cataracts after that age, when cataracts increase naturally in prevalence (NCHS, 1983).

Table 9. Relative Risk of Cataracts Among Veterans
by Age and Occupation

Age	Diagnosis	Radar Workers	Nonradar Workers	Relative Risk	x^2
50-54	Cataract	9	699	1.02	0.08 NS
	Other	4	316		
40-49	Cataract	7	1517	0.39	3.39 NS
	Other	13	1101		
20-39	Cataract	3	418	0.94	0.09 NS
	Other	4	522		

From Cleary et al. 1965

Numerous ocular surveys have been made since the late 1950s involving personnel in military and industrial settings. They have been largely cross-sectional and prevalence studies with the principal aim of determining the significance of minor lens changes as possible early markers of microwave exposure or precursors of cataracts. These occupational studies have generally emphasized careful eye examinations including the use of slit-lamp biomicroscopy, without comparable attention to study design, selection bias, age comparabilty of study groups, interaud intra-observer bias, and followup plans for exposed and comparison groups.

Lens imperfections have been found to occur normally even during the childhood years and to increase markedly with age (Zydecki, 1974). By about age 50, lens defects have been reported in most comparison subjects, based on data from various studies (Silverman, 1980). Many efforts have been made to classify, grade and score minor lens changes (Zaret and Eisenbud, 1961; Appleton and McCrossan, 1972; Odland, 1972; Siekierzynski et al., III 1974; Shacklett et al., 1975). Although a few suggestive differences between microwave workers and comparison groups have been reported (Cleary and Pasternack, 1966; Majewska, 1968; Zydecki, 1974),

there is no clear indication that minor lens defects are a marker
for microwave exposure in terms of type or frequency of lens
changes, exposure factors or occupation. Clinically significant
lens changes, which would permit selection of individuals to be
followed, have not been identified nor is there evidence from
ophthalmic surveys to date that minor lens opacities are
precursors of clinical cataracts. Reported retinal changes
(Aurell and Tengroth, 1973) have not been confirmed.

Congenital Anomalies and Reproductive Effects

Microwave radiation can be teratogenic in experimental animals
exposed at specific times during gestation to levels that raise
maternal body temperatures (WHO, 1981). In humans there is no
evidence to date of congenital defects following exposure in
utero. There have been two preliminary and inconclusive
epidemiologic investigations of the effect of paternal occupational exposure to radar on the occurrence of congenital
malformations in their offspring, one concerning fathers of
children with Down's syndrome and the other with births to
military personnel.

A case-control study of Down's syndrome and parental exposure
to ionizing radiation in the city of Baltimore (Sigler et al.,
1965) yielded an unexpected and provocative finding regarding
paternal exposure to microwave radiation. Fathers of children
with mongolism gave more frequent histories of work as radar
operators or technicians during military service than did fathers
of unaffected children, a difference that was of borderline
statistical significance. Exposure during military service
occurred prior to the birth of the index child. The study was
expanded from 216 matched pairs of children to 344 pairs, and
additional followup of all fathers and search of available armed
forces records were undertaken to obtain more detailed information
about radar exposure (Cohen et al., 1977). The original
suggestive excess of radar exposure among fathers of Down's
syndrome children was not confirmed on further study. It turned
out to be very difficult to document occupational exposures to
radar and impossible to obtain any measurement data. A chromosome
study of peripheral blood of exposed and unexposed fathers showed
some suggestive but inconclusive changes; results of the analysis
are not yet available.

A study of congenital malformations in the State of Alabama
(Peacock et al., 1971) noted an excess of clubfoot (talipes) cases
reported from an area in which a U.S. Army helicopter training
base was located. The excess related to the number of cases
expected from birth certificate notifications for the State during
a three-year period 1968-1971. A more detailed investigation of a

larger geographic area for the same time period revealed a substantially higher rate of anomalies (diagnosed within 24 hours after birth) to military personnel than in the State as a whole (Burdeshaw and Schaffer, 1976). The military base was situated near many radar stations and low flying helicopter pilots were thought to be heavily exposed. Errors in malformation data on birth certificates and probable overreporting from the base led to the conclusion that the evidence was not convincing for radar-associated congenital anomalies. Further study was not possible.

Microwave diathermy, once used frequently as treatment for women with menstrual and pelvic disorders, sometimes resulted in exposures before or during early pregnancy. Early case reports (Rubin and Erdman, 1959) indicated no interference with ovulation and conception. The use of microwave heating as diathermy to relieve the pain of uterine contractions during labor has been reported among several thousand women in Belgium as beneficial but followup of cases and controls has not been reported (Daels, 1976). Recent studies have been made of occupational exposures of physiotherapists to diathermy, suggesting a possible increase in congenital defects among offspring of female therapists who used radiofrequency (shortwave) equipment (Kallen et al., 1982), and heart disease among male therapists who used shortwave equipment (Hamburger et al., 1983).

Reproductive efficiency in male laboratory animals may be temporarily reduced by microwave exposures that increase testicular temperatures to a moderate degree, and may be permanently changed by very high testicular temperatures. In man, reports of loss of libido and interference with spermatogenesis have appeared in accounts of the neurasthenic syndrome (Baranski and Czerski, 1976) as well as in case reports of high level exposures (Rosenthal, et al., 1968). The study in Yugoslavia referred to earlier (Djordjevic et al., 1978) found no difference in loss of libido between long term radar workers and a nonexposed comparison group. In Romania a study was carried out to find objective evidence of the symptoms reported as part of the neurasthenic syndrome (Lancranjan et al., 1975). The study involved 31 microwave technicians, average age 33 years, who had a mean exposure of eight years (range 1-17 years) to frequencies between $10,000$ and $3,600$ MHz and fields in the range of tens to hundreds mW/cm^2. The comparison group was composed of 30 men of similar mean age and no known exposure to microwaves. About 80 percent of the exposed men had signs of the neurasthenic syndrome and 70 percent had a decrease in libido and had orgasm disturbances. In 74 percent there were alterations of spermato-genesis such as decreases in the number of sperm, percent of motile sperm, and percent of normal sperm. Three months after

450

removal from the source of exposure, spermatogenesis was improved
in two-thirds of the technicians. No effect on testicular
endocrine function was detected.

Cancer

Microwave radiation has not induced cancer experimentally but
its role as a possible co-carcinogen has been suggested
(Szmigielski et al., 1982; Kunz et al., 1984). Case reports in
humans of clusters of tumors associated with high occupational
levels have not been validated, nor have geographic associations
between nearness to airport radar and cancer incidence (Lester and
Moore, 1982). The cohort studies of U.S. naval personnel
(Robinette et al., 1980) and U.S. employees at the American
Embassy in Moscow (Lilienfeld et al., 1978) found excesses of some
forms of cancer but none could be interpreted as microwave-related
in terms of morbidity or mortality. Recent analyses of occupational mortality statistics have reported increased proportional
mortality ratios for leukemia among workers in occupations with
potential exposure to electric amd magnetic fields (Milham, 1982;
McDowall, 1983) and similar findings have been reported for
proportional incidence ratios (Wright et al., 1982; Coleman et
al., 1983). Some of the occupational classes could involve
microwave exposure but there are no exposure data. Reports of
increased cancer mortality rates among residential populations
living near high voltage overhead transmission lines (Wertheimer
and Leeper, 1979) concern alternating electric current and its
magnetic fields, not microwave radiation..

PROBLEMS OF QUANTITATION

Dose

As in other environmental situations (Maclure and MacMahon,
1980), the principal source of uncertainty in epidemiologic
studies of microwave effects is the limited, unobtainable or
nonexistent information about human exposures. In investigations
involving prior exposures, it is a formidable and sometimes
impossible task to reconstruct exposure data from available
records or recall by study subjects. In investigations with some
exposure measurements, it has not been possible to assign exposure
intensities to individual study subjects. Exposure to microwave
radiation, unlike ionizing radiation, cannot be measured by a
personal device such as a film badge. Exposures over a period of
years cannot be evaluated within reasonable limits because of the
complexities of measurement, movement of persons in the irradiated
fields, and changing fields. Whether repeated exposure results in
cumulative doses to critical organs is not known. Dosimetry,
literally the measurement of dose, generally refers to measurement

of the intensity of exposure fields. Within recent years, empirical formulas have been developed to calculate the specific absorption rate (SAR) as a measure of the rate of energy absorption but its application is still limited.   Apart from accidental overexposures or the deliberate use of high doses for medical treatment such as diathermy for deep heating and hyperthermia for cancer therapy, the exposures to which study populations have been exposed are often described as consistent with national guidelines or standards.

Effects

Biologic or health effects in humans are not yet clearly defined. The bulk of investigations consists of cross-sectional studies which provide prevalence data without determination of the temporal sequence of exposure and effect and without longitudinal followup. In the two recent cohort studies, effects have been measured in terms of total number of cases in specified populations over a period of time, that is, a cumulative incidence rate in the persons initially at risk (Robinette et al., 1980), and as the number of cases that occur per unit of population time, person-years at risk (Lilienfeld et al., 1978).

Latent Period

The time between exposure and the appearance or detection of an effect is an element of quantitation about which there is little information. Whether the duration of latency is influenced by dose is not known. A case report of cataract formation suggests a short latency period of several days after exposure to very high intensity fields (Cleary, 1980). Other factors such as specific microwave frequency (wavelength) and ambient humidity and temperature may affect latency. It is conceivable that in the case of endpoints such as cataract or cancer, the latent period may be the time required to reach the age when cataracts or certain cancers become naturally prevalent.

Dose-Response

The uncertainties of dose, of response and of temporal factors make dose-response considerations very speculative. Animal models differ among the various species and are generally not applicable to man. It seems likely that acute cataract induction is a threshold phenomenon in man, as it appears to be in the rabbit, but there are only a few individual case reports to support this (Cleary, 1980). While there is universal agreement about the heating effects of high dose microwave radiation, controversy continues about detectable responses to low, so-called nonthermal doses. At the clinical level, only eastern European

investigators have reported the neurasthenic syndrome, not only
for microwave exposures but also in somewhat similar form for
radiofrequencies and magnetic fields.

Interactions

There is considerable uncertainty about the action of environmental agents that are present in the work environment of microwave personnel. In many industrial settings there are other
physical and chemical agents present whose action or interaction
with microwaves is not known. In the hyperthermia treatment of
cancer, microwaves appear to enhance the effects of ionizing
radiation therapy. Susceptibility to adverse effects of microwave
radiation according to age and sex cannot be determined. Study
populations are overwhelmingly male in the 20-45 year age range
with no followup into older ages. Within these limits, there
appears to be no dependence of clinical symptoms on age. Observations on females generally concern a therapeutic situation and
infrequently involve work settings. Nothing is known of the
susceptibility of children to microwave radiation.

SUMMARY

Microwave radiation is a form of nonionizing electromagnetic
radiation that is biologically active although of very low photon
energies. The uses of microwave energy have increased dramatically during the past few decades with the result that unknown but
increasing numbers of persons are exposed at their work and
general populations are potentially exposed everywhere. General
population exposure is long-term (for some, probably a lifetime),
very low level and intermittent; it varies with technologic
development, geographic location, urban-rural characteristics and
other features of communities. In contrast to other environmental
"pollutants", microwaves and radiowave are necessary because of
our dependence on radio communications. In U.S. cities it is
estimated that 99 percent of the population is exposed to less
than 0.1 mW/cm^2 (Tell and Mantiply, 1978). Persons occupationally
exposed have been mainly adult males in industry or the military
who are exposed for the work day or part of it under controlled
conditions. Occupational exposure limits vary widely from 0.01 to
10 mW/cm^2 in various countries; some efforts are underway to
narrow the gap.

Biologic effects in humans are not yet clearly defined and
most of the postulated health effects have yet to be tested
adequately or appropriately. Acute effects from high intensity
exposures in accidental situations are due to tissue heating and
may result in burns of any severity, cataract formation and
testicular damage. The effects of exposures that are long-term,

low-level or both are still a matter of dispute because of inadequate investigation, differences in concepts of nonthermal mechanisms of action and problems of extrapolation from experimental studies. It is difficult to identify exposed populations, select suitable controls and obtain exposure data. Some study groups already characterized can be improved by the acquisition of additional exposure data, some groups should be followed for longer periods of time, and some should be investigated for additional endpoints. In addition, exposed groups not yet investigated should be considered for study. Specific endpoints which require further study are cataracts, mental and behavioral changes, congenital anomalies and reproductive effects, and malignancies. The problems of quantitation in epidemiologic studies of microwave effects are numerous and include uncertainties about "dose", effects, latent periods, dose-response relationships and interactions.

REFERENCES

Appleton, B., and McCrossan, G.C., 1972, Microwave lens effects in humans, Arch. Ophthal., 88:259-262.

Aurell, E. and Tengroth, B., 1973, Lenticular and retinal changes secondary to microwave exposure, Acta Ophthal., 51:764-771.

Baranski, S. and Czerski, P., 1976, "Biological Effects of Microwaves," Dowden, Hutchinson and Ross, Inc., Stroudsburg, PA.

Barron, C.I., and Baraff, A.A., 1958, Medical considerations of exposure to microwaves (Radar). J. Am. Med. Ass., 168: 1194-1199.

Barron, C.I., Love, A.A., and Baraff, A.A., 1955, Physical evaluations of personnel exposed to microwave emanations. J. Aviat. Med., 26:442-452.

Burdeshaw, J.A., and Schaffer, S., 1976, "Factors Associated with the Incidence of Congenital Anomalies: A Localized Investigation:, Environmental Protection Agency, Final Report, Contract No. 68-02-0791, March 31.

Cleary, S.F., 1980, Microwave cataractogenesis. Proc. IEEE, 68:49-55.

Cleary, S.F., and B.S. Pasternack, 1966, Lenticular changes in microwave workers: A statistical study. Arch. Environ. Health, 23:23-29.

Cleary, S.F., Pasternack, B.S. and Beebe, G.W., 1965, Cataract incidence in radar workers, Arch. Environ. Health, 11:179-182.

Cohen, B.H., Lilienfeld, A.M., Kramer, S., and Hyman, L.C. 1977, Parental factors in Down's syndrome: Results of the second Baltimore case-control study, in: "Population Cytogenetics-- Studies in Humans," Hook, E.B. and Porter, I.H., eds., Academic Press, New York, New York. pp. 301-352.

Coleman M; Bell J.; Skeet R., 1983, Leukemia incidence in
    electrical workers, Lancet, pp 982-983, April 30.
Czerzki, P., Sierkierzynski, M. and Gidynski, A., 1974. Health
    surveillance of personnel occupationally exposed to
    microwaves. I. Theoretical considerations and practical
    aspects. Aerospace Med., 45:1137-1142.
Czerski, P., Ostrowski, K., Silverman, C., Shore, M.L., Suess,
    M.J. and Waldeskog, B, Eds, 1974, "Biologic Effects and
    Health Hazards of Microwave Radiation" Polish Medical
    Publishers, Warsaw, Poland, p. 334.
Daels, J., 1976. Microwave heating of the uterine wall during
    parturition, J. Microwave Power, 11:166-168.
Djordjevic, Z., Kolak, A., Stojkovic, M., Rankovic, N., and
    Ristic, P., 1979. A study of the health status of radar
    workers, Avait. Space Environ. Med., 50:396-398.
Glaser, Z.R., Cleveland, R.F. and Kielman, J.K., 1979, Physical
    principles and extent of exposure, Chapter 2, "NIOSH Draft
    Criteria Document on Radiofrequency and Microwave Radiation",
    National Institute for Occupational Safety and Health,
    Washington, D.C. (Director's Draft). pp.14-27.
Gordon, Z. V., 1966, "Biological Effect of Microwaves in
    Occupational Hygiene", Translated fron Russian, NASA
    TTF-633, TT 70-50087, NTIS N71-14632, 1970.
Hamburger, S., Logue, J. N. and Sternthal, P.M., 1983,
    Occupational exposure to nonionizing radiation and an
    association with heart disease: An exploratory study, J.
    Chronic Dis., 36:791-802.
Kallen, B., Malmquist, G., and Moritz, U., 1982, Delivery outcome
    among physiotherapists in Sweden: Is non-ionizing radiation a
    fetal hazard?, Arch. Environ. Health, 37:81-85.
Kunz, L.L., Johnson, R.B., Chou, C.K., Guy, A.W., 1984. Patho-
    biological effects of low-level lifetime exposure of rats to
    pulsed, radio frequency radiation: Final report (Part II).
    Presented at 6th Annual Meeting of Bioelectromagnetics
    Society, July 15-19, Atlanta, Georgia.
Lancranjan, I., Maiconescu, M., Rafaila, E., Klepsch, I., Popescu,
    H.I., 1975, Gonadic function in workmen with long-term
    exposure to microwaves, Health Physics, 29:381-383.
Lester, J. R., and Moore, D. F., 1982, Cancer incidence and
    electromagnetic radiation, J. Bioelectricity, 1:59-76.
Lilienfeld, A. M., Tonascia, J.,Tonascia, S., Libauer, C. A., and
    Cauthen, G. M., 1978, "Foreign Service Health Status Study--
    Evaluation of Health Status of Foreign Service and Other
    Employees from Selected Eastern European Posts", Final
    Report, Contract No. 6025-6190973 (NTIS PB-288163), Dept. of
    State, Washington, D.C.
Maclure, K. M., and MacMahon, B., 1980, An epidemiologic
    perspective of environmental carcinogenesis, Epidemiol.
    Reviews, 2:19-48.

Majewska, K., 1968, Study of effects of microwaves on visual organs, Klin. Oczna (Polish) 38:323-328.

McDowall M. E., 1983. Leukemia mortality in elecrical workers in England and Wales, Lancet, p. 29, Jan. 29.

Milham, S., Jr., 1982, Mortality from leukemia in workers exposed to electrical and magnetic fields, New England J. Med, 307:249.

Moss, E., Murray, W., Parr, W., and Conover, D., 1977, Physical hazards: Radiation, In: Key, M. M., Henschel, A. F., Butler, J., R. N., Tabershaw, I. R., Eds, "Occupational Diseases: A Guide to Their Recognition", DHEW (NOISH), Publication No. 77-181, Washington, D.C., p. 479.

NCHS, 1983, Ganely, J. P., Roberts, J., "Eye Conditions and Related Need for Medical Care Among Persons 1-74 Years of Age, United States, 1971-72", National Center for Health Statistics, Vital and Health Statistics, Series 11 No. 228, DHHS Pub No.(PHS)83-1678, Washington, D.C.

NCRP, 1981, "Radiofrequency Electromagnetic Fields: Properties, Quantities and Units, Biophysical Interaction, and Measurements", NCRP Report No. 67, National Council on Radiation Protection and Measurements, Washington, D.C.

Odland, L. T., 1972, "Observations on microwave hazards to USAF personnel," J. Occup. Med. 14:544-547.

Peacock, P. B., Simpson, J. W., Alford, C. A., and Saunders, F., 1971, Congenital anomalies in Alabama, J. Med. Assoc. State Ala, pp. 42-50.

Petrov, I. R., ed. 1970, "Influence of Microwave Radiation on the Organism of Men and Animals", "Meditsina" Press, Leningrad, NASA, TTF-708, 1972.

Robinette, C. D., and Silverman, C., 1977, Causes of death following occupational exposure to microwave radiation (Radar), in: "Symposium on Biological Effects and Measurements of Radiofrequency/Microwaves", D. G. Hazzard, ed. HEW Publication (FDA) 77-8026, Rockville, Maryland, pp. 338-344.

Robinette, C. D., Silverman, C., and Jablon, S., 1980, Effects upon health of occupational exposure to microwave radiation (R) Am. J. Epidemol., 112:39-53.

Rosenthal, D.S. and Berring, S.C., 1968, Hypogonadism after microwave radiation, JAMA, 205:245-248.

Rubin, A. and Erdman, W.J., 1959, Microwave exposure of the human female pelvis during early pregnancy and prior to conception, Am. J. Phys. Med., 38:219-220.

Sadchikova, M. N., 1974, Clinical manifestations of reactions to microwave irradiation in various occupational groups, in: " Biologic Effects and Health Hazards of Microwave Radiation," Czerski, P., Ostrowski, K., Silverman, C., Shore, M. L., and Waldeskog, B., Eds., Poland, Polish Medical Publishers, pp. 261-267.

Shacklett, D. E., Tredici, T. J., and Epstein, D. L., 1975, Evaluation of possible microwave-induced lens changes in the United States Air Force, Aviat. Space Environ. Med., 46: 1403-1406.

Siekierzynski, M., Czerski, P., Milczsert, H., Gidynski, A., Czarecki, C., Dziuk, E., and Jedrzejczak, W., 1974, Health surveillance of personnel occupationally exposed to micro-waves, II Functional disturbances. Aerospace Med. 45: 1143-1145.

Siekierzynski, M., Czerski, P., Milczsert, H., Gidynski, A., Czarecki, C., Dziuk, E., and Jedrzejczak, W., 1974, Health surveillance of personnel occupationally exposed to microwaves, III. Lens translucency. Aerospace Med. 45:116:1148.

Sigler, A.T., Lilienfeld, A.M., Cohen, B.H., and Westlake, J.E., 1965, Radiation exposure in parents of children with mongolism (Down's Syndrome). Bull. J. Hopkins Hosp., 117:374-399.

Silverman, C., 1980, Epidemiologic studies of microwave effects. Proc. IEEE, 68:78-84.

Silverman, C., 1973, Nervous and behavioral effects of microwave radiation in humans, Amer. J. Epidemiol. 97-219-224.

Szmigielski, S., Szymdzinski, A., Pietraszek, A., Bielac, M., Jamiak, M. and Wrembel, J.K., 1982, Accelerated development of spontaneous and benzopyrene-induced skin cancer in mice exposed to 2450MHz microwave radiation. Bioeletromagnetics, 3:179-191.

Tell, R.A. and Mantiply, E.D., 1978, "Population Exposure to VHF and UHF Broadcast Radiation in the United States", Report No. ORP/EAD 78-5 (U.S. Environmental Protection Agency, Las Vegas).

U.S. Senate, 1977, "Radiation Health and Safety", Hearings before the Committee on Commerce, Science, and Transportation, 95th Congress, First Session on Oversight of Radiation Health and Safety, June 16,17, 27, 28, and 29, 1977, Serial No. 95-49, pp. 284, 1195, 1196.

U.S. Senate, 1979, Committee on Commerce, Science, and Transportation. Committee Print, "Microwave Irradiation of the U.S. Embassy in Moscow", April 1979, U.S. Government Printing Office, Washington, D.C., (43-949).

Wertheimer, N., and Leeper, E., 1979, Electrical wiring configurations and childhood cancer. Am J Epidemiol 109:273-284.

WHO, 1981, "Environmental Health Criteria 16, Radiofrequency and Microwaves", World Health Organization, Geneva.

Wright W. E., Peters, J. M., Mack, T. M., 1982. Leukemia in workers exposed to electrical and magnetic fields, Lancet, pp 1160-1161, Nov. 20.

Zaret, M.M. 1974, Selected cases of microwave cataract in man associated with concomitant annotated pathologies, in: "Biologic Effects and Health Hazards of Microwave Radiation", Czerski, P., Ostrowski, K., Shore, M.L., Silverman, C., Suess, M.J. and Waldeskog, B., eds. Polish Medical Publishers, Warsaw, Poland. pp. 294-301.

Zaret, M.M., and Eisenbud, M., 1961, Preliminary results of studies of the lenticular effects of microwaves among exposed personnel. in: "Biological Effects of Microwave Radiation", Vol. I, Proceedings of the 4th Tri-Service Conference, M.F. Peyton, ed. Plenum Press, New York, New York. pp. 293-308.

Zydecki, S. 1974, Assessment of lens transluceny in juveniles, microwave workers, and age-matched groups, in: "Biologic Effects and Health Hazards of Microwave Radiation", Czerski, P., Ostrowski, Silverman, C., Shore, M.L., Suess, M.J., and Waldeskog, B., Eds., Poland, Polish Medical Publishers, pp. 306-308.

ESTABLISHING THE LINK BETWEEN HUMAN PROTO-ONCOGENES

AND GROWTH FACTORS

Keith C. Robbins, Hisanaga Igarashi, Arnona Gazit,
Ing-Ming Chiu, Steven R. Tronick and Stuart A. Aaronson

Laboratory of Cellular and Molecular Biology
National Cancer Institute
Bethesda, Maryland 20205

Investigations of acute transforming retroviruses have led
to important insights concerning a small group of cellular genes
with transforming potential. Acute retroviruses have arisen in
nature by recombination of replication competent type C retroviruses
with cellular genes, termed proto-oncogenes. The transduced
cellular (onc) sequences confer to the virus properties essential
for the induction and maintenance of transformation (Weiss et al.,
1982; Duesberg, 1983; Bishop, 1983).

Proto-oncogenes are well conserved in evolution, implying that
they possess important functions in basic normal cellular processes.
In the present review, we summarize studies that have led to
identification of the first normal cellular function of a proto-
oncogene and present evidence suggesting how this gene may be
involved in certain kinds of human cancer.

THE sis TRANSFORMING GENE

The sis oncogene was first identified as the transforming gene
of the simian sarcoma virus (SSV). SSV is the only primate-derived
acute transforming retrovirus (Theilen et al., 1971). SSV, like
other sarcoma viruses, transforms cultured fibroblasts (Aaronson,
1973) and induces fibrosarcomas and glioblastomas in appropriate
host animals (Wolfe et al., 1971; Wolfe et al., 1972).

The cloning of biologically active SSV DNA made possible a
detailed analysis of this transforming viral genome (Robbins et al.,
1981). When the cloned 5.8-kbp SSV genome was compared to the

genome of its helper virus, SSAV, by restriction enzyme mapping and heteroduplex analyses, a restriction fragment, approximately 1 kbp in length, that was not detectably related to SSAV sequences could be localized towards the 3' end of the SSV genome. In accordance with convention, this segment was designated sis.

In order to determine the origin of the sis sequence, retroviral DNAs and normal cellular DNAs were analyzed by Southern blotting using a molecularly cloned v-sis specific probe. Retroviral genomes failed to hybridize with sis; however, sis-related restriction fragments were found to be present at low copy number in the DNAs of species as diverse as humans and quails. These findings suggested that recombination between SSAV and a normal cellular gene led to the creation of SSV (Robbins et al., 1982a). DNAs derived from New World primates annealed with this probe to a significantly greater degree than the DNAs isolated from any other species tested. Furthermore, hybrids formed between sis and woolly monkey cellular DNA exhibited the same thermal stability as that of the homologous v-sis DNA duplex. These results strongly implied that v-sis arose from the woolly monkey genome (Robbins et al., 1982a).

V-sis IS REQUIRED FOR THE ONCOGENIC ACTIVITY OF SSV

In order to determine whether v-sis was required for the transforming activity of SSV, a series of deletion mutants was constructed from molecularly cloned SSV DNA. These DNAs were then tested for their ability to transform NIH/3T3 cells in transfection assays. All constructs that resulted in the deletion of sis sequences were unable to transform NIH/3T3 cells (Robbins et al., 1982b). For example, deletion of the 3' LTR had no effect on transforming efficiency. However, when the deletion was extended to all but 82 base pairs of sis, no activity could be detected. Similarly, a mutant that lacked 250 bp at the 5' end of sis also was inactive. By this analysis, the transforming gene of SSV could be localized to v-sis.

NUCLEOTIDE SEQUENCE ANALYSIS OF SSV

The potential coding capacity of v-sis was revealed by the determination of the complete nucleotide sequence of SSV (Devare et al., 1983). An open reading frame 271 codons long encompassed v-sis and also included helper sequences (254 bp) 5' to v-sis. The termination codon was located 347 bp upstream from the 3' end of sis. By sequence comparison with Moloney MuLV and SSAV, the 5' end of the open reading frame was identified as the amino terminus of the SSAV env gene. The carboxyl terminus of the SSAV env gene encoding p15E was found to flank sis at its 3' end. Thus, creation of SSV involved a large deletion of the SSAV env gene and substitution of v-sis.

460

How might a sis gene product or products be synthesized? In addition to the first methionine of the open reading frame at position 3657, two methionines are predicted to occur prior to the start of v-sis sequences (positions 3969 and 3792). RNA splicing acceptor sites reside near each of these methionines. One of the ATG codons corresponds to that proposed as the initiator of the Moloney MuLV env gene product (Shinnick et al., 1981). Thus, an intriguing possibility is that the sis gene uses the same sequences for the initiation of its transcription and trans- lation as the env gene it replaced. In fact, the SSV genome codes for a 2.7-kb mRNA that contains LTR and sis sequences, but does not hybridize with gag-specific probes (Robbins et al., unpublished observations). A message of this size could accommodate enough information to code for proteins of 33,000, 30,000, or 28,000 MW predicted to initiate from the first three methionines, respectively, in the v-sis open reading frame.

IDENTIFICATION OF THE SSV TRANSFORMING PROTEIN

The task of identifying a sis protein(s) could now be readily attempted by synthesizing peptides predicted by the nucleotide sequence and preparing antibodies to them (Robbins et al., 1982b). One such antibody, directed towards amino terminal sequences of the predicted sis protein specifically precipitated a 28,000 dalton polypeptide from extracts of SSV-transformed cells. In contrast, antibodies against the SSAV env gene product did not precipitate this protein. These findings suggested that the trans- lation of the sis protein commenced at the third ATG of the open reading frame. Further confirmation that the 28,000 MW polypeptide (p28^{sis}) is coded for by the v-sis open reading frame was obtained by the demonstration that partially purified p28^{sis} possessed cyanogen bromide cleavage fragments which were predicted from its sequence. Additionally, a carboxyl terminal peptide antiserum specifically precipitated p28^{sis} from SSV-transformed cells. The structural features of the SSV genome showing its gene products are summarized in Fig. 1.

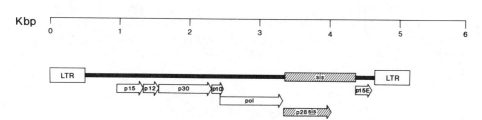

Fig. 1. The genome of SSV. The figure depicts the structural organization of biologically active SSV DNA and also indicates its gene products.

Having identified the SSV transforming protein, attempts were made to identify its function. Studies on the origin of oncogenes carried out over the last few years have shown in every case that oncogene sequences are highly conserved among eucaryotic species. Thus, mammalian v-onc probes detect specific restriction fragments in the genomes of evolutionarily distant species such as flies and worms (Shilo and Weinberg, 1981), and most recently, even in yeasts (DeFeo-Jones et al., 1983). Such evolutionary conservation must imply that proto-oncogene function is critical in cellular processes such as growth and development.

Elucidation of the molecular structure of retroviral onc genes has led to the detection, in many instances, of their protein products. The prototype of one group of onc genes, the src gene of Rous sarcoma virus, was found to possess tyrosine-specific protein kinase activity (Collett and Erikson, 1978; Levinson et al., 1978). Several other v-onc encoded proteins, although lacking in detectable protein kinase activity nevertheless share partial amino acid sequence similarities with the known retroviral tyrosine kinases (Bishop, 1983). The ras oncogene family encodes proteins possessing GTP-binding activity (Scolnick et al., 1979), and other onc proteins are thought to interact with substrates in the cell nucleus, due to their localization in this cell compartment (Alitalo et al., 1983; Hann et al., 1983; Curran et al., 1984). The transforming protein of SSV displayed none of the known properties of other characterized transforming gene products.

THE SSV TRANSFORMING PROTEIN IS RELATED TO
HUMAN PLATELET-DERIVED GROWTH FACTOR

The rapid proliferation of nucleotide sequence data, and thus predicted amino acid sequences for numerous proteins, in combination with the development of sequence data banks and computer programs for rapidly searching for similarities among these sequences (Wilbur and Lipman, 1983), has recently led to a number of striking observations. One such discovery was that the amino acid sequence of a peptide chain of platelet-derived growth factor, PDGF, a potent human connective tissue cell mitogen, showed a high degree of match with a segment of the predicted v-sis sequence (Doolittle et al, 1983; Waterfield et al., 1983). Thus, for the first time, the normal function of a proto-oncogene had been identified.

In active PDGF preparations, two peptides have been identified, designated PDGF-1 and PDGF-2 by Antoniades and Hunkapiller (1983). At their amino terminal ends, these peptides share 8 out of 19 residues without the introduction of gaps in their sequences. The predicted sis coding sequence, starting at residue 67, demonstrated an 84% match to PDGF-2 over this same stretch. Furthermore, in the total of 70 PDGF-2 residues identified, 87.1% corresponded to the p28^{sis} sequence. Taking into account the New World primate origin of v-sis (Robbins et al, 1982a), it was concluded that the v-sis transforming gene arose by recombination between the SSAV genome and a host cell gene for PDGF or a very highly related protein. Thus, all the observed amino acid differences between human PDGF-2 and v-sis could be accounted for by the known degree of divergence between the genomes of humans and cebids (Wilson et al., 1977).

Efforts were undertaken to directly establish that the v-sis gene product and human PDGF shared structural, immunological, and biological properties (Robbins et al., 1983). We utilized antibodies directed against peptides synthesized on the basis of the predicted N-and C-termini of p28^{sis} (Devare et al., 1983) to study its biogenesis. Marmoset cells infected with SSV were pulse-labeled with ^{35}S-methionine for various times, extracted, and then immunoprecipitated with the appropriate antisera. The immunoprecipitates were then analyzed on SDS-gels in the presence or absence of reducing agent. The following events in the biogenesis and post-translational modification of the SSV transforming protein were shown to occur. First, a 28,000 dalton single peptide chain is synthesized and rapidly undergoes disulfide-bond mediated dimerization to a 56,000 dalton species. The 56 K dimer is then cleaved at its amino terminal end. The products of these proteolytic events detected under reducing conditions are single chains of 11 K (amino terminal) and 20 K (C-terminal) peptides (designated p11^{sis} and p20^{sis}, respectively).

Other steps involved in the processing of p28^{sis} were uncovered by studies utilizing anti-PDGF serum. Under nonreducing conditions, the same sized species as precipitated by the anti-sis C-terminal serum were detected. In addition, the PDGF antiserum detected a 24 K protein that was not recognized by the sis N- and C-terminal specific antisera. This species appeared to be the most stable processed form of the sis gene product. These results demonstrated that the sis protein also undergoes cleavage at its 3' end.

In addition to the close structural homology between p28^{sis} and PDGF demonstrated by the antibody studies, the intracellular forms of the sis protein bear striking similarities to protein species in biologically active PDGF preparations. Thus, PDGF is comprised of a range of molecules from 28,000 to 35,000 daltons that upon reduction are converted to peptides ranging from 12,000 to 18,000 daltons (Antoniades et al., 1979; Heldin et al., 1981; Deuel et al., 1981; Raines and Ross, 1982). In fact, a proteolytic cleavage signal (Lys-Arg) is present at residues 65-66 in the v-sis sequence, and the next residue commences the homology between v-sis and PDGF-2. Cleavage here results in an approximately 20,000 dalton peptide which corresponds closely in size to PDGF-2.

THE HUMAN sis PROTO-ONCOGENE

The demonstration of striking structural and immunological similarities between a known human growth factor and a viral oncogene product presented the opportunity to define, at the molecular level, the role of the sis proto-oncogene in human malignancies. Sis-related mRNAs have been detected in human tumor cells originating from connective tissue, but not in epithelial tumor cells (Eva et al., 1982). Moreover, human glioblastoma and osteosarcoma cell lines have been reported to produce PDGF-like polypeptides (Heldin et al., 1980; Nister et al., 1982; Graves et al., 1983). Genetic alterations affecting the transcription and/or translation of the sis proto-oncogene might induce sustained, inappropriate cell division of human cells responsive to the mitogenic activity of a PDGF-like molecule. Thus, activation of the sis locus might be implicated in the malignant transformation of certain types of human cells.

In order to characterize the sis/PDGF-2 locus, we isolated v-sis-related sequences from a bacteriophage library of normal human DNA (Chiu et al., 1984). These clones represented a continuous stretch of approximately 30 kbp. By Southern blotting analysis and hybridization with a v-sis probe, five v-sis-homologous restriction fragments were identified which could be localized within a 15-kbp region. Nucleotide sequence analysis of the v-sis-related regions was performed and demonstrated that an open reading frame was contained within the first five c-sis (human) exons. The 5'-most exon lacked a translation initiation codon in its open reading frame (Josephs et al., 1983; Chiu et al., 1984). Thus, c-sis coding sequences are incompletely represented in SSV. This conclusion is further supported by the observation that a 4.2-kbp sis-related transcript is present in human cells (Eva et al., 1982). When the predicted c-sis (human) coding sequence was compared with that of the polypeptides representing PDGF-2, there was complete homology except at two of a total of 104 residues (Chiu et al., 1984) (Fig. 2). These findings strongly imply that c-sis (human) is the structural gene for PDGF-2.

EXPRESSION OF THE NORMAL CODING SEQUENCE FOR HUMAN PDGF-2/sis CAUSES CELLULAR TRANSFORMATION

The transcription of c-sis (human) was studied by using probes representing 30 kbp of the human sis/PDGF-2 locus. A 4.2-kbp mRNA in the A2781 human tumor cell line was detected by a v-sis probe and by c-sis probes representing each of the c-sis exons (Igarashi et al., unpublished observation). The only other probe that hybridized to the same sized message was derived from the region from 0 to 0.6 kbp on the c-sis map. This probe (pc-sisl) did not detect v-sis RNA, and could represent a non-sis-related exon

```
                →(v-sis-helper virus junction)                                  →(exon 2)              60                →(exon 3)
p28sis MTLTWQGDPI PEELYKMLSG HSIRSFDDLQ RLLQGDSGKE DGAELDLNMT RSHSGGELES LAPGKRSLGS LSVAEPAMIA
c-sis  *****  ******E***D ***H**P*E* ************ ************ ************ *****R***** *TI********
PDGF-2                                                                      **** *TI********

                                                          120              →(exon 4)
p28sis ECKTRTEVFE ISRRLIDRTN ANFLVWPPCV EVQRCSGCCN NRNVQCRPTQ VQLRPVQVRK IEIVRKKPIF KKATVTLEDH
c-sis  ********** ************ ************ ********** ********** ********** ********** **********
PDGF-2 ********** ************ ************ ********** ********** ********** ***?*?***** ***?*?*****

                      →(exon 5)                                          226
p28sis LACKCEIVAA ARAVTRSPGT SQEQRAKTTQ SRVTIRTVRV RRPPKGKHRK CKHTHDKTAL KETLGAtrm
c-sis  ******T*** **P*******G **********P* T********** ********** ********** *******trm
PDGF-2 ******?***** *
```

Fig. 2. Comparison of amino acid sequences of p28sis, c-sis (human), and human PDGF-2. The predicted amino acid sequence of p28sis, shown in the one-letter amino acid code, is given in the top line. Shared residues are indicated by *. The location of c-sis (human) exons relative to the v-sis nucleotide sequence is indicated as well as the 5' helper virus v-sis junction. The PDGF-2 sequence is taken from Waterfield et al. and Hunkapiller (1983). One letter code: A = alanine; R = arginine; N = asparagine; D = aspartic acid; C = cysteine; Q = glutamine, E = glutamic acid; G = glycine; H = histidine; I = isoleucine; L = leucine; K = lysine; M = methionine; F = phenylalanine; P = proline; S = serine; T = threonine; W = tryptophan, Y = tyrosine; V = valine.

of the c-sis transcriptional unit (Igarashi et al., unpublished observation; Gazit et al., unpublished observation).

Nucleotide sequence analysis of pc-sis1 was performed and revealed the presence of three open reading frames initiated by a methionine codon. Donor splice sites were found at positions within pc-sis1 that would allow for in-phase translation of each reading frame when spliced to the acceptor splice site in the first v-sis-related exon.

The DNA of a c-sis (human) phage clone (ω-c-sis clone 8) that contained all of the PDGF-2 coding sequences (Chiu et al., 1984) was introduced into NIH/3T3 cells via transfection in order to study the structural requirements for c-sis gene expression. The sequences contained within clone 8 were incapable of transforming cells nor did they synthesize transcripts as determined by cotransfection experiments using a selectable marker gene (pSV2-gpt). Positioning a retroviral LTR upstream of the ω-c-sis clone 8 coding regions failed to confer transforming activity.

Since the putative upstream exon of c-sis (human) contained a potential amino terminal sequence for a PDGF/sis precursor, but not identifiable promoter signals, this segment was ligated in the proper orientation between the retroviral LTR and first exon of c-sis (human) clone 8. Upon transfection of NIH/3T3 cells with this molecular construct, transforming activity comparable to that observed for SSV DNA was observed (10^5 ffu/pmol). The foci induced by the human construct and by SSV DNA were morphologically indistinguishable. These findings established that the normal human gene encoding PDGF-2/sis is capable of acquiring transforming activity when expressed in a cell susceptible to the effects of PDGF. As such, they provide direct proof for a model in which the constitutive expression of the gene for a normal growth factor in a cell susceptible to its growth promoting actions can result in cell transformation.

IMPLICATIONS

The pathways leading toward the malignant state are rapidly becoming better understood. Identification of the function of the sis proto-oncogene as a human growth factor has been followed by the discovery that amino acid sequences of human epidermal growth factor receptor are highly related to those predicted for the v-erb-B oncogene product (Downward et al., 1984). Thus perturbations in at least two of the steps by which growth factors exert their proliferative effects may lead to transformation.

The number of steps in the neoplastic process may be relatively limited as indicated by studies on the effects of the simultaneous addition of oncogenes to cells either by transfection or virus

466

infection. Rat embryo fibroblasts in culture can be successfully
transformed when transfected by ras and myc or ras and the adenovirus Ela gene, but do not become malignant when transfected by
only one (Land et al., 1983; Ruley, 1983). These findings also
suggest the existence of complementing groups of oncogenes. It
is likely that more proto-oncogenes will be discovered. The
identification of such genes, their normal functions and mechanisms
of activation as oncogenes in human malignancies may be of critical
importance in devising clinically applicable strategies for
cancer diagnosis, detection, and hopefully prevention.

REFERENCES

Aaronson, S. A., 1973, Biologic characterization of mammalian cells
    transformed by a primate sarcoma virus, Virol, 52:562.
Alitalo, K., Ramsay, G., Bishop, J. M., Pfeifer, S. O., Colby,
    W. W., and Levinson, A. D., 1983, Identification of nuclear
    proteins encoded by viral and cellular myc oncogenes,
    Nature, 306: 274.
Antoniades, H. N., Scher, C. D., and Stiles, C. D., 1979, Purifi-
    cation of human platelet-derived growth factor, Proc.
    Natl. Acad. Sci. USA, 76:1809.
Antoniades, H. N., and Hunkapiller, M. W., 1983, Human platelet-
    derived growth factor (PDGF): Amino terminal amino acid
    sequence, Science, 220:963.
Bishop, J. M., 1983, Cellular oncogenes and retroviruses, in: "Ann.
    Rev. Biochemistry, Vol. 52," E. E. Snell, P. D. Boyer,
    A. Meister, and C. C. Richardson, eds., Academic Press,
    Palo Alto.
Chiu, I.-M., Reddy, E.P., Givol, D., Robbins, K.C., Tronick, S.R.,
    and Aaronson, S. A., 1984, Nucleotide sequence analysis
    identifies the human c-sis proto-oncogene as a structural
    gene for platelet-derived growth factor, Cell, 37:123.
Collet, M. S., and Erickson, R. L., 1978, Protein kinase activity
    associated with the avian sarcoma virus src gene product,
    Proc. Natl. Acad. Sci. USA, 75:2021.
Curran, T., Miller, A. D., Zokas, L., and Verma, I. M., 1984, Viral
    and cellular fos proteins: a comparative analysis. Cell,
    36:259.
DeFeo-Jones, D., Scolnick, E. M., Koller, R., and Dhar, R., 1983,
    Ras-related gene sequences identified and isolated from
    Saccharomyces cerevisiae, Nature, 306:707.
Deuel, T. F., Huang, J. S., Proffit, R. T., Baenziger, U. U.,
    Chang, D., and Kennedey, B. B., 1981, Human platelet-derived
    growth factor. Purification and resolution into two active
    protein fractions, J. Biol. Chem., 256:8896.
Devare, S. G., Reddy, E. P., Law, J. D., Robbins, K. C., and
    Aaronson, S. A., 1983, Nucleotide sequence of the siman
    sarcoma virus genome: Demonstration that its acquired

cellular sequences encode the transforming gene product,
p28$\underline{sis}$. Proc. Natl. Acad. Sci. USA, 80:731.

Doolittle, R. F., Hunkapiller, M. W., Hood, L. E., Devare, S. G.,
Robbins, K. C., and Aaronson, S. A., and Antoniades, H. N.,
1983, Simian sarcoma virus onc gene, v-sis, is derived
from the gene (or genes) encoding a platelet-derived
growth factor, Science, 221:275.

Downward, J., Yarden, Y., Mayes, E., Scrace, E., Totty, N.,
Stockwell, P., Ullrich, A., Schlessinger, J., and
Waterfield, M. D., 1984, Close similarity of epidermal
growth factor receptor and v-erb-B oncogene protein
sequences, Nature, 307:521.

Duesberg, P. H., 1983, Retroviral transforming genes in normal
cells?, Nature, 304:219.

Eva, A., Robbins, K. C., Andersen, P. R., Srinivasan, A., Tronick,
S. R., Reddy, E. P., Ellmore, N. W., Galen, A. T.,
Lautenberger, J. A., Papas, T. S., Westin, E. H., Wong-
Staal, F., Gallo, R. C., and Aaronson, S. A., 1982, Cellular
genes analogous to retroviral onc genes are transcribed in
human tumor cells, Nature, 295:116.

Graves, D. T., Owen, A. J., and Antoniades, H. N., 1983, Evidence
that a human osteosarcoma cell line which secretes a
mitogen similar to platelet-derived growth factor requires
growth factors present in platelet-poor plasma, Cancer
Res., 43:83.

Hann, S. R., Abrams, H. D., Rohrschneider, L. R., and Eisenman,
R, N., 1983, Proteins encoded by v-myc and c-myc oncogenes:
identification and localization in acute leukemia virus
transformants and bursal lymphoma cell lines, Cell, 34:789.

Heldin, C. H., Westermark, B., and Wasteson A., 1980, Chemical
and biological properties of a growth factor from human-
cultured osteosarcoma cells: Resemblance with platelet-
derived growth factor, J. Cell. Phys., 105:235.

Heldin, C. H., Westermark, B., and Wasteson, A., 1981, Demonstration of antibody against platelet-derived growth
factor. Exp. Cell. Res., 136:255.

Josephs, S. F., Dalla Favera, R., Gelmann, E. P., Gallo, R. C., and
Wong-Staal, F., 1984, 5' viral and human cellular sequences
corresponding to the transforming gene of simian sarcoma
virus, Science, 219:503.

Land, H., Parada, L. F., and Weinberg, R. A., 1983, Tumorigenic
conversion of primary embryo fibroblasts requires at least
two cooperating oncogenes, Nature, 304:596.

Levinson, A. D., Opperman, H., Levintow, L., Varmus, H. E., and
Bishop, J. M., 1978, Evidence that the transforming gene
of avian sarcoma virus encodes a protein kinase aasociated
with a phosphoprotein, Cell, 15:561.

Nister, M., Heldin, C. H., Wateson, A., and Westermark, B., 1982,
A platelet-derived growth factor analog produced by a

human clonal glioma cell line, <u>Ann. NY Acad. Sci.</u>, 397:25.

Raines, E. W., and Ross, R., 1982, Platelet-derived growth factor I. High yield purification and evidence for multiple forms, <u>J. Biol. Chem.</u>, 257:5154.

Robbins, K. C., Devare, S. G., and Aaronson, S. A., 1981, Molecular cloning of integrated simian sarcoma virus: genome organization of infectious DNA clones, <u>Proc. Natl. Acad. Sci. USA</u>, 78:2918.

Robbins, K. C., Antoniades, H. N., Devare, S. G., Hunkapiller, M. W., and Aaronson, S. A., 1983, Structural and immunological similarities between simian sarcoma virus gene product(s) and human platelet-derived growth factor, <u>Nature</u>, 305: 605.

Robbins, K. C., Devare, S. G., Reddy, E. P., and Aaronson, S. A., 1982a, <u>In vivo</u> identification of the transforming gene product of simian sarcoma virus, <u>Science</u>, 218:1131.

Robbins, K. C, Hill, R. L., and Aaronson, S. A., 1982b, Primate origin of the cell-derived sequences of simian sarcoma virus, <u>J. Virol.</u>, 41:721.

Ruley, H. E., 1983, Adenovirus early region 1A enables viral and cellular transforming genes to transform primary cells in culture, <u>Nature</u>, 304:602.

Scolnick, E. M., Papageorge, A. G., and Shih, T. Y., 1979, Guanine nucleotide-binding activity as an assay for src protein of rat-derived murine sarcoma viruses, <u>Proc. Natl. Acad. Sci. USA</u>, 76:5355.

Shilo, B. Z., and Weinberg, R. A., 1981, DNA sequences homologous to vertebrate oncogenes are conserved in Drosophila Melanogaster, <u>Proc. Natl. Acad. Sci. USA</u>, 78:6789.

Shinnick, T. M., Lerner, R. A., and Sutcliffe, J. G., 1981, Nucleotide sequence of Moloney murine leukemia virus, <u>Nature</u>, 293:543.

Theilen, G. H., Gould, D., Fowler, M., and Dungworth, D. L., 1971, C-type virus in tumor tissue of a woolly monkey (<u>Lagothrix spp.</u>) with fibrosarcoma, <u>J. Natl. Cancer Inst.</u>, 47:881.

Waterfield, M. D., Scrace, G. T., Whittle, N., Stroobant, P., Johnsson, A, Wasteson, A., Westermark, B., Heldin, C. H., Huang, J. S., and Deuel, T. F., 1983, Platelet-derived growth factor is structurally related to the putative transforming protein p28^{sis} of simian sarcoma virus, <u>Nature</u>, 304:35.

Weiss, R. A., Teich, N., Varmus, H., and Coffin, R. J., "Molecular Biology of Tumor Viruses, RNA Tumor Viruses. 2nd edit.," Cold Spring Harbor, New York (1982).

Wilbur, W. J., and Lipman, D. J., 1983, Rapid similarity searches of nucleic acid and protein data banks. <u>Proc. Natl. Acad. Sci. USA</u>, 80:726.

Wilson, A. C., Carlson, S. S., and White, T. J., 1977, Biochemical evolution, <u>Ann. Rev. Biochem.</u>, 46:573.

Wolfe, L. G., Deinhardt, F., Theilen, G. J., Rabin, H., Kawakami, T., and Bustad, L. K., 1971, Induction of tumors in marmoset monkeys by simian sarcoma virus, type 1 (lagothrix) a preliminary report, J. Natl. Cancer Inst., 47:1115.

Wolfe, L. G., Smith, R. K., and Dienhardt, F., 1972, Simian sarcoma virus type 1 (Lagothrix): Focus assay and demonstration of nontransforming associated virus, J. Natl. Cancer Inst., 48:1905.

MELANOMA AND OTHER SKIN CANCERS: A CONTRAST IN SOLAR RADIATION

CARCINOGENESIS

John A.H. Lee

Department of Epidemiology, SC-36
University of Washington
Seattle, Washington 98195

SUMMARY

Exposure to sunlight of the poorly pigmented skin of people of
European descent leads to neoplastic change in both the cells that
give rise to the squamous cell and basal cell carcinomas, to the
lentigo maligna melanomas, and to the nodular and superficial
spreading melanomas. However, the dose relationships, timing, and
precursor lesions are quite different. Thus an opportunity for
studying carcinogenesis in humans where different cell types are
exposed to the same carcinogen.

The Physical Background: Our Nakedness

Homo sapiens is a strange sort of great ape, and the European
variety is a strange sub-set of Homo. The characteristics that make
Europeans so unusual also on occasion get them into difficulties – the
risk of skin cancers that we are to discuss today is one of the more
prominent. Humans are clearly mammals, beings who maintain a constant
temperature that is usually higher than that of the environment; who
bring forth their young alive (an oversimplification, but a kitten is
more like a cat than an egg is like a hen); and who then nourish them
with milk, derived from specialized sweat glands. But if you think
about mammals, your generalized impression is of a rather hairy or
furry sort of creature. If they are close to us, their hairiness is a
sort of caricature – the orangutan as one's kindly grandfather. If an
animal is really without much hair, they are very different from us,
for example, the elephant or the rhinoceros. Horses, if left outside
in the Canadian winter, suprisingly survive if kept supplied with
liquid water. They get most unfamiliarly furry. Hairiness – fur –

471

is clearly a heat retaining device. Mammals, with their active metabolism, have, for most of the time, to dump excess heat the environment.

Along the way, humans diverged from the great apes, and shed the bulk of their body hair. This looks like a response to a need to avoid an overload of metabolic heat. Man has numerous sweat glands, as does the horse. Both get wet when exerting themselves and exploit the very large latent heat of vaporization to keep within a tolerable temperature.

Once hair has been given up, for whatever reason, there is nothing particulartly human, or even difficult, about getting skin tumors. These tumors do occur in animals; our experimental friends produce them with ease by permitting mice to bask in the gentle rays of sunlamps, and if we select cats to make phaeomelanin, the resulting marmalade-tinted animals get skin cancers. White-faced bovines do so as well, and even, after years of Australian life, does that toughest of animals, the sheep. All these animals get their tumors on parts of themselves where the skin surface is directly exposed - the ears of the mice, the cats´ noses, the perineums of the docked sheep.

The Physical Background: Our Colored Skin

Once hair was lost, humans in Africa and Southern Asia got the function of their pigment-producing cells; the melanocytes were modified and the people became not only nude but brown or black. The advantage of this is not completely clear. Thus a pigmented person standing in the sun will absorb more heat than a white one. Camouflage is an obvious possibility. Avoiding vitamin D toxicity due to over-synthesis was a theoretical possibility, but white people living in the Tropics turn out not to the troubled by this. The selection pressure must be quite strong - Tropical peoples are all pigmented. In contrast, at least on casual observation, the color of the skin of a furry or feathered animal does not seem to bear much relationship to the color of the animal as produced by its fur. Part the fur on a black dog and you may find a black dog or a white dog underneath.

The Physical Background: Our Uncolored European Skin

Comfortably and efficiently hairless and brown, human beings extended their range, adapting little by little to cooler conditions. Fire was tamed, skins were fashioned into effective clothing. Reverse evolution - the recapturing of a previous state, in this case hairiness, as usual, did not occur. There was no reversion, as far as we know, to primitiveness hairiness in order to keep warm.

People were moving slowly into Europe from the south and east, always finding new hunting grounds to the cooler wetter and less sunny northwest. They were moving towards a climatic anomaly - an area where the warm Gulf Stream enabled the land to support animals and people (compare Scandinavia with Labrador) in latitudes where sunlight is weak. When living in the Tropics, the vitamin D requirements had been met by synthesis in the skin under the influence of utraviolet light. Once you put pigmented people in high latitudes they have to have a good source of vitamin D in their diet - marine fish or mammals - or they will suffer from delayed hardening of bones - rickets (1). The change in skull shape, and the bow legs are bad enough, but the severe problem is the decline in reproductive capacity from the flat pelves of the growing girls. Fast, classical Darwinian selection for the ability to allow photons to penetrate deeply enough to be useful is the most plausible cause of the pale complexions of the European people. The British had effectively removed rickets from their population through fortification of milk, butter and margarine with vitamin D only to see the disease recur with the arrival of dark skinned Indian people who did not use these products. Oriental peoples also depigmented, but less completely than the Europeans. The Eskimos have no difficulty because of dietary sources of vitamin D from fish and marine mammals. The inland Indians of the North presumably had enough animal food, even if it was not marine.

So, we Europeans gave up our fur, and then in the cold invented clothes; we gave up our skin pigment, and avoided rickets. There was a price; energy from photons penetrated to the living cells of the skin, and damaged them. Persons unable to repair DNA damage - xeroderma pigmentosum - suffered misearbly damaged skins and all the varieties of skin malignancy on those areas exposed to light. Skin exposed to enormous doses of sunlight by a combination of clothing habits, the occupation of the subject, and the his age developed squamous cell and basal cell carcinomas. These were reported in sailors, farmers, etc. Such tumors can almost always be cured by simple modern surgery; without that they are in the end fatal. However, from the age at which they occur, their impact on the gene pool must have been slight. Squamous cell carcinomas of skin are, of course, produced without much difficulty, and not at a great age, in pigmented persons with burn scars or in chronically irritated skin.

The Physical Background: The European Diaspora

Staying at home in Bergen or Aberdeen and balancing the reproductive future of the community's little girls against a few spectacularly nasty tumors in old men is one thing, but setting up large white populations in places like Texas, Queensland, or South Africa where the advantages of the specific European pigmentary arrangements are of no utility is quite another. The problem is, of course, compounded by social systems which make it unlikely that people will be protected by having a pigmented grandparent.

The germinal layer of the skin contains melanocytes which produce the melanin pigment that diffuses in various ways through the horny layer, producing the various degrees of pigmentation. These, too, can become lethally malignant. The lentigo maligna or Hutchinson's malignant freckle is very similar to the squamous cell carcinoma in its development on a pale skin subjected to prolonged exposure. They are histologically distinct from the other melanomas, and are regularly reported to have a better prognosis than the commoner melanomas.

The common melanomas - the superficial spreading and the nodular varieties, which do seem to be distinct from each other - are quite different because of their liability to early and lethal metastasis. Prognosis, for a tumor which is visible on the skin, and usually readily diagnosed, is about as bad as that for breast cancer. Both the non-melanoma skin cancers and the melanomas have been increasing in incidence in recent decades. Although earlier diagnosis has improved prognosis considerably, the death rate continues to rise.

Rates for both the skin melanomas and the non-melanoma tumors of the skin are higher the nearer to the Equator the affected persons live. There have been exceptions and puzzles, but these seem to be related to variations in the behavior of populations living in different places. The data have been reviewed in (2,3,4). Migrants to sunny places do better than the native-born of European stock. However, a most important observation is that this protection is related to age at migration. Adults keep their natal risk, whatever they do; child migrants acquire the risks of their new neighbors (5).

The incidence of the malignant melanomas of the skin is rising rapidly in almost every white population in which it has been studied. This rise appears to be driven by year-of-birth or cohort effects. The rising incidence rate is not homogeneous - rates for melanomas of the head and neck are only going up slowly, while those for the trunk and limbs are rising more rapidly. There is general agreement among epidemiologists that this rising rate is a result of an increase in the lifetime risk of persons born in successively later years. Risk at any age is determined by age and year of birth. Such a year-of-birth effect, or cohort effect, implies that the level of lifetime risk is established early. Examples include tuberculosis risk after primary infection in childhood, and lung cancer risk after the acquisition of cigarette addiction in adolescence. Such cohort effects, if they are in the direction of increasing risk with later year of birth, reduce the mean age of the patients being diagnosed or dying. The age distributions are correct, they merely do not correctly represent the influence of age on the incidence or mortality of the disease. Stevens and Moolgavkar (6) have shown that for the different anatomic sites, the influence of age on the incidence of malignant melanoma is the same, when account is taken of different rates of change of the incidence rates with time.

The different parts of the human torso are exposed, in very different ways. The areas covered by the underpants are hardly exposed at all, and are covered by two layers of clothing. The back is often exposed at work or play, the female breast much less so. Mr. Frank Westrom, a graduate student in our school, reclassified seven hundred melanomas of the trunk from the Western Washington Cancer Surveillance System, into what may be described as functional areas (Table 1). The tumors of the underpants area were older than the average in males and females, suggesting either that the latent period was longer for this protected site, or, more economically, that the incidence there is rising slowly.

The low mean age of the melanomas occurring on the skin of the female breast was unexpected. These were identified as such by a comment in the original charts. To explore the finding, we searched the literature with the help of our colleague Dr. Robert F. Jones of the Department of Surgery, University of Washington. We have so far found five published series. In four of these the mean age is given as an incidental finding, without comment. All were close to our own, and low in comparison with melanoma of other sites (Table 2). Either the incidence of melanomas on the female breast is increasing very rapidly indeed, or the biology is different.

Table 1 MEAN AGE AT DIAGNOSIS OF MELANOMAS
OF SKIN BY SITE AND SEX
WESTERN WASHINGTON 1974-84*

	MALE	FEMALE
HEAD & NECK	57.0	49.7
TRUNK	48.2	44.4
BACK	48.1	44.3
ANTERIOR CHEST	49.2	42.1
BREAST	-	33.6
UNDERPANTS	54.0	47.7
ABDOMEN	45.6	48.4
TRUNK N.O.S.	43.6	40.2
UPPER LIMB	49.7	47.9
LOWER LIMB	49.7	47.9
ANY SPECIFIED	51.0	50.3
SITE UNSPECIFIED	55.1	58.3
ALL CASES	51.5	51.4

* from (7)

475

Table 2 MEAN AGE AT DIAGNOSIS OF MELANOMAS
OF SKIN OF FEMALE BREAST

Present Western Washington Series	34
Ariel & Caron 1972 (NYU)	35
Lee, Sparks & Morton 1977 (UCLA)	36
Roses, Harris, Stern & Gumport 1977 (NYU)	36
Papachristou & Fortner et al 1978 (S-K CC)	34

Melanomas of the uveal tract, away from the flux of ultraviolet light, are not increasing over time. They were not thought to have a latitude gradient (8). It turns out, however, that their incidence is greater in blue-eyed than in brown-eyed people. Eye color does have a latitude gradient in the U.S., and when this is allowed for, the incidence of the eye melanomas does increase from north to south (Dr. Margaret Trueman, personal communication).

The melanomas, apart from the lentigo maligna ones, are not concentrated on the head and neck in the same way that the non-melanoma skin cancers are. However, they do have a predilection for the exposed sites. The non-melanomas require enormous doses, the melanomas much smaller ones.

The precursor lesions of the melanomas and the non-melanoma skin cancers are different. Solar keratoses are nearly tumors, and are treated as such. Like the tumors, they occur in elderly persons and on anatomic sites permanently exposed to the sun. Their occupational relationship is clear. In contrast, the common acquired nevi appear in childhood and adolescence. Only a tiny proportion become melanomas – too few for prophylactic surgery. As with the keratoses, the nevi appear to have a similar site distribution to their associated tumor. The dysplastic nevi, whether familial or sporadic, are much more likely to undergo malignant change than ordinary nevi, or probably than congenital ones. Their description and natural history continues to be under vigorous study.

In summary, sunlight, and presumably its ultraviolet component, strike the different cells of the germinal layer of the skin. Large doses accumulating over a lifetime produce much visible and histologic damage to the skin – solar keratoses, a large fraction of which turn into cancers. In contrast, much smaller doses, delivered at a particular time of life, produce nevi, few of which become malignant. Some of these nevi are dysplastic, and these become malignant with a much higher frequency. The nature of neoplastic change can be explored in the contrasted response of two types of cell to the same insult.

References

1. Murray FG. Pigmentation, sunlight, and nutritional disease.
   Am Anthropologist 1934;36:438-45.

2. Mackie RM. The role of sunlight in the aetiology of cutaneous
   malignant melanoma. Clin and Experiment Dermatol 1981;6:407-410.

3. Lee JAH. Melanoma and exposure to sunlight. Epidemiologic Rev
   1982;4:110-136

4. Lee JAH. Epidemiology of Malignant Melanoma: 10 Year's Progress.
   In Pigment Cell Vol.6 (ed. RM Mackie) 1983 Basel Karger.

5. Holman CDJ, Armstrong BK. Pigmentary traits, ethnic origin,
   benign nevi and family history. Risk factors for cutaneous
   cutaneous malignant melanoma. J Natl Cancer Inst 1984;72:257-266.

6. Stevens RG, Moolgavkar SH. Malignant melanoma: dependence of
   site-specific risk on age. Am J Epidemiol 1984;119:890-5.

7. Westrom F, Lee JAH. In preparation.

8. Scotto J, Fraumeni JF, Lee JAH. Melanoma of the eye and other
   noncutaneous sites: epidemiologic aspects. J Natl Cancer Inst
   1976; 56:489-491.

EPIDEMIOLOGICAL APPROACH

TO BREAST CANCER ETIOLOGY

Paolo Bruzzi

Clinical Epidemiology and Trials Unit
Istituto Nazionale per la Ricerca sul Cancro
Viale Benedetto XV n.10- Genova, Italy

INTRODUCTION

So far, approaches to breast cancer control based on secondary prevention (early diagnosis and treatment) have failed to provide satisfactory results, and substantial improvements are not expected in the near future: in fact, the impact on mortality attainable by early detection programs appears to be limited, and almost counter-balanced by the high costs and the negative effects associated with these programs (psychological stress, fear, surgical procedures on false-positive women, etc). However, the most important considera-tion is that, in Western Countries,breast cancer control by means of secondary prevention implies acceptance of the fact that one out of 13-14 women will develop breast cancer (unless she dies before it), during her lifetime, with good chances to undergo mastectomy.

On the other hand, primary prevention, due to the substantial improvements in our understanding of breast cancer etiology which have taken place over the last decades, is no longer an unrealistic goal. These improvements were and are possible through the contribu-tions of scientists working in various fields, and, in order to fully grasp the present understanding of this disease, a multidisci-plinary approach is necessary.

Breast cancer is probably the most extensively studied cancer, but, because of the complexity of its pathogenetic mechanisms, a unified view of its etiology is still lacking. The following is an attempt to present an etiologic model based on what is generally agreed upon by most students of the problem, and reflects, with some modifications, the ideas put forth by Russo[1], and by Moolgavkar[2], which are based on quite different, but complementary, sets of observations. As any etiologic model, it has obvious limitations, but has the aim to provide a plausible biological background to the existing experimental, epidemiologic and clinical evidence, to allow testable predictions and to suggest new areas of investigation. Only a selection of the available literature will be discussed in this instance: for more extensive reviews see Kelsey[3], Thomas[4] and Petrakis et al[5].

EPIDEMIOLOGIC EVIDENCE

Environmental vs genetic factors

The relevance of environmental factors in breast cancer etiology is supported by a) geographic comparisons, b) migrant studies and c) twin studies.
a) Internationally breast cancer incidences show large differences, with a ratio of the highest to the lowest rates of almost 8 to 1[6]. The distribution of these rates tends to be related to socio-economic "Westernization" and affluence. Large differences are observed, within racial groups, among populations living in different countries. Mortality studies within countries show a direct relationship with the degree of urbanization and with the average income of a county[7]. It must be anticipated that the international variation in incidence cannot be accounted for by variation in personal factors connected to childbearing practices, a major determinant of breast cancer risk[8,9].
b) Migrants from countries at low incidence to countries at high incidence show an increase in breast cancer risk. The rates approach those of the host country within one to three generations, depending on the cultural similarity between the country of origin and the host country[10,11].
c) Twin studies have shown that, even though a higher degree of concordance for breast cancer does exist for monozygotic than dizygotic twins, the attributable risk of genetic factors is modest[12].

Breast cancer: one disease of two?

Several lines of evidence point toward the presence of two distinct pathological entities, which should have, at least in part, a different etiology: a) the shape of the age-incidence curves for female breast cancer differs in countries at different risk; b) The distribution of specific tumor characteristics shows differences in

480

different areas; c) several breast cancer risk factors have a different importance depending on age.

a) Breast cancer incidence rates rise steadily with age between the usual ages of menarche and menopause, and then decline slightly, nearly level off or increase more slowly, with age, in areas of low, intermediate and high breast cancer risk, respectively[13]. Thus, most of the international variation would be accounted for by differences in post menopausal incidence. This has suggested a different etiology for premenopausal and postmenopausal disease, the latter being associated with the environmental factors which are responsible of the high risk in Western countries[14]. It has been argued[15] that this hypothesis is based on cross-sectional incidence rates, which would be influenced by the cohort effect, due to the increased lifetime risk of more recent cohorts of birth. Different sets of data have been used to support either hypothesis, but it seems clear that, also in countries with stable incidence, the rate of increase in the incidence rates with age shows a marked change around the age of 40-50 years; the extent of this change may differ in areas at different risk[16].

b) It has been observed that the prognosis of breast cancer patients is somewhat better in several low-risk areas, such as Japan, even after adjustment for stage at diagnosis. Also the distribution of the histologic types shows differences in different areas, the medullary type being more common in Japan than in U.S.[17]. Furthermore, recent studies indicate that the frequency of premenopausal cancers in which estrogen receptors are detected is similar in Japan and U.S., while it is higher in U.S. than in Japan among postmenopausal cases[18]. It has to be pointed out that, according to some authors[19,2] receptors for sex hormones are present in all cancers during their early developmental stages: the amount of circulating hormones would determine a clonal advantage either to receptor-positive cells or to cells which, as a consequence of their neoplastic transformation, have lost their ability to bind sex-hormones.

c) Contrasting evidence is available with regard to the presence of a different role of known breast cancer risk factors at various ages: several studies indicate that premenopausal (or younger) cases are more commonly associated with a family history of breast cancer and with inbalances in ovarian secretion, while dietary or constitutional (e.g. obesity) factors would be more relevant in postmenopausal years[21,22]. However, most known risk factors seem to exert a lifetime effect.

Specific risk factors

There is only one environmental agent which has been shown to cause breast cancer in humans, namely ionizing radiation. Most of the known risk factors for breast cancer are rather indirect indicators of underlying, poorly known, mechanisms, than true carcinogens or co-carcinogens. This short review is limited to those factors on which enough evidence is available, or which are particularly relevant because of their implications.

Reproductive factors: with few exceptions, most studies have found breast cancer risk to be associated with age at first full-term pregnancy. Women who bear their first full-term child before age 18 years have about one-third the risk of women whose first full-term delivery occurs after age 35 years. Nulliparous women experience a risk comparable to that of women who had their first child in their late twenties. There is strong evidence that further protection is afforded by births after the first, especially when occurring at a young age. The increased risk associated with a delayed pregnancy seems not to be related to reduced fertility, which implies a direct protective effect of an early first pregnancy[23]. Presently, breast feeding does not appear to have any protective effect.

Menstrual factors: a weak, but consistent association between early menarche and increased breast cancer risk has been found by most studies in various parts of the world. A more striking relationship is seen between breast cancer risk and age at either natural or artificial menopause. The earlier the menopause, the lower the lifetime breast cancer risk.[24]

Other aspects of mestrual activity, such as menstrual irregularity, length of cycle, menstrual pain, history of swelling and tenderness during menstruation, have been investigated with inconclusive or frankly negative results.

Nutrition: the relationship between breast cancer risk and dietary habits and/or nutritional status has been widely investigated, on the grounds that dietary differences could explain the marked geographic and racial variations in breast cancer incidence. Ecological comparisons are strongly suggestive of this relationship, showing a positive correlation between breast cancer and consumption levels of fats and proteins. Case-control studies have not provided clear-cut evidence on this issue, but their results support the relevance of dietary animal fats and proteins as determinants of breast cancer risk. It is noteworthy that the overall dietary pattern, rather than single food items, seems to influence the risk[25,26]. Many studies have investigated the relationship between breast cancer and height, weight, and obesity, with strikingly inconsistent results; however, the role of body size, if any, is probably more marked in (or limited to) postemenopausal years[27,28].

Endocrine factors: the dependence of breast tissue on various hormones for growth, differentiation, and maintenance has led to speculate that endocrine factors could be involved in breast cancer etiology. Differences in incidence between males and females (sex ratio is < 1/100), the fact that oophorectomy can induce dramatic regression in the growth of human breast cancer, its relationship with menstrual and reproductive history, give indirect but convincing support to this hypothesis.

The presence on breast epithelial cells of receptors for estrogens, progesterone and prolactin provides molecular evidence of the dependence of breast tissue on hormonal stimulation. The presence, in many tissue samples of breast tumors, of analogous receptors substantiates the hypothesis of a role of hormones in cancer growth as well, even though it has been shown that a proportion of "receptor positive" breast cancer cases do not respond to hormonal manipulation, while several "negative" cases do[29]. However, many attempts to find an association between breast cancer and serum levels, metabolism, urinary excretion, or relative balance of various hormones have failed, so far, to produce consistent and/or interpretable results. Available evidence seems to indicate that there is no difference, between high risk and low risk populations, in the endogenous rate of synthesis of the various estrogens, but that differences could be present in the available quota. The hypothesis of an unopposed estrogen carcinogenic action due to insufficient progesterone production soon after menarche and around menopause (two windows hypothesis) has presently less credit.

Also the influence of exogenous hormones on breast cancer risk remains an open question[30]. Most studies failed to show an association with contraceptive use, with few exceptions for specific subgroups. The effect of menopausal estrogens, which is plausible on theoretical grounds, has not yet been clearly demonstrated, with most studies showing no association; there are, however, some indications that long-term users, particularly when affected by benign breast diseasen, could experience an increased risk.

Benign breast disease (BBD): two main problems hinder the investigation of the relationship between breast cancer and the various chronic breast affections which are lumped together under the label of Benign Breast Disease:

a) The lack of a universally adopted protocol for the pathological classification of this heterogeneous and intriguing group of affections, which often are present together in the same breast, and which range from minimal benign changes to frankly preneoplastic lesions, and from isolated cysts or solid tumors to massive infiltrating or sclerosing processes.
b) The lack of reliable information about the prevalence of these lesions among the general healthy population.

However, it has been clearly demonstrated that women who undergo one or more biopsies for a benign breast lesion are at increased risk of developing breast cancer for at least 20 years. The relative risk is in the order of 2-3. Sufficient evidence is available that the risk of subsequent cancer differs depending on the histopathologic type of the benign lesion, even though disagreement exists as to which type: fibrocystic lesions, ductal atypia, epithelial proliferative lesions, have been, in turn, indicated as the components of BBD which are responsible for the increased risk.

Uncertainty exists also as to whether particular types of BBD represent an intermediate step of the sequence of events that leads to carcinoma, or, alternatively, benign lesions and cancer are concomitant lesions which may share common causes, or a similar early ancestry, but which diverge at a very early stage of their development[31]. An important observation is that, in women with BBD, both breasts are similarly at an increased breast cancer risk.

Studies trying to correlate BBD with known risk factors for breast cancer have reported conflicting results, which is not surprising, since few studies focused on specific histopathologic BBD subtypes. Available data suggests an association between BBD and low parity, rather than age at 1st birth, and late menipause[32]. A striking finding of several recent studies is the above mentioned interaction of BBD and exogenous estrogens in increasing breast cancer risk[33].

Family history: first degree relatives of breast cancer patients are at increased risk of breast cancer. The presence of a second-degree relative with breast cancer in the family, either paternal or maternal, increases the risk in a comparable manner. The magnitude of the increased risk, which ranges from two to fourfold, depends strongly on the number, age at diagnosis and tumor laterality of the affected relatives. Cases with a family history of breast cancer tend to occur at a younger age and to be more often bilateral[34]. Present epidemiological evidence suggests that this increased risk does not depend only on environmental exposures shared by members of the same family but also on genetic factors. It is not known whether the familiar predisposition is due to heritability of predisposing conditions, such as hormonal anomalies, altered immunity, DNA-repair deficiency, or to direct genetic causes, such as intercalation of an oncogenic virus into a chromosome.

Environmental factors: Radiation: exposure of the breast to ionizing radiation increases the risk of breast cancer after a latent period which can range from 5 up to at least 40 years. The excess risk shows a strong dose-response relationship. The most relevant aspect of this association is its dependence on age at exposure: the relative risk of radiation-induced breast cancer is highest for exposures in the age range 0 to 20 years, then decreases dramatically, and is close to unity for exposures after age 40[35]. Radiation-induced breast cancer appear to be indistinguishable, from a morphological viewpoint, from other breast cancers[36].

To date, no other environmental factor has been demonstrated to increase breast cancer risk.

The most important recognized risk factors for breast cancer, which have been found in epidemiological studies are summarized in Tab. 1. As it can be seen, the clues and the indications provided by the epidemiological literature are many, yet the etiology of breast cancer seems to elude an easy and unified explanation. This becomes, at least in part, possible, if the the evidence deriving from other areas of research is taken into account.

ANIMAL STUDIES

The results of animal studies are of utmost importance for understanding the underlying mechanisms of breast carcinogenesis. Only few relevant aspects will be mentioned of the large amount of evidence which has been derived from studies of mammary carcinogenesis in laboratory animals.

Carcinogenesis

In the most widely accepted model of carcinogenesis, normal cells are transformed to neoplastic cells by the two steps of initiation and promotion. The first of these two steps, initiation, is thought to be a discrete and irreversible event, in which the content or the flow of genetic information coded in the base sequence of DNA is modified. The susceptibility of a cell to undergo malignant trasformation correlates with the rate of DNA synthesis and cell proliferation, and with the cellular competency in DNA excision repair.

TAB. 1   BREAST CANCER RISK FACTORS

1)Established factors

Age	Rapid increase in risk from puberty to menopause - then increase at a lower rate
Place of birth	Lowest risk in Asian and developing countries - highest in U.S.and West Europe
Age at 1st pregnancy	Increasing risk with increasing age at 1st pregnancy - nullipariry = 1st pregnancy in late 20's
Early menarche	Increased risk
Age at menopause	Increas.risk with incr. age at menop.
Family hist.of br.cancer	Increas.rsk,partic. if multiple rel. premenop.relat. rel.with bilat. dis.
Pre-existing B.B.D.	Increased risk for specific subtypes
Ionizing radiation	Incr.Risk if before age 40, particularly if before 1st pregnancy

2) Suspected factors

High-fat,high-protein diet	Increased risk
Obesity	Incr. risk, if any, only postmenopause
Exogenous estrogens	Only long-term users, particularly when affected by B.B.D.
Oral contraceptives	Teen-agers ? premenopausal women ?
Endogenous hormones	Low androgens ? available quota of estrogens ?

Susceptibility: mammary carcinomas induced in Sprague-Dawley
rats by dimethylbenz (a) anthracene (DMBA), appear to be a model
which mimics the most significant aspects of human breast cancer.
They are hormone-dependent adenocarcinomas, and are histologically
similar to human breast cancer. The incidence is higher when the
carcinogen is administered to nulliparous rats. A full-term pregnancy prior to DMBA administration protects against tumor development,
while tumor growth is stimulated by pregnancy.

The process of differentiation of the mammary gland appears
to be crucial in determining susceptibility to neoplastic transformation in female rats. The least differentiated structures, tubular
end buds (TEB), which are present at birth and increase in number
and density up to the end of the 3rd week, slowly differentiate into
intermediate structures, the alveolar buds (AB), which, in turn,
under the influence of ovarian hormones, begin to differentiate
into lobules. In the virgin female rat the mammary glands never
develop totally, and by 3 months of life they have acquired a steady
population of TEB, AB, and lobules. After 14 months of age, the
mammary gland undergoes involution. Pregnancy occurring at a young
age induces in the mammary gland a rapid differentiation of TEB
into AB, and of these into lobules. By the end of the pregnancy, TEB
have almost completely disappeared; following cessation of nursing,
although involutional processes bring the gland to its previous size
and structures, some morphological changes can still be detected:
in particular, very few TEB can be observed. Estrogens have been
shown to evoke ductal growth and the sprouting of TEB, while progesterone is required for the completion of the lobuloalveolar development in the virgin female.

The administration of DMBA to young virgin rats stops the
normal process of differentiation TEB-AB-lobule, producing instead
the sequence TEB-intraductal proliferation-carcinoma. AB, under the
influence of DMBA, do not develop carcinomas, but form benign lesions
such as fibroadenomas or cysts. After administration of DMBA to female rats of various ages and parity, the incidence of carcinomas
is directly proportional to the density of DEB which are ready to
differentiate to AB and which have a high DNA-labelling index. The
epithelial cells of the differentiated structures have a longer cell
cycle, less avidity for DMBA, and possess a more efficient DNA
excision repair capacity. The development of the human breast shows

strict analogies with what described in female rat. Under the influence of cyclic ovarian stimulation, mammary gland development and differentiation slowly take place from menarche until about age 35. Pregnancy induces an intense growth and a full differentiation, even though repeated pregnancies are needed in order to extend lobular development and differentiation to the totality of the gland. In vitro studies of the undifferentiated stuctures of human breast of women of different age and parity have confirmed their analogy with the TEB, which are believed to be the target tissue for neoplastic transformation under the influence of chemical carcinogens.

Nutrition[37]:enhanced mammary tumorigenesis, as a result of increasing dietary fat, has now been demonstrated in many experimental murine, benign and malignant, mammary tumor models, including chemically and radiation-induced carcinomas. In general, when animals are fed a high fat diet, mammary tumor incidence is sharply increased and/or the latent period markedly reduced, in comparison with animals fed an isocaloric, low-fat diet. Unsaturated fats appear superior to saturated fats in increasing the yield of mammary carcinomas. The effect is stronger when the high-fat diet is fed after carcinogen treatment than when it is fed before it. Studies of transplants of either carcinogen-treated mammary glands or mammary tumors have clearly shown that dietary fat is a potent promoter in mammary tumorigenesis, but a role in the initiation phase has been demonstrated as well. Lifetime high-fat diet can enhance the decreasing sensitivity of aging rats to carcinogenesis, and lowers the threshold dose of carcinogens. There is a strong correlation between duration of high-fat diet (before or after carcinogen administration) and effect on mammary tumor induction [38].

The mechanisms of action of high-fat diet on mammary tumorigenesis are unclear, and several hypotheses have been proposed: high fat diets induce prolonged estrous cycles and early puberty, but enhancement of prolactin and ovarian hormone secretion has not yet been clearly demonstrated. Furthermore, high-fat diets stimulate development of a number of rodent mammary tumors known to be nonresponsive to hormones. The hypothesis that the effect of high-fat diet is mediated through alterations of the immune system has not been adequately investigated. A particularly attractive hypothesis is that high levels of dietary fat affect the lipid composition of the mammary cell membranes and/or cell-to-cell communication. The mammotropic effects of hormones may be mediated through alterations of lipid membrane composition.[39] Since the enhancement is observed both with fat-soluble carcinogens which require metabolic activation and with water-soluble and direct acting carcinogens it does not appear that the co-carcinogenic effect of high-fat diet is related to uptake or metabolism of carcinogens by mammary tissue.

INITIATION AND PROMOTION IN HUMAN BREAST CANCER

Moolgavkar et al [2] proposed a two-stage model for human breast carcinogenesis which views carcinogenesis as the end results of two discrete, heritable and irreversible events in the target cell. This model takes into account variations in breast cellular turnover with age, and attains good fitting with available data. It also provides plausible explanations for most of the effects of menstrual and repro-ductive events, and for the role of genetic factors. Day [40], in a later paper, demonstrates how the epidemiological evidence used in constructing the model can be fitted into the lines of well-esta-blished principles of carcinogenesis, and implies the exstence of promoting effects which are responsible of the shape of the age-specific incidence curve of breast cancer. This shape, after adjust-ment for temporal trends (cohort effect) is similar in populations at different overall risk.

In the following discussion the available evidence derived from epidemiological, clinical and animal studies will be fitted in a framework slightly at variance with the views of Moolgavkar. No formal translation of the model into mathematical terms has been attempted.

Initiation

Initiation in human breast cancer requires the presence in the breast of adequate structural targets, that are probably represented by terminal ducts and/or intralobular terminal ducts, which are pre-sent at birth, increase in number and density until menarche and shortly thereafter, then slowly start to differentiate into more mature states under the influence of cyclic progesterone stimulation. Thus, susceptibility to initiating agents is highest around menarche and decreases with increasing age. Pregnancy induces a marked dif-ferentiation, and repeated pregnancies are necessary in order to complete the development of the whole gland. The protection affor-ded by early pregnancy is due to the reduction of the duration of potential "effective" exposure to initiators, i.e. to the reduction in the number of susceptible cells. Late pregnancies afford little, if any, protection against initiation, compared to nulliparity, because the breasts have already been susceptible for many years and have undergone, to a certain extent, differentiation under ovarian progesterone stimulation. The reason why early menarche is associated with increased risk is less clear: it is possible that an early menarche increases the time span during which susceptible cells actively replicate without differentiating, and therefore are more susceptible to initiation. Another explanation is that a third factor both increases breast cancer risk and anticipates menarche. Increased fat intake, which has been shown to anticipate puberty and to increase subsequent susceptibility to carcinogens, is a good candidate for this role.

As to the initiatiors, little is known: ionizing radiation is the only recognized factor, and the behaviour of its effects with increasing dose and age at exposure perfectly fits the proposed model: it is worth reporting that nulliparous women appear more susceptible to radiation induced breast cancer than parous women of similar age[41]. However, the attributable risk of exposure to ionizing radiation is probably low in the general population,even though accurate data on the effects of diagnostic x-rays during adolescence is still lacking.

Despite our ignorance about initiating agents in human breast cancer, migrant studies indicate that early events, which probably are related to initiation, are crucial in determining the international variation in breast cancer incidence: western women, by early adulthood, have probably more cells which have undergone initiation than women from countries at low risk. While it is not known if, in western countries, there is an increased exposure to environmental carcinogens during the first 20 years of life, it is plausible that the high-fat diets which are more common in high risk countries do exert a co-carcinogenic effect, enhancing the initiating capacity of low-level enviromental pollutants. The effects of initiation, which are irreversible and heritable, are life-long, as it has been observed for the increased risk due to ionizing radiation and delayed pregnancy.

The mechanism of action of familiar susceptibility to breast cancer is probably of two, or more types: members of the same family tend to share aspects of lifestyle such as diet, and are likely to commonly share environmental exposures. They tend to be similar in various genetically-determined physiological and biochemical functions, such as hormonal functions, DNA-repair capacity, enzimatic systems (including those necessary for the metabolic activation of carcinogens). However, it is believed by several authors[42,2] that in a significant proportion of families with multiple cases of breast cancer, as suggested by Knudson[43], the initiating event has occurred in an ancestral germ-cell,and is inherited as a cancer gene. The earlier occurrence and frequent bilaterality of familiar cases supports this hypothesis.

Interesting indications are provided by animal studies also with regard to Benign Breast Disease. The proliferative benign changes which are induced by carcinogenic stimuli on partially differentiated structures, resemble some types of human BBD, and are completely different in evolution from the intraductal proliferation which arises from undifferentiated structures and can progress to carcinoma.This observation, which is in agreement with the views of Azzopardi (31), suggests that the incresed risk of breast cancer in BBD patients may be due to previous carcinogenic stimuli which have caused, in the same woman, different lesions depending on the degree of differentiation of the various parts of her breasts. Specific BBD subtypes, however, may represent true pre-neoplastic stages.

Promotion

In the model proposed by Moolgavkar, both stages are assumed to be discrete and irreversible; furthermore, it is suggested that lobular carcinoma in situ may represent the intermediate stage, i.e. a cellular clone which has undergone the first but not the second event.

However, several lines of evidence seem to indicate that the second stage is more adequately described according to the promotion phase in mouse skin experiments, where repeated exposures to promoting agents at frequent intervals are required, and effects are reversible if the interval between exposures is prolonged; induced changes appear progressive and stable, intermediate and reversible stages can be observed prior to malignancy.

Acceptance of this model for breast cancer promotion is suggested by the available epidemiological evidence. By early adulthood, the number of initiated cells has been largely determined, but the risk of breast cancer continues to increase for the rest of the life, with only a change in the rate of increase around menopause. This fact seems to indicate the presence of a continuous, progressive process which leads to neoplastic transformation over a period which can be very long, and can be accelerated or slowed by various factors and events.

The most important promoting factors in human breast cancer are probably dietary fat and hormones. As previously noted[38], it is possible that hormones act with a lipid-mediated mechanism. On the other hand, obese postmenopausal women have high estrogen levels, due to peripheral conversion of surrenal androgens by adipose tissue, and and possibly low hormone-binding protein levels[44]; therefore it is possible that high-fat diets, contributing to obesity, act with an hormone-mediated mechanism as well. The crucial point is that promotion must continue for many years, and that progression to frankly neoplastic lesion can be accelerated or slowed down by several factors or events. The common clinical observation that breast cancer tends progressively to show a more aggressive biological and clinical behaviour while it progresses to more advanced stages (loss of hormonal receptors, loss of differentiation, increased frequency of cellular aberrations) is in support of this hypothesis.

During premenopausal years, promoting stimuli are provided by ovarian function and by dietary fat.

A late pregnancy, as shown by animal experiments, can accelerate the process; it must be noted that the increased risk associated with a late pregnancy is a long term one, which is difficult to explain with the two-discrete-events model.

At menopause, after cessation of ovarian function, promotion is still provided by dietary fat, but the estrogens produced peripherally in the adipose tissue become more necessary for progression to cancer, since human breast cancer is believed to be almost always hormone-dependent in its early stages. While this explains the change in the rate of increase of breast cancer incidence at menopause, it is, again, difficult to account for the long-term increase in risk associated with a late menopause unless promotion is regarded as a long, multistage process.

The increased risk associated with exogenous hormones, which is seen only in long-term users, particularly when affected by Benign Breast Disease, perfectly fits the model.

There are, however, several lines of evidence which cannot be easily accomodated within this framework; among these, particularly interesting is the relationship between various risk factors and specific tumor characteristics. The level of estrogen receptors seems to be related to age and/or menopausal status, older patients being more commonly positive. Racial groups at high risk for breast cancer show higher proportions of "receptor positive" cancers than low-risk groups. Reproductive breast cancer risk factors and obesity tend to be associated to more frequent positivity. Furthermore, differences in the histologic distribution and the agressiveness have been reported between high and low-risk racial groups,[45,46,47]. These findings are consistent with an etiological heterogeneity which is not considered in the previous model, even though alterative explanations are possible.

CONCLUSIONS

This hypothesis on breast cancer etiology is more based on assumptions and extrapolations than actual facts and figures. However, it accomodates most of the available epidemiological evidence, and suggests several areas of potential investigation.

According to it, the high incidence of breast cancer in Western countries is largely determined by high dietary fat intake, and possibly by unknown enviromental carcinogens. Differences in hormonal patterns are not needed in order to explain the international variation in breast cancer incidence.[48] Potentially, dietary fat can act with three mechanisms: it can enhance the initiating potency of low-level mutagens or procarcinogens during the first 20-30 years of life; it continuously promotes malignant transformation of the initiated cells; finally, it can contribute to obesity which, in turn, can provide estrogenic stimulation in postmenopausal years.

It must be pointed out that, in high risk areas, high-fat diets are so common that it is difficult to detect remarkable dose-effect gradients; nevertheless, case-control studies have reported increased fat consumption among breast cancer cases. Conversely, the relationship between fat intake during adolescence and lifetime breast cancer risk has never been investigated, and it is unlikely that the large, long-term follow-up study which would be necessary in order to answer this question will ever be undertaken. The same holds for exposure to mammotropic carcinogenic substances, which is also much more difficult to measure and monitor.

Thus, it is unlikely that this etiologic hypothesis, like others, will be proved true or discarded in the near future, unless strenuous efforts are devoted to the study of environmental factors in breast carcinogenesis. On the other hand, verification of etiological hypotheses which imply a crucial role of environmental factors in breast carcinogenesis might be rewarded by the possibility of preventing what is considered the number one cancer, in terms of mortality, mutilating consequences, and induced fear, among Western women.

REFERENCES

1. J. Russo, L. K. Tay, and I. H. Russo, Differentiation of the mammary gland and susceptibility to carcinogenesis, Breast Cancer Res. Treat. 2, 5-73, (1982)

2. S. H. Moolgavkar, and N. E. Day, Two-stage model for carcinogenesis: Epidemiology of breast cancer in females, JNCI, 65:3, 559 (1980)

3. J. L. Kelsey, A review of the epidemiology of breast cancer, Epidemiologic Revs, 1:74-109, (1979).

4. D. B. Thomas, Epidemiologic and related studies of breast cancer etiology, in "Reviews in Cancer Epidemiology" A. M. Lilienfeld ed. Elsevier/New York, (1980).

5. N. L. Petrakis, V. L. Ernster, and MC King, Breast, in "Cancer Epidemiology and Prevention" , D.Shottenfeld and J.F.Fraumeni eds., W.B.Saunders Company,Philadelphia, (1982).

6. J. Waterhouse, C. Muir et al., "Cancer Incidence in 5 Continents", Vol. IV, Lyon, IARC Scientific Publications No. 42, (1982).

7. W. J. Blot, J. F. Fraumeni, and B. J. Stone, Geographic patterns of breast cancer in the United States, J.N.C.I., 59:1407-11, (1977).

8. G. Hems, A. Stuart, Breast cancer rates in populations of single women, Br.J.Cancer, 31:118-123, (1975).

9. A. M. Y. Nomura, et al., Breast cancer in two populations with levels of risk for the disease, Am. J. Epidemiol., 119/4:496/502, (1984).

10. A. M. Lilienfeld, M. L. Levin and I. I. Kessler, "Cancer in the United States", Harvard University Press, Cambridge, (1972).

11. P. Buell, Changing incidence of breast cancer in Japanese-American women, J.N.C.I., 51:1479, (1972).

12. A. G. Knudson, L. C. Strong and D. E. Anderson, Heredity and cancer in man, Prog. Med. Genet., 9:113, (1973).

13. O. Bjarnason et al., The effect of year of birth on the breast cancer age-incidence curve in Iceland, J.N.C.I., 13:689, (1984).

14. F. de Waard, Premenopausal and Postmenopausal Breast Cancer: one disease or two ?, J.N.C.I., 63/3:549, (1979).

15. S. H. Moolgavkar, R. G. Stevens, J. A. H. Lee, Effect of age on incidence of breast cancer in females, J.N.C.I., 62:493, (1979).

16. F. de Waard, Epidemiology of Breast Cancer: a Review, Eur.J.Clin. Oncol., 19/12:1671, (1983).

17. A. B. Chabon, S. Takeuchi, and S. C. Sommers, Histological Differences in breast carcinoma of Japanese and American women, Cancer, 33:1577, (1974).

18. Y. Nomura et al., Estrogen receptor and endocrine responsiveness

in Japanese versus American breast cancer patients, Cancer Res. 37:106, (1977)

19. Y. Nomura, et al., Relationship between estrogen receptors and risk factors of breast cancer in Japanese pre- and postmenopausal patients, Breast cancer Research and Treatment, 4:37, (1984)

20. S. M. Thorpe, et al., Estrogen and progesteron receptoer profile patterns in primary breast cancer, Breast Cancer Research and Treatment, 3:103, (1983).

21. J. H. Lubin, et al., Risk factors for breast cancer in women in Northern Alberta, as related to age at diagnosis, J.N.C.I. 68/2 :211, (1982).

22. D. T. Janerich, M. B. Hoff, Evidence for a cross-over in breast cancer risk factors, Am.J.Epid., 116:737, (1982)

23. L. Brinton, R. Hoover, and J. F. Fraumeni, Reproductive factors in the aetiology of breast cancer, Br.J.Cancer, 47:757, (1983)

24. B. Armstrong, and R. Doll, Environmental factors and cancer incidence and mortality in different countries with special reference to dietary prectices, Int.J.Cancer, 15:617, (1975).

25. A. B. Miller, et al., A study of diet and breast cancer, Am. J. Epidemiol., 107:499, (1978).

26. J. H. Lubin, et al., Dietary factors and breast cancer risk, Int. J. Cancer,28:685, (1981).

27. R. Talamini, et al., Social factors, diet and breast cancer in a northern Italian population, Br.J.Cancer, 49:723, (1984).

28. F. deWaard, J. Poortman, and H. J. A. Collette, Relationship of weight to the promotion of breast cancer after menopause, Nutr. Cancer 2:237,(1981).

29. M. E. Lippman, Efforts to combine endocrine and chemotherapy in the management of breast cancer: do two and two equal three?, Breast Cancer Research and Treatment, 3:117, (1983).

30. L. A. Brinton, The relationship of exogenous estrogens to cancer risk, Cancer Detection and Prevention, 7:159, (1984)

31. J.G. Azzopardi, Benign and Malignant Proliferative Epithelial Lesions of the Breast; a Review, Eur.J.Cancer Clin.Oncol. 12: 1717 (1983).

32. V. L. Ernster, The epidemiology of benign breast disease, Epidemiologic Reviews, 3:184, (1981).

33. R. Hoover, et al., Menopausal estrogens and breast cancer, N.Engl. J.Med., 295:401, 41976).

34. G. R. Howe, Epidemiology of Radiogenic Breast Cancer, in "Radiation Carcinogenesis: Epidemiology and Biological Significance", J.D.Boice and J.F.Fraumeni eds., Raven Press, New York, (1984).

35. T. J. Craig, Comstock G.W., and P. B. Geiser, Epidemiologic Comparison of breast cancer patients with early and late onset of malignancy and general populations controls, J.N.C.I., 53:1577 (1974).

36. S. Tokuoka, Histologic Review of breast cancer cases in survivors of atomic bombs in Hiroshima and Nagasaki, Japan, Cancer, 54:849, (1984).

37. C. W. Welsch, and C. F. Aylsworth, Enhancement of mureine mammary carcinogenesis by feeding high levels of dietary fat: a hormonal mechanism ?, J.N.C.I., 70/2:215, (1983).

38. T. L. Dao, and P. Chan, Effect of duration of high fat intake on enhancement of mammary carcinogenesis in rats, J.N.C.I., 71/1:201, (1983).

39. L. P. Yotti, C. C. Chang and J. E. Trosko, Elimination of metabolic cooperation in Chinese Hamster cells by a tumor promoter, Science, 206: 1089, (1979).

40. N. E. Day, Epidemiological evidence of promoting effects-the example of breast cancer, Carcinogenesis, 7:183, (1982)

41. J. D. Boice, B. J. Stone, Interaction between radiation and other breast cancer risk factors, in " Late biological effects of ionizing radiation", Vol.I:231, International Atomic Energy Agency, Vienna, (1978).

42. M. C. King, et al., Allele increasing susceptibility to human breast cancer may be linked to the glutamate-pyruvate transaminase locus, Science, 208:406, (1980).

43. A. G. Knudson, H. W. Hethcote and Brown B. W., Mutation and childhood cancer: a probabilistic model for the incidence of retinoblastoma, Proc.Natl.Acad.Sci., 72:5116,(1975).

44. P. K. Siiteri, Extraglandular estrogen formation and serum binding of estradiol:relationship to cancer, J. Endocrinol.

45. A. S. Morrison, et al., Some international differences in histology and survival in breast cancer, Int.J.Cancer, 11:261, (1973)

46. E. L. Winder, et al., A comparison of survival rates between American and Japanese patients with breast cancer, Surg.Gynecol. Obstet., 117:196, (1963).

47. T. Nemoto, et al., Differences in breast cancer between Japan and the United States, J.N.C.I., 58:193, (1977).

48. M. C. Pike, et al.,'Hormonal' risk factors, 'breast tissue age' and the age-incidence of breast cancer, Nature, 303:767, (1983).

EPIDEMIOLOGIC STUDIES OF CHEMOTHERAPY-RELATED ACUTE LEUKEMIA

Mark H. Greene

Environmental Epidemiology Branch
National Cancer Institute
Bethesda, Maryland 20205

INTRODUCTION

Virtually all patients with disseminated malignancy, and a substantial fraction of those with more localized disease, are destined to die of their cancers in the absence of proper treatment. Unfortunately, effective cancer therapy often results in exposure of patients to cytotoxic drugs with carcinogenic potential. Many anticancer drugs are known to be carcinogenic in experimental animals (1). The systematic exposure of large numbers of patients to these potentially hazardous compounds has created a unique opportunity to (a) evaluate and quantify the risk of various malignancies following exposure to specific compounds; (b) identify unusually hazardous or unusually safe treatment regimens; and (c) elucidate mechanisms of radiation and drug carcinogenesis in man. Over the last several decades, an enormous anecdotal literature has developed describing in case report form the development of a malignancy as an apparent complication of anticancer treatment. However, such relationships can only be explored systematically and scientifically through the use of various epidemiologic techniques. In this review, I will concentrate my discussion upon studies which have been done using the techniques of analytic epidemiology. The following research strategies have been employed:

1) Follow-up of cohorts of patients with a specific index disease (malignant or non-malignant) and treatments of interest. Data on the patients and treatments are collected; after stratification by therapy, observed numbers of subsequent cancers are compared with expected numbers derived from appropriate general population

incidence or mortality data. Life-table techniques are used to estimate the cumulative risk of subsequent cancer.

2) Follow-up of patients with a specific index disease treated in randomized clinical trials. In addition to the analytic approaches cited above, this strategy permits the evaluation of subsequent cancers in comparable groups of patients, some randomized to receive the treatment of interest and some not so exposed. This allows assessment of treatment-related cancer risk without reliance upon general population rates.

3) Case-control studies. In this approach, patients who develop a subsequent cancer of interest are compared to patients with the same initial disease who do not develop a subsequent cancer. These special studies may be done within a defined cohort or may represent a separate study in which subjects are drawn from other sources, such as population-based tumor registries. This strategy is particularly efficient in collecting detailed dosimetry data, since it generally requires data abstraction from considerably fewer patient records than does the cohort approach. In contrast to isolated case reports or case series, informative analytic studies designed to address the relationship between the treatment of an initial cancer and the development of subsequent neoplasia include the following characteristics. First, metastasis as an explanation for subsequent cancer must be ruled out. The chronology of tumors must be considered; formal analysis of malignancies occurring prior to the index cancer is uninformative. The studies must be of sufficient size to permit detection of risks of what ever magnitude might be anticipated. The analysis of subsequent cancers should be conducted in a site-specific fashion rather than aggregating cancers of all kinds into a single category. Quantitative analytic techniques of the types outlined above must be applied and details of cancer therapy must be taken into account to determine whether excesses of subsequent cancers can be reasonably attributed to tumor therapy administered for an initial malignancy or some other explanation.

TREATMENT-RELATED LEUKEMIC CONDITIONS

The development of acute leukemia as a complication of therapy administered to patients with cancer is well known. The vast majority of the acute leukemias which occur in this setting are of the acute nonlymphocytic type (ANL) (2). This rubric is comprised of acute myelogenous leukemia and its variants (FAB types M1 through M6) (3). While occasional reports of other forms of leukemia have been presented following anticancer therapy, ANL is

the only type that has been systematically linked to the administration of cytotoxic chemotherapy. Thus, in the present discussion, other types of leukemia will not be considered. The ANL
which occurs following cancer therapy has a variety of characteristics which distinguish it from its spontaneous counterpart.
The treatment-related form of ANL is nearly always heralded by a
period of prolonged pancytopenia. On histologic examination, the
bone marrow reveals dysplasia of one or more cell lines and
establishing a definitive diagnosis can be very difficult. Some
studies have suggested that there may be an excess of particular
ANL subtypes, i.e., acute myelomonocytic leukemia and acute ery-
throleukemia. Cytogenetic abnormalities (particularly monosomy 5
or 7) are seen in the vast majority of treatment-related ANL
patients. These leukemias appear to have a very short latent
period: the first cases appear at approximately two years following initiation of therapy rising to an apparent peak at about five
years post-treatment. Compared with spontaneous ANL, the treatment-related variant is exceedingly refractory to therapy; most
patients die within six months of diagnosis. The vast majority of
patients developing ANL in this context have received prolonged
therapy with cytotoxic drugs; the class of drugs most frequently
implicated are the alkylating agents. Treatment-related ANL appears
to be part of a broader spectrum of myelodysplastic syndromes (MDS)
which include, in order of progressive severity, refractory anemia
(RA), RA with sideroblasts, RA with excess blasts (RAEB), chronic
myelomonocytic leukemia, and RAEB "in transformation" (4). These
conditions, often designated "preleukemia," occur with significant
frequency in patients receiving cytotoxic chemotherapy. Until
recently, however, difficulties in establishing a precise diagnosis
in these patients has led to their not being included in formal
analyses of the leukemic complications of cytotoxic chemotherapy.
However, it is clear that these conditions (which fall short of the
required diagnostic criteria for full-fledged ANL) are nonetheless
an important source of morbidity and mortality (5). In one series
of 37 preleukemic patients, 19 (51%) terminated in ANL; all 37
patients were dead within four years (6). In another series of
26 patients with MDS, 14 (54%) terminated in ANL. Three patients
with RA progressed to RAEB while eight patients remained stable.
One patient with RA died (2). Finally, a survey of 42 patients
with preleukemia revealed that 90% of the 10 patients exposed
previously to alkylating agent therapy developed ANL while only 25%
of 32 patients not exposed developed ANL (7). Thus, the entities
RAEB, RAEB in transformation, and ANL represent a spectrum of bone
marrow injury all of which should be included in formal analyses
of the leukemogenic effects of anticancer therapy whenever possible.
One limitation must be kept in mind: general population incidence
rates do not include MDS; thus, when making comparisons between
observed cases of leukemic conditions and expected numbers derived
from general population rates, the MDS cases cannot be included.
They can, however, be included in analyses which do not rely upon

population-based incidence or mortality data, such as internal
comparisons within the context of a randomized clinical trial or
life-table analyses. In the review which follows, I will summarize
quantitative epidemiologic studies of the relationship between
cytotoxic therapy and the development of ANL/MDS in humans. I will
be selective in citing representative reports for specific primary
cancer types with the goal of illustrating the various types of
studies that can be performed as well as indicating which specific
chemotherapeutic agents have been shown to be leukemogenic in man.

ACUTE LEUKEMIA FOLLOWING HODGKIN'S DISEASE

The occurrence of ANL in patients receiving chemotherapy
and/or radiation therapy for Hodgkin's disease is perhaps the most
extensively studied example of the carcinogenic effects of anticancer therapy. In a particularly careful study of a large group
of patients with Hodgkin's disease followed for a substantial
period of time, Coleman, et al quantify the risk of ANL (8). In
their series of 1,222 patients with Hodgkin's disease (median
follow-up: 5.4 years), 23 patients developed ANL; 0.33 cases were
expected, yielding a ratio of observed to expected cases (O/E) of
70. When this group was stratified on the basis of the therapy
administered for Hodgkin's disease, the authors observed one
patient with ANL among 441 patients treated with radiation therapy
alone, 16 patients with ANL among 525 patients receiving radiation
therapy (XRT) and adjuvant chemotherapy, one patient with ANL
among 147 patients treated with XRT plus salvage chemotherapy,
three patients with ANL among 65 patients receiving XRT plus
colloidal gold (all three leukemia patients received salvage
chemotherapy with MOPP), and two cases of ANL among 44 patients
treated with chemotherapy alone. The cumulative risk of acute
leukemia at ten years following diagnosis of Hodgkin's disease
was 3.5% in the entire cohort, and ranged from 0.6% in patients
treated with radiation alone to 15.6% among patients treated with
chemotherapy alone. The differences in risk between patients
receiving adjuvant chemotherapy compared to those receiving XRT
alone and those receiving chemotherapy alone compared to XRT were
both highly significant. Furthermore, intensity of radiation
therapy was unrelated to ANL risk in this series. A review of the
large quantitative studies of acute leukemia occurring in patients
treated for Hodgkin's disease reveals that of 166 reported ANL
cases, 159 (96%) occurred in individuals treated with chemotherapy.
The vast majority of these developed following treatment with the
four drug chemotherapy regimen known as "MOPP," (mustargen,
oncovin, procarbazine, and prednisone). These findings have been
replicated in many similar studies, documenting the leukemogenic
potential of MOPP chemotherapy. Many studies have suggested that
the addition of radiation therapy to MOPP leads to a substantial
increase in the risk of ANL (9-11). However, more recent studies
have tended to suggest that the differences are not as great as

originally believed. It is now generally accepted that the bulk
of the ANL risk observed in patients with Hodgkin's disease can be
attributed reasonably to the intensive chemotherapy with which
these patients are treated, and that this risk includes an excess
of MDS as well (5). Several studies have indicated that the risk
of ANL increases as the age at Hodgkin's disease diagnosis increases. In the study of Coleman et al (8), the cumulative risk
of ANL at ten years was 1.3% among individuals who were less than
age 20 at Hodgkin's disease diagnosis compared with 12.7% among
patients who were age 50 or greater. Several groups have observed that combination chemotherapy regimens such as ABVD (adriamycin,
bleomycin, vinblastine, and actinomycin D) (10) or PAVe (procarbazine, alberan, velban) (8) have not shown (thus far) the high
risk of ANL associated with MOPP. These studies are based on
relatively small numbers of patients followed for relatively
short intervals; this is a question which requires further study.
Based on the available data, the risk of MOPP-associated ANL
appears to persist for at least 10 years following treatment.
In summary, there appears to be a dramatic excess of ANL in
patients receiving intensive chemotherapy for Hodgkin's disease.
The risk of ANL is not elevated following the administration of
radiation therapy alone. While the MOPP combination is clearly
leukemogenic in man, the specific drugs within this combination
to which the ANL/MDS risk can be attributed have not been
identified on the basis of analytic studies. Nitrogen mustard
and procarbazine, either alone or synergistically, are the leading
candidates. Among the important unanswered questions in Hodgkin's
disease are: 1) Does the combination of XRT and chemotherapy have
a higher risk of ANL than chemotherapy alone? 2) Does the risk of
ANL decline after ten years of treatment? 3) Is there a relationship between chemotherapy dose and risk of ANL? 4) Does the
sequencing of XRT and/or chemotherapy affect the risk of ANL? and
5) Do alternative chemotherapy regimens (ABVD; PAVe) have lesser
leukemogenic potential than MOPP?

ACUTE LEUKEMIA FOLLOWING NON-HODGKIN'S LYMPHOMA

In a cohort study of patients with non-Hodgkin's lymphoma
(NHL) treated at the U.S. National Cancer Institute, 517 patients
accrued 2,203 person-years of observation (12). In this cohort,
27 subsequent cancers were observed compared with 11.4 expected
(O/E = 2.4; 95% CL = 1.6; 3.5). This excess was accounted for
entirely by ANL (O = 9; E = 0.08; O/E = 105). The excess risk of
ANL in this cohort was 4.1 cases per 1,000 persons per year.
Treatment data were available readily only on the initial treatment administered to each of the patients in this cohort. When
stratified on the basis of whether they had received chemotherapy,
radiation therapy, or both, the risk of ANL seemed greatest in
patients treated with radiation therapy (O = 7; O/E = 209).
Further, the risk was greatest among those patients who received

intensive XRT in the form of total nodal or total body irradiation. As was noted among patients with Hodgkin's disease, the risk of ANL among patients with NHL was positively correlated with age at lymphoma diagnosis. The rate of ANL rose from 2.9 per 1,000 person per year among individuals less than 35 at diagnosis to 5.7 per 1,000 per year among patients who were age 50 or older. Similarly, the risk of ANL persisted for at least ten years following additional treatment. However, we were concerned that the apparent strong relationship between initial XRT and risk of ANL might be misleading, since the main data file used for this cohort analysis contained neither complete treatment histories nor information on dose of either drugs or radiation therapy. In an effort to clarify this situation, a case-control study nested within the larger cohort was performed. Cases were defined as NHL patients who developed ANL; controls were NHL patients who did not develop ANL. Four controls were matched to each case on the basis of sex, race, and duration of survival. We then abstracted detailed treatment data from the 45 patient records involved in this smaller study. With this information, patients were classified as ever having been exposed to chemotherapy alone, radiation alone, or both. Six cases (67%) compared to eight controls (22%) received both radiation and chemotherapy, a distribution which is significantly different from chance. Thus, when full treatment histories were available, combined modality therapy rather than XRT alone was most closely relative to ANL risk. Furthermore, patients who developed ANL were more intensively treated than were controls. For example, the average radiation dose to active bone marrow was significantly greater for cases (1180 rads) compared to controls (490 rads). With regard to chemotherapy dose, exposed cases received an average of three times more cyclophosphamide than did exposed controls (71,000 mg. versus 23,300 mg.). To further assess dose response relationships and drug radiation interactions in ANL risk, each patient was classified into one of nine radiation-chemotherapy exposure levels. This revealed roughly equal proportions of cases and controls in each of the three chemotherapy exposure categories, in contrast to increasing numbers of cases and decreasing numbers of controls as one progressed from low to high radiation exposure groups. The relative risk of ANL in the high radiation exposure group (total dose > 700 rads) compared to the two lower exposure groups combined was 8.1 (95% CL = 1.8; 36). Controlling for duration of chemotherapy, there was significant trend of increasing ANL risk with increasing cumulative bone marrow radiation dose. In contrast to the data on cyclophosphamide dose cited earlier, no association between duration of chemotherapy and risk of ANL was observed. Duration of treatment was chosen as the exposure measure because of the difficulties entailed in making comparisons between patients who received multiple different drugs. There is, at present, no accepted method for combining data on multiple drugs into a single, aggregate measure of dose. However, duration of chemotherapy may not have accurately reflected the total cyto-

toxic drug exposure of patients. Thus, for example, cases
exceeded controls with regard to mean duration of cytoxan treatment, mean dose of cytoxan, and both mean duration of treatment
and mean dose at each level of exposure. These observations
suggest that using duration of treatment as an index of chemotherapy exposure may mask important dose trends which might be
evident were there a reasonable method for aggregating doses of
different drugs into a single dose parameter for each patient.
This study demonstrated that there is a significant risk of ANL
in patients treated with combined modality therapy for non-
Hodgkin's lymphoma. This risk showed a male/female excess (2/1),
an increasing risk within increasing age at first treatment, and
a predominance in patients with indolent NHL histologies. The
risk of ANL increased significantly with increasing cumulative
radiation dose to the bone marrow; cases received higher doses
of cyclophosphamide over a longer duration than did controls.
The risk of ANL in this study was greatest among patients with
indolent NHL subtypes who received multiple courses of combined
modality therapy. These data suggested that induction regimens
for indolent NHL should minimize both the duration and quantity
of therapy in an effort to reduce the risk of ANL.

ACUTE LEUKEMIA FOLLOWING MULTIPLE MYELOMA

Several studies have documented a dramatic excess of ANL
following the administration of chemotherapy to patients with
multiple myeloma. Perhaps the most impressive series is that
reported by Bergsagel, et al in which 14 of 364 patients with
multiple myeloma developed ANL (13). The risk of ANL in this
cohort was over 200 times that expected on the basis of general
population incidence rates. The cumulative risk of ANL in this
cohort reached a staggering 17.4% at 50 months of follow-up.
All of these patients were treated with the alkylating agent
melphalan. However, undefined proportions of the cohort also
received cyclophosphamide and/or BNCU, making it difficult to
implicate a specific agent in the pathogenesis of the ANL observed.
In general, however, melphalan appears to be the drug most
frequently associated with the development of ANL in patients
with multiple myeloma. One possible explanation for what appears
to be an unusally high risk of ANL is the possibility that there
may be an underlying predisposition to the development of leukemia
in patients with multiple myeloma, a predisposition which is
unrelated to therapy. In support of this possibility, there are
at least 41 case reports of patients with plasma cell neoplasms
who developed ANL without having been exposed to cytotoxic chemotherapy. Thus, alkylating agents appear largely responsible for
the ANL excess observed in patients with multiple myeloma. The
tendency to expose such patients to multiple drugs makes it
difficult to single out a particular agent as the key one. The
risk of ANL in patients with multiple myeloma seems considerably

higher than that observed among other cancer patients. This might possibly be attributed to an intrinsic predisposition to leukemia which is exacerbated by exposure to an exogenous carcinogen.

ACUTE LEUKEMIA FOLLOWING POLYCYTHEMIA VERA

In a study of 431 patients participating in a randomized clinical trial of the treatment of polycythemia vera, 26 patients developed acute leukemia (14). When stratified by treatment, only one of 134 patients treated with phlebotomy alone developed ANL compared with 16 (11%) of 141 patients treated with the alkylating agent chlorambucil. An intermediate risk was observed among patient treated with the radioisotope P^{32}. This analysis revealed that the risk of ANL in patients receiving chlorambucil was 13.5 times greater than that observed in patients treated with phlebotomy only; the corresponding comparison for chlorambucil versus P^{32} was 2.3. This study also suggested that the risk of ANL was greater among patients exposed to higher doses of chlorambucil. Depending upon the measure of dose employed, the risk of ANL in "high dose" patients ranged from 4 to 5 times greater than that observed in "low dose" patients. In another survey, the piperazine derivative pipobroman was linked with the development of ANL in patients being treated for p. vera (15). Among 73 patients receiving pipobroman, 5 developed ANL, an incidence rate of 13 cases per 1,000 per year. The lack of a pipobroman-unexposed group in this study prevented a definitive association of this compound with ANL. These studies of ANL risk in patients with p. vera are of particular importance since they provide the first quantitative data documenting that chlorambucil is a cause of human leukemia. Further, they suggest that the risk of ANL appears to be dose-related. An alkylating agent of a novel type, pipobroman, may be leukemogenic as well.

ACUTE LEUKEMIA FOLLOWING OVARIAN CANCER

In a study of five randomized clinical trials, 1,399 women with ovarian cancer accrued 3,458 person-years of observation (16). In this cohort, twelve women developed ANL compared with 0.18 cases expected (O/E = 67). The excess risk of ANL was 3.5 cases per 1,000 women per year with a seven year cumulative risk of ANL equal to 4.7% ($\pm$1.6). However, when this cohort was stratified on the basis of treatment, all twelve patients with ANL were among the 998 women exposed to alkylating agent chemotherapy (O/E = 110). The ANL rate of this subgroup was 5.8 cases per 1,000 per year, with a cumulative ANL risk at seven years equal to 9.6%. No cases of ANL were observed among women who were unexposed to alkylating agent therapy. In addition, this ANL risk could be directly linked to the alkylating agents melphalan and chlorambucil; ten ANL patients received the former, while two received the latter. The risks associated with these two specific drugs were similar. The risk of ANL persisted for at least seven years following the initial exposure to alkylating agent therapy. Evaluation of the risk of ANL as a function of <u>initial</u> drug dose in the three single agent trials revealed that all cases of ANL occurred in a high dose category, except for one woman whose initial treatment was radiation therapy; she subsequently received high dose melphalan. The absence of ANL cases in the one trial which employed a very low cumulative dose melphalan regimen is consistent with a dose response effect. All ten melphalan related cases occurred in patients receiving twelve or more cycles of therapy, while the two chlorambucil-related cases developed in women who received daily therapy for more than eighteen months. Dose and duration of treatment were so highly correlated that the separate effects of each could not be distinguished in this relatively small cohort. This survey was of particular importance since it was the first to quantitatively document the risk of ANL in patients receiving <u>adjuvant</u> chemotherapy. In a Danish survey, 553 women treated with the alkylating agent Treosulfan (dihydroxybusulfan) accrued 1,159 woman-years of observation (17). Seven cases of ANL developed, compared with 0.04 cases expected, for an O/E = 175. The cumulative risk of ANL in this cohort was 7.6% at five years, with an ANL rate of 6.0 cases per 1,000 women per year. Although not statistically significant, there was a suggestion that women receiving higher doses of chemotherapy were at greater risk of ANL in this series as well. In summary, women with ovarian cancer are at increased risk of alkylating agent-induced ANL. These studies have documented the leukemogenicity of melphalan and Treosulfan and provided further confirmation of the relationship between chlorambucil and risk of ANL. In this context, the addition of radiation therapy to chemotherapy does not further increase the risk of ANL. These studies also provide additional evidence for a dose-response relationship in ANL risk.

ACUTE LEUKEMIA FOLLOWING GASTROINTESTINAL CANCER

In a series of 1,402 white men treated for colorectal cancer between 1958 and 1964, 10,902 person-years of observation were accrued (18). Overall, six patients developed acute leukemia compared with 3.8 cases expected (O/E = 1.6; n.s.). When stratified by therapy, three patients treated with surgery alone had developed ANL (2.1 cases expected) while three patients treated with the alkylating agent thio-tepa developed ANL (1.2 cases expected). A very low dose of chemotherapy was employed in this clinical trial; thus, it is not surprising that an excess of leukemia was not observed even though an alkylating agent was employed. In a more recent survey of patients enrolled in nine randomized clinical trials designed to assess the effectiveness of adjuvant chemotherapy for gastric, colon or rectal cancer, 2,067 of 3,633 study participants were exposed to the nitrosourea alkylating agent methyl-CCNU (19). The end point in this survey was the development of either ANL or MDS (together defined as "leukemic disorders". A total of 18 leukemic disorders were observed: RAEB = 5, RAEB in transformation = 3, and ANL = 10. Seventeen leukemic disorders occurred during 7,009 person-years of observation among patients exposed to methyl-CCNU. Nine of these cases were ANL, compared with 0.8 cases expected (O/E = 10.8). In contrast, only one patient developed ANL during 5,448 person-years of observation among patients unexposed to methyl-CCNU. The relative risk of ANL in patients exposed to methyl-CCNU compared to those unexposed was 15.9 (95% CL = 2; 320). The risk of ANL was very low within the first year after initiation of chemotherapy, and appeared to increase during the seven years of observation. The rate of ANL was 0.3 cases per 1,000 per year less than two years after initiation of treatment compared to 3.1 cases per 1,000 per year during years four through seven (p = 0.02). The cumulative risk at seven years was 2.3% ($\pm$1.3) for ANL and 3.2% ($\pm$1.4) for ANL plus MDS. A review of observed and expected numbers of ANL following gastrointestinal cancers in data derived from the Connecticut Tumor Registry during the pre-nitrosourea era revealed no excess of ANL: 28 cases observed, 27.5 cases expected. Thus, we can say with confidence that ANL is not part of the natural history of untreated gastrointestinal cancer. In summary, this study demonstrates that chloroethyl nitrosourea drugs are leukemogenic in man. Although similar quantitative data are not yet available on other nitrosourea compounds (i.e., BCNU, CCNU, streptozotocin) it seems plausible to anticipate that they may prove to be leukemogenic as well. The cumulative risk of leukemic conditions (3.2% at seven years) is similar to that observed following exposure to other alkylating agents. Since all nine trials were designed to assess the benefits of adjuvant chemotherapy for gastrointestinal cancer, and since very little evidence of therapeutic efficacy has yet to emerge from these studies, the benefit of adjuvant alkylating therapy must be carefully weighed against the risk of therapy associated ANL and MDS. Finally, very low doses of thio-tepa do not seem to be leukemogenic.

ACUTE LEUKEMIA FOLLOWING BREAST CARCINOMA

Utilizing the National Cancer Institute's network of population-based cancer registries, the risk of acute leukemia associated with the first course of cancer treatment was evaluated in 59,115 women with breast cancer diagnosed between 1973 and 1980 (20). During 166,491 woman-years of follow-up for the entire cohort, 27 patients developed ANL compared with 13.2 cases expected (O/E = 2.1). The rate of ANL in the total cohort was 0.23 cases per 1,000 women per year. Fourteen of these cases developed during 117,547 woman-years of observation among patients initially treated with surgery alone (9.8 cases expected; O/E = 1.4). Eight patients developed ANL following initial treatment with radiation alone while five developed ANL following initial treatment with chemotherapy alone, for O/E = 3.7 and 27.8 respectively. The risk of ANL was greatest between years three through seven of follow-up. This survey provided the first quantitative evidence that women with breast cancer are at increased risk of ANL. This risk is linked to chemotherapy and to radiation therapy in the only analytic study published, a finding which must be regarded with caution since data were not available on subsequent treatments administered to these patients. It seems likely that many women treated initially with radiation therapy were subsequently exposed to chemotherapy. In this survey, specific drugs could not be linked with risk of ANL. Given the very large number of women exposed to chemotherapy for carcinoma of the breast, particularly since much of this treatment is in the adjuvant setting, this is an area in urgent need of additional, more precise data.

ACUTE LEUKEMIA FOLLOWING LUNG CARCINOMA

Among 5,000 patients with lung cancer treated at Memorial Sloan-Kettering Hospital in the pre-chemotherapy era, 56 patients survived for ten years (21). Eleven of these individuals developed a second cancer; none developed acute leukemia. Thus, ANL does not appear to be part of the natural history of untreated carcinoma of the lung. In a randomized clinical trial of lung cancer, 0 of 249 placebo-treated patients developed ANL compared with 4 of 243 patients receiving the alkylating agent busulfan (22). All four busulfan-related cases developed within a subset of 19 busulfan treated patients who experienced prolonged pancytopenia, further supporting the relationship between ANL and MDS. This study provides the only quantitative human data regarding the leukemogenic potential of busulfan in humans. More recently, a survey of 158 patients receiving intensive combined modality therapy (including XRT, CCNU, procarbazine and cytoxan) for small cell carcinoma of the lung revealed three patients with ANL compared with 0.01 cases expected (O/E = 316; 95% CL = 76; 818) (23). The cumulative risk of ANL was 25% (±13) at 3.1 years, and the ANL incidence rate was 17.2 cases per 1,000 persons per year. These two studies demonstrate that busulfan (like dihydroxy-busulfan) is leukemogenic in man and that aggressive combined modality therapy for small cell cancer of the lung may have an exceedingly high risk of ANL.

ACUTE LEUKEMIA FOLLOWING TESTICULAR CANCER

In the previously cited study by Curtis et al (20), ANL was observed in 0 (0.2 cases expected) of 883 patients with surgically-treated testicular cancer. In contrast, two patients developed acute leukemia (0.39 cases expected; O/E = 5.1) among 1,821 testicular cancer patients treated with radiation and/or chemotherapy. Another survey revealed the presence of five patients

with ANL among 1,150 patients with germ cell tumors of the testis
(24). Unfortunately, no quantitative estimate of ANL risk was
computed in this latter study. While good epidemiologic data
regarding the risk of ANL in patients treated for testicular cancer
are not yet available, the non-quantitative literature suggests
that an ANL excess may well exist. Sufficient numbers of long-term
survivors of testicular cancer are now available to permit an
analytic study. Studies of this particular tumor site would
provide an opportunity to assess the leukemogenicity of an as-yet
unstudied class of therapeutic agents: the platinum compounds.

ACUTE LEUKEMIA FOLLOWING ANTI-METABOLITE THERAPY

In a survey of 457 women with gestational trophoblastic
neoplasms receiving the anti-metabolite methotrexate, two second
cancers developed (3.5 cases expected; O/E = 0.6) during 3,522
woman-years of observation (25). One patient developed breast
cancer and one developed ANL. The latter patient received
multiple cytotoxic drugs (cytoxan, actinomycin D, adriamycin,
platinum, VP16, vincristine, and hydroxyurea) in addition to
mexotrexate. No overall cancer excess was observed in this cohort
in spite of the fact that approximately half the patients also
received other cytotoxic drugs. In the previously-cited survey
of low dose adjuvant chemotherapy in patients with colorectal
cancer (18), 470 patients received the anti-metabolite 5-fluoro-2-
deoxyuridine. No cases of ANL were observed. In the survey of
ANL following adjuvant chemotherapy with methyl-CCNU (19), 404
patients received as a single agent the anti-metabolite 5-fluor-
ouracil. Again, no cases of ANL developed in this subgroup. Only
limited epidemiologic data are available regarding the leukemogenicity of anti-metabolites, partly owing to their predominant
use in combination chemotherapy regimens which also include
alkylating agents. The available data indicate that methotrexate
and 5-FU are not leukemogenic, confirming experimental data
derived from laboratory studies of these drugs (1).

SOLID TUMORS FOLLOWING CHEMOTHERAPY

The risk of subsequent malignancy other than ANL has not
been extensively evaluated, in part because the latent period of
the solid tumors is presumed to be much longer than the two to five
year latent period observed for ANL. In addition, most potential
study populations have not yet accrued sufficiently large numbers
of greater than ten year survivors to permit reliable estimates of
the risk of solid tumors. However, if the experience in radiation
carcinogenesis applies, one may reasonably anticipate the emergence
of excess solid tumors after the administration of chemotherapy and
prolonged survival. This is a matter which will require careful
monitoring and detailed evaluation as time passes. Nonetheless,
there are several noteworthy examples of post-chemotherapy solid

tumors. In the early 1960's, Danish investigators reported a dramatic excess of carcinoma of the urinary bladder among patients receiving chlornaphazine for the treatment of polycythemia vera (26). (This compound is closely related to the well-known bladder carcinogen beta-naphthylamine.) In a series of 61 patients receiving this drug, ten developed carcinoma of the bladder and an additional five developed "abnormal urine cytology." These observations lead to the withdrawal of this chemotherapeutic agent from clinical practice. Several studies have demonstrated an excess risk of bladder cancer among patients receiving the alkylating agent cyclophosphamide for various malignant and non-malignant conditions (27-29). These studies have documented that cyclophosphamide is a carcinogen in humans. There is an enormous case literature suggesting that this compound also causes ANL (1) but, at the moment, no good epidemiologic data have been produced to quantify this association which, in my opinion, certainly does exist. Finally, several studies of the immunosuppressive drug azathioprine have documented a dramatic excess of non-Hodgkin's lymphoma following its administration to renal transplant recipients (30) or patients with other immunologic conditions (29). A glimpse into what lies ahead in non-ANL second cancers as longer term follow-up accrues can be obtained from studies of subsequent malignancy in survivors of childhood cancer (31). Among 9,170 survivors of childhood cancer, 167 subsequent malignancies developed (11.4 cases expected; O/E = 15). In addition to a 28-fold excess of ANL, this survey documented substantial excesses of second primary cancers of bone (O/E = 133), thyroid (O/E = 53), connective tissue (O/E = 41), and digestive tract (O/E = 38). The relationship between the cancer excesses at these particular sites and the chemotherapy received for the initial malignancy is currently under analysis. One striking observation is the persistence in the risk of subsequent malignancy as the duration of follow-up is extended. In this survey, the rate of subsequent cancers among children followed for twenty years of more after initial diagnosis was 15 cases per 1,000 person per year compared with 1.5 cases per 1,000 per year among children followed less than five years. The cumulative risk of subsequent neoplasia among children in this cohort climbed steadily to 12.1% at 25 years. Thus, it seems inevitable that as follow-up of other exposed cohorts is extended, excesses of cancers other than ANL will emerge.

SUMMARY

The International Agency for Research on Cancer (IARC) has a program under which various chemicals are assessed formally to determine their carcinogenic risk for humans. Compounds are classified into one of three broad categories: Group 1 - the chemical is carcinogenic to humans; Group 2 - the chemical is probably carcinogenic to humans; and Group 3 - the chemical cannot be classified as to its carcinogenicity in humans (1). According to their most recent summary, the following anticancer drugs are classified as definite human carcinogens: azathioprine, busulfan, chloranaphazine, chlorambucil, cyclophosphamide, melphalan, "MOPP," and treosulfan. Data reviewed above suggests that methyl-CCNU (and probably the other nitrosoureas) should be added to this list as well. Compounds classified as probable human carcinogens include nitrogen mustard and procarbazine. No epidemiologic data permit evaluating these compounds on an individual basis. Based upon the information reviewed above, pipobroman should be added to this group. Compounds regarded as probable human carcinogens with a lower degree of certainty (Class 2B) include actinomycin D, adriamycin, BCNU, CCNU, cis-platinum, DTIC, thio-tepa, and uracil mustard. While methotrexate and 5-FU are listed in Class 3, the data currently available for these two agents suggests that they are not carcinogenic.

In this review, I have attempted to illustrate the variety of epidemiologic techniques which are available for the formal assessment of the carcinogenic risks associated with chemotherapeutic agents. Such studies have documented the leukemogenicity of at least eight different drugs and several multi-drug combinations. As a class, alkylating agents are clearly human leukemogens. Combined modality therapy (that is, radiation therapy plus chemotherapy) may, in some cases, have a greater leukemogenic risk than that associated with chemotherapy alone. The risk of ANL has been documented in patients receiving adjuvant chemotherapy. This is of particular importance since a significant (albeit unknown) fraction of these patients are destined not to develop recurrence of their primary disease. Thus, these individuals are being exposed to significant potential long-term toxicity without therapeutic benefit. The risk of ANL/MDS seems to persist for at least ten years following chemotherapy exposure. There are insufficient data available at present to determine whether the risk persists or declines beyond that time. There may be a positive correlation between age at chemotherapy exposure and risk of developing ANL/MDS. A moderate amount of data suggest a positive relationship between drug dose and risk of ANL. This indicates that clinical practice should, insofar as possible, use the minimum dose of chemotherapy consistent with therapeutic benefit. Host susceptibility may contribute to the risk of ANL in certain cases (e.g., multiple myeloma). The limited data currently available suggest that anti-metabolite chemotherapeutic agents may not be leukemogenic. To the extent that they are clinically effective, these drugs might reasonably be substituted for more toxic agents. Chemotherapy-induced ANL is a distinctive clinical pathologic entity, which is part of a spectrum of myelodysplastic disorders. These myelodysplastic conditions are events worthy of analysis in the setting of chemotherapy exposure. The enormous relative risks of ANL described in the studies reviewed here occur primarily in the long-term survivors of patients with advanced neoplastic

disease. Overall, ANL is a minor contributor to mortality in
these patients; the vast majority die of their primary cancer.
It is highly probable that the benefit of these agents outweighs
the risk of ANL in patients treated for advanced malignancy.
However, the use of these drugs in the adjuvant therapy of cancer
patients at low risk of recurrence and the treatment of non-
neoplastic diseases is another matter. Alkylating agents should
be avoided it at all possible in these settings. When they must
be used, the dose and duration of administration of drug should
be kept to an absolute minimum. Insofar as future research in
this area is concerned, subsequent studies should be conducted to
clarify questions related to drug dose, drug schedule and differences in ANL risk between specific agents or drug combinations.
These latter issues are of particular importance in Hodgkin's
disease, in which no studies to date have addressed the issue of
drug dose as a determinant of ANL risk and in which several groups
have suggested that non-MOPP combination drug regimens (e.g., ABVD;
PAVe; VBM [belban, bleomycin, methotrexate]) may have a lower risk
of ANL. Primary cancer sites in need of study in order to determine whether patients with these tumors are at increased risk of
ANL/MD S include carcinomas of the breast and testis. Breast
cancer is of particular importance given the large number of women
currently receiving adjuvant chemotherapy for this condition. Data
regarding the carcinogenicity of adriamycin and cis-platinum are
urgently needed. Studies of these particular compounds have been
hampered by their routine use in combination regimens which include
other chemotherapeutic agents already known to be carcinogenic.
There are virtually no data available on other drugs currently
being used rather widely including VP16, bleomycin, and the vinca
alkaloids. Finally, as indicated above, long term surveillance
of cohorts exposed to treatment regimens of interest will be
required in order to assess the risk of solid tumors in such
patients.

REFERENCES

1. IARC Monogr Eval Carcinog Risk Chem Hum 1981: Vol 26.
2. Pedersen-Bjergaard J, et al: Blood 57: 712-723, 1981.
3. Bennett JM, et al: Brit J Haematol 33: 451-458, 1976.
4. Bennett JM, et al: Brit J Haematol 51: 189-199, 1982.
5. Pedersen-Bjergaard J, et al: N Engl J Med 307: 965-971,
    1982.
6. Economopoulos T, et al: Acta Haematol 65: 97-102, 1981.
7. Anderson RL, et al: Leuk Res 6: 175-181, 1982.
8. Coleman CN, et al: Cancer Surveys 1: 733-744, 1982.
9. Toland DM, et al: Cancer Clinical Trials 1: 27-33, 1978.
10. Valagussa P, et al: Brit Med J 280: 216-219, 1980.
11. Tester WJ, et al: J Clin Oncol 2: 762-769, 1984.
12. Greene MH, et al: Cancer Res 43: 1891-1898, 1983.
13. Bergsagel DE, et al: N Engl J Med 301: 743-748, 1979.

14. Berk PD, et al: N Engl J Med 304: 441-447, 1981.
15. Brausamolino E, et al: J Clin Oncol 2: 558-561, 1984.
16. Greene MH, et al: N Engl J Med 307: 1416-1421, 1982.
17. Pedersen-Bjergaard J, et al: Cancer 45: 198-29, 1980.
18. Boice JD, et al: J Natl Cancer Ist 64: 501-511, 1980.
19. Boice JD, et al: N Engl J Med 309: 1079-1084, 1983.
20. Curtis RE, et al: J Natl Cancer Inst 72: 531-544, 1984.
21. Watson WL, et al: Diseases Chest 53: 65-75, 1968.
22. Scott H, et al: Brit Med J 2: 1513-1517, 1977.
23. Chak LY, et al: J Clin Oncol 2: 385-390, 1984.
24. Cockburn , et al: Proc ASCO 2: 139 (Abstr. #C546), 1983.
25. Rustin GJS, et al: N Engl J Med 308: 473-476, 1983.
26. Thiede T, et al: Acta Med Scand 185: 133-137, 1969.
27. Wall RL, et al: N Engl J Med 293: 271-273, 1975.
28. Plotz PH, et al: Ann Intern Med 91: 221-223, 1979.
29. Kinlen LJ, et al: Brit Med J 282: 474, 1981.
30. Kinlen LJ, et al: Brit Med J 2: 1461-1466, 1979.
31. Tucker MA, et al: in Radiation Carcinogenesis: Epidemiology
    and Biological Significance, JD Boice Jr. and JF Fraumeni Jr.
    eds; Raven Press, New York, pp 211-224, 1984.

THE CENTRAL NERVOUS SYSTEM AND IN UTERO EXPOSURE TO IONIZING
RADIATION: THE HIROSHIMA AND NAGASAKI EXPERIENCES

William J. Schull and Masanori Otake

The Epidemiology Center
School of Public Health, UT Health Science Center
Houston, Texas

INTRODUCTION

An extensive literature speaks to the deleterious effects of
in utero exposure to ionizing radiation. Much of the evidence
stems from studies of the survivors of the atomic bombing of
Hiroshima and Nagasaki. It is clear too that ionizing radiation
used therapeutically in the treatment of brain tumors or acute
leukemia can have damaging effects on the developed central
nervous system (e.g., Meadows et al., 1981; Hochberg, and
Slotnick, 1980; Raimondi and Tomita, 1979).   Meadows and her
colleagues (1981) have reported "Significant reductions were found
in overall IQ score for the majority of children, younger patients
being most affected." The exposures involved in these instances
are high, tens of Grays. Most of the individuals were also
receiving chemotherapy. The apparent effect of ionizing radiation
could, therefore, confound the effect of the latter. However, Ron
and her colleagues (1982) have reported a similar finding among
individuals treated for tinea capitis who were not on adjuvant
therapy and received much lower brain doses, possibly 130 cGy, on
the average. They have stated that "The irradiated children had
lower examination scores on scholastic aptitude, intelligence
quotient (IQ) and psychologic tests, completed fewer school
grades, and had an increased risk for mental hospital admissions
for certain disease categories." Epilepsy was among these
diseases.

Earlier clinical investigations have revealed an increased
prevalence of mental retardation in survivors exposed in utero to
the atomic bombs in Hiroshima and Nagasaki (Plummer, 1952; Miller,
1956; Wood, Johnson and Omori, 1967; Wood, Johnson, Omori,

515

Kawamoto, and Keehn, 1967; Miller and Blot, 1972; Blot and Miller, 1972; Blot, 1975; Miller and Mulvihill, 1976; Yamazaki, Wright and Wright, 1954). Recently, we have presented the results of a reevaluation of the prevalence of mental retardation among the latter survivors (Otake and Schull, 1983, 1984). In this analysis, a mentally retarded individual was defined as one "unable to perform simple calculations, to make simple conversation, to care for himself or herself, or if he or she was completely unmanageable or had been institutionalized" (Wood et al., 1967a, b). This definition, although clearly sociologically important, is arbitrary. It dichotomizes a continuous distribution of levels of intellection based upon the capacity to perform a series of socially significant tasks. It is obviously important, therefore, to determine whether less profound impingements on forebrain development may have occurred; whether these also exhibit critical periods of sensitivity; and lastly, whether such critical periods correlate with intrauterine events that may explain their occurrence.

MATERIALS AND METHODS

Over the years, the Atomic Bomb Casualty Commission and its successor, the Radiation Effects Research Foundation, have established several overlapping samples of individuals exposed in utero to the atomic bombings. They were chosen to serve different purposes, e.g., as the bases for clinical examinations, or mortality surveillance. These ends imposed limitations on the size of the sample and the nature of its selection. Mortality surveillance in Japan is relatively simple, inexpensive, entails no intrusion on the subject's life and followup can be readily effected wherever an individual might currently reside. Clinical examinations are, however, impracticable if an individual lives too far from the examination site; they may be intrusive, and their cost can be substantial. As earlier stated, these considerations have led to the definition of different samples at different times and as a result, there is not always a continuity of observation prior to the time of the sample selection.

Attention here is restricted to the in utero clinical sample known as the Revised PE-86 (Beebe and Usagawa, 1968; see also Otake and Schull, 1984). The latter presently numbers 1608 individuals. All were born between 6 August 1945 and 31 May 1946 (Hiroshima) or between 9 August 1945 and 31 May 1946 (Nagasaki). The manner of their identification, the followup procedures used in their study, and the like have been described in other publications (Burrow et al., 1960; Burrow et al., 1961; Wood et al., 1967a, b). Briefly, the sample is divided into three portions -- (a) a group of individuals exposed within 2000 meters of the hypocenters in Hiroshima and Nagasaki, (b) a group of individuals exposed in Hiroshima within 3000-5000 meters (in Nagasaki beyond 2,500 meters) and matched by age, city and sex to group (a), and finally, (c) a group of individuals who were not exposed to the atomic bombings and are age, city and sex matched to group (a).

Gestational age (weeks)

Gestational age within the sample is based on a special item, "the estimated days of pregnancy at the time of the bomb (ATB)," in Section 5 of the ABCC Major Medical Examination Record (CD #319, revised 18 February 1960). In this record, the days of pregnancy ATB have been determined from the first day of the last menstrual period by the following procedure:

Days of pregnancy (ATB) = 280 - (Date of birth* - 6 or 9 August 1945)

where the mean duration of pregnancy calculated in this manner is taken to be 280 days, and * denotes the date of birth obtained by interview with the individual or his or her mother, not the koseki record. To obtain the age after conception, fourteen days have been subtracted from the "days of pregnancy ATB". Age in days was changed to age in weeks by dividing by seven and the latter quotient was presumed to be zero if it was negative.

Different functions in the primate central nervous system are localized into different structures, and the differentiation of the latter takes place at different times and for different durations. These discontinuities in development provide a basis for grouping the in utero exposed. Four categories have been recognized, namely, 0-7, 8-15, 16-25 and 26 or more weeks of age (after conception) at the time of exposure. In the first, the precursors of the neurons and neuroglia are mitotically active and presumably able to replace lost cells (Martinez Martinez, 1982). In the second, a rapid increase in the number of neurons occurs; the latter migrate to their ultimate developmental sites and lose their mitotic ability. In the third, in situ differentiation accelerates, synaptogenesis that has begun about the eighth week increases and the definitive cytoarchitecture of the brain unfolds. The fourth interval is largely one of continued differentiation and growth in connectivity between cells.

Dosimetry

The revised T65 dosimetry has been used to estimate fetal absorbed doses (Milton and Shohoji, 1968; Kerr and Salomon, 1976; Kerr, 1979). Although this dosimetry is presently suspect (Kerr, 1981; Loewe and Mendelsohn, 1981), it is likely to remain for some time the only one applicable to most survivors, shielded and

517

unshielded. Elsewhere the effect of alternative estimates of tissue dose on the frequency of mental retardation has been examined (Otake and Schull, 1983); it is not large and presumably the same would obtain with respect to intelligence testing. Under any circumstance, alternative exposure estimates should not impinge upon the search for periods of maximum sensitivity; these are independent of questions of dosimetry.

The samples

Mental retardation:--Wood et al. (1967a,b) list 30 individuals, 22 in Hiroshima and 8 in Nagasaki, with mental retardation among 1608 children, 1260 in Hiroshima and 348 in Nagasaki, nonexposed and exposed in utero to the A-bombs. Nine of these children, all in Hiroshima and none mentally retarded, have been excluded because the information on the exposure of their mothers is incomplete.

Intelligence test scores:--In the years in which the individuals in the Revised PE-86 sample were in seen in the clinical facilities of the Atomic Bomb Casualty Commission two tests were in vogue in Hiroshima and Nagasaki in the assessment of intelligence -- the Tanaka-B and the Koga test. The former is a Japanese standardized version of the Stanford-Binet (Tanaka, 1947, 1975; see also Tanebashi, 1972), and the latter is a test developed by Professor Yukiyoshi Koga (Koga, 1956). The analysis is limited to the Koga Test for it involves the larger sample of tested persons. Some of these were evaluated on more than one occasion, and so to enhance comparability further, the data have been restricted to those tests performed in the months from July 1955 to May 1956, inclusive.

RESULTS

Mental retardation

The distribution of mentally retarded individuals among the in utero exposed by gestational age categories (weeks) for the cities combined is shown in Table 1. The risk of mental retardation increases with increasing dose for ages 8-15 weeks and also, but to a lesser extent, in the age group 16 weeks and over. No mentally retarded subjects were exposed at less than 8 weeks of gestational age although one was seen in the numerically much larger control group. Most of the retarded individuals are in Hiroshima (22 of 30) and were exposed at 8-15 weeks after the supposed day of conception; indeed, the relative risk for exposure at these weeks is four times that for exposure at 16 weeks or later.

Table 1. Mentally retarded individuals exposed in utero to the atomic bombings of Hiroshima and Nagasaki. The cities have been combined and the cases distributed by gestational age at exposure and fetal absorbed dose, based on the T65 revised dosimetry. The absorbed doses are based on Kerr's body shielding factors. [After Otake and Schull, 1984.]

Ages	Dose Categories (cGy)				
	< 1	1-9	10-49	50-99	100+
All gestational ages:	Cities combined				
Subjects	1085	292	169	34	19
Retarded	9	4	4	6	7
Percent	0.8	1.4	2.4	17.6	36.8
0-7 Weeks:					
Subjects	156	42	19	2	1
Retarded	1	0	0	0	0
Percent	0.6	0.0	0.0	0.0	0.0
8-15 Weeks					
Subjects	253	64	48	11	8
Retarded	1	2	3	4	5
Percent	0.4	3.1	6.3	36.4	62.5
16-25 Weeks					
Subjects	324	94	49	14	6
Retarded	3	2	1	2	1
Percent	0.9	2.1	2.0	14.3	16.7
26 Weeks or more					
Subjects	352	92	53	7	4
Retarded	4	0	0	0	1
Percent	1.1	0.0	0.0	0.0	25.0

Table 2 summarizes the statistical findings. The frequency of mental retardation increases significantly with dose for all gestational ages, for 8-15 weeks and for 16 weeks or greater. The ratio of the slope of occurrence on dose for 8-15 weeks and for 16 weeks or greater varies about four fold. Finally, the variation in occurrence in the 8th through the 15th week is largely accounted for by a linear model. Evidence for a relationship between exposure and mental retardation in the other age groups is weak, particularly after the 25th week of conception. Perusal of the observations themselves discloses very few cases at fetal absorbed doses of less than 50 rad.

Table 2. The relationship of mental retardation to absorbed fetal dose. [Abridged from Otake and Schull, 1984, Table II.]

| Gestational Age | Cities Combined | | | | | |
	a	b	s_b	Reg.	Res.	P_{Res}
All gestational ages	0.476	0.212	0.030	49.94*	5.97	0.11
8-15 weeks	0.779	0.393	0.039	101.54*	1.18	0.76
16 weeks or more	0.665	0.107	0.022	23.56*	2.06	0.56
Relationship of mental retardation to dose: 'controls' excluded						
8-15 weeks	0.177	0.400	0.055	52.89*	1.53	0.47
16 weeks or more	-0.116	0.119	0.026	20.95*	3.78	0.15
Relationship of mental retardation to dose: 'controls' combined						
Pooled control	0.749	0.416	0.040	108.16*	1.26	0.54

The chi-square for regression (Reg) has one degree of freedom; the chi-square for the residual (Res) has three or two degrees of freedom; the P value is the probability (two tailed) of exceeding the residual chi-square by chance under the null hypothesis. a is the estimated number (intercept) of cases of mental retardation (per 100 individuals) in the zero dose group; b is the increase in the frequency of mental retardation with dose expressed in grays (100 rad) and s_b is its standard error.

* Significant at the 1% level.

To assess the internal consistency of the data, regressions were fitted after the removal of the zero dose group. Within the period of maximum sensitivity, 8-15 weeks after conception, the regression coefficient does not change much and the values predicted from the latter coefficient do not differ significantly from the frequencies actually observed (see Table 2). Since the frequency of mental retardation does not vary with gestational age in the various zero dose groups, the "control" data have been pooled and a new regression fitted to dose within the sensitive period. Again, this pooling (see Table 2) does little to change the regression coefficient.

Three observations could compromise these assertions. First, some of the mentally retarded have health problems, presumably nonradiation related, which could account for their status; second, there are other mentally retarded individuals among the in utero exposed outside the study population; and third, there is an apparent difference between Hiroshima and Nagasaki in the frequency of radiation-related mental retardation. Their impact has been examined elsewhere (Otake and Schull, 1983), and will only be summarized here. Exclusion of individuals with health problems that could conceivably account for their mental retardation does not alter the findings appreciably.

Some 601 children (428 in Hiroshima and 173 in Nagasaki) were exposed in utero at 2000-2999 meters (Burrow, Hrubec and Hamilton, 1960). Of these approximately 190 (145 in Hiroshima; 45 in Nagasaki) were under 16 weeks of gestation ATB. At the distances these individuals were exposed, their doses would place them in the less than one rad group and thus in the "control." The inclusion of the mentally retarded among these 601 could diminish the sampling error associated with the observed value. These individuals have not, however, been systematically studied clinically and it is not clear exactly how many are mentally retarded. A variety of lines of reasoning suggest that the frequency of mental retardation is not different from that found in the present "control" group.

Finally, there is the inter-city difference. Here, comparison of the "control" groups in Nagasaki with those in Hiroshima failed to reveal a statistically significant difference. A significant difference between the cities does exist, however, in the proportion of survivors exposed in the most critical gestational period, i.e., 8-15 weeks. Only 23 individuals of the 348 in the in utero cohort in Nagasaki were exposed at these weeks of development and 16 received absorbed doses of less than 50 rad.

Intelligence test scores

Table 3 identifies the relationship of individuals within the Revised PE-86 sample on whom intelligence test data are available with the members of the same sample studied clinically. The largest discrepancy involves the "control" many of whom, particularly in Hiroshima, were not identified until after collection of the intelligence test data had stopped. Presumably data were available on many, but not collected for they were not a part of the sample at that time.

Table 3. An accounting of the number of rejected observations and the cause of the rejection among the individuals who comprise the clinical, that is, the PE-86 sample.

	Hiroshima	Nagasaki	Total
Total individuals in sample	1260	348	1608
Unknown exposure	9	0	9
Subjects selected after 1959* (no test data collected)	521	32	553
Potentially available for analysis	726	316	1042
No test data found	66	2	68
Used in the analysis	660	314	974

* Among these individuals, in Hiroshima, are 194 exposed within 2000 meters, 327 exposed at distances of 3000 meters or more, and 34 not exposed; in Nagasaki, the comparable figures are 2, 25 and 4.

Four questions have been addressed. First, within an age group, do the test scores appear to be drawn from more than one population: that is to say, is there evidence of inhomogeneity? Second, do the means (or variances) of the distribution of test scores differ significantly and systematically between exposure categories in the different age groups? Third, do individual exposures within an age group 'explain' a significant amount of test score variation? Finally, if so, what is the form of the dose-response relationship?

Heterogeneity within age groups

To address the issue of a mixed distribution of individuals, the result of a bimodality of effects, the skew of each distribution of test scores has been examined within age and age-exposure groups using Fisher's estimate (1950) and the cumulative distribution plotted to search for inflections that might suggest a bimodality. Of the sixteen measures of skew in the age-exposure cells in Table 4a seven are positive, seven are negative

Table 4a. Mean intelligence score (Koga) by fetal or embryonic
age at exposure and tissue absorbed dose for those individuals
within the clinical, the Revised PE-86 sample based upon the T65DR
estimate of tissue kerma and Kerr's 1979 organ dose estimates.
Individuals diagnosed as mentally retarded clinically are
included.

Dose category (cGy)		Age in weeks after conception				
		0-7	8-15	16-25	26+	Total
less than one	N	120	151	203	203	677
	mean	107.3	107.6	111.3	108.6	109.0
	st.d.	13.70	13.86	15.46	15.82	14.98
1-9	N	17	32	53	48	150
	mean	101.8	111.2	105.2	101.3	104.9
	st.d.	15.20	14.06	17.61	15.07	16.11
10-99	N	18	39	41	37	135
	mean	107.8	98.6	104.2	105.5	103.4
	st.d.	15.42	19.73	17.35	15.91	17.58
100+	N	2	5	2	3	12
	mean	95.0	82.6	71.5	108.0	89.2
	st.d.	42.43	16.52	16.26	8.89	21.92
All	N	157	227	299	291	974
	mean	106.6	106.0	109.0	107.0	107.3
	st.d.	14.46	15.87	16.62	15.83	15.89

Significance of the differences among dose means within an age
group

Age group	F (df1,df2)	Sign.
0-7	1.192 (3,153)	n.s.
8-15	8.910 (3,223)	.001
16-25	7.115 (3,295)	.03
26+	2.967 (3,287)	.01
All	11.889 (3,970)	.001

Table 4b. Mean intelligence score (Koga) by fetal or embryonic
age at exposure and tissue absorbed dose for those individuals
within the clinical, the Revised PE-86 sample based upon the T65DR
estimate of tissue kerma and Kerr's 1979 organ dose estimates.
Individuals diagnosed as mentally retarded clinically are
excluded.

Dose category (cGy)		Age in weeks after conception				
		0-7	8-15	16-25	26+	Total
less than one	N	120	150	203	202	675
	mean	107.3	107.9	111.3	108.9	109.1
	st.d.	13.70	13.24	15.46	15.48	14.74
1-9	N	17	32	53	48	150
	mean	101.8	111.2	105.2	101.3	104.9
	st.d.	15.20	14.06	17.61	15.07	16.11
10-99	N	18	37	39	37	131
	mean	107.8	100.7	106.4	105.5	104.7
	st.d.	15.42	17.96	14.68	15.91	16.14
100+	N	2	4	1	3	10
	mean	95.0	87.8	83.0	108.0	94.8
	st.d.	42.43	13.67	-	8.89	19.38
All	N	157	223	296	290	966
	mean	106.6	106.8	109.5	107.2	107.7
	st.d.	14.46	14.71	15.98	15.62	15.36

Significance of the difference among dose means within an age
group

Age group	F (df1,df2)	Sign.
0-7	1.192 (3,153)	n.s.
8-15	5.954 (3,219)	.001
16-25	4.376 (2,293)	.01
26+	3.282 (3,286)	.02
All	7.731 (3,962)	.001

and two are zero. They range from -0.790 to 0.755 and none
deviate significantly from zero at the one percent level.
Insofar as the marginal cells are concerned, skew is significant
in one instance, i.e., within the 8-15 week age group (4%). It is
negative. When the clinically diagnosed mentally retarded are
excluded (Table 4b), the 8-15 week group is no longer significant.
Skew remains negative in the age group 8-15 weeks but is
substantially reduced, from -0.342 to -0.216. Measured in terms
of a normal deviate this is a fall from 2.02 to 1.66.

The cumulative age-group specific probability distributions
differ little, if at all from that expected of a homogeneous
sample from a normal distribution (data not shown). This suggests
that the significant changes described reflect a general
phenomenon, a shift in the distribution of scores with exposure,
rather than the inclusion of a qualitatively different group of
individuals, possibly, unrecognized cases of mental retardation.

Means and variances

Tables 4a and b present estimates of mean test scores (and
standard deviations) for the same four categories of embryonic or
fetal age used in the analysis of the clinical data, namely, 0-7,
8-15, 16-25 and 26 weeks or more, and four of exposure -- less
than 1, 1-9, 10-99, and 100 cGy or more. Table 4a includes data
on those eight mentally retarded children (5 in Hiroshima; 3 in
Nagasaki) who were clinically examined in the year in which the
tests occurred; Table 4b does not. These eight children, whose
diagnoses of mental retardation were made without reference to the
intelligence tests, had scores that ranged from 56 to 64 and of
the eight, two had estimated exposures of 1 Gray or more and four
exposures of 0.10 through 0.99 Gray. Their presence has an
important effect on the mean scores among the individuals of all
gestational ages with exposures of 0.1 Gray or more, and it is for
this reason they have been excluded from one of the analyses to
ascertain whether a more pervasive effect on intellection exists.

The exposure means within an embryonic or fetal age group are
significantly different for the age groups 8-15, 16-25 and 26+
weeks; the latter two are less strikingly heterogeneous than the
first (see Table 4a). At the sex and city levels (data not
shown), males are different only in the age group 8-15 weeks (1%
level), and females in the group 16-25 weeks (1%). Within cities
(sexes pooled), all four age groups are significantly
heterogeneous among dose categories in Hiroshima [0-7 weeks (7%);
8-15 (1%); 16-25 (2%); 26+ (5%)] but in Nagasaki the only
significant difference involves doses within 0-7 weeks (8%), 8-15
(1%), and 16-25 (1%). These further subdivisions make the
individual sample sizes smaller, of course, and thus the possible
distorting effect of the clinically mentally retarded greater.

Table 4b exhibits the same age-dose means when the eight clinically diagnosed, mentally retarded children are excluded. Note that the only age groups that are significantly heterogeneous are the ages 8-15 (0.1%), 16-25 (2%) and 26+ (5%).

Examination of the homogeneity of the variances among age-groups for fixed exposure categories fails to reveal significant differences in any of the four dose categories with or without inclusion of the eight retarded individuals previously described. When the variances were examined among exposure categories for fixed ages, chi-squares (Bartlett's Test; 3 df) of 5.65, 8.70, 1.79 and 1.04 were obtained for 0-7, 8-15, 16-25 and 26+ weeks, respectively. Of these chi-squares only the one for 8-15 weeks is significant, and then only at the 0.03 level. Removal of the mentally retarded reduces this chi-square to 5.82 which is no longer significant. Thus, no compelling evidence emerges that the variances are different either among doses for fixed age, or among ages for fixed doses.

Regression analysis

A better method of analysis than that previously described, one that does not depend upon grouped data, is to fit a regression of test scores on the individual estimates of exposure within an age group. This has been done with and without inclusion of the clinically diagnosed cases of mental retardation. Table 5 presents the regression coefficients obtained when a linear dose-response model is fitted; the latter removes significant variability among individuals within the age groups 8-15, and 16-25. Significant heterogeneity does exist among the four regression coefficients although all are negative. When the eight clinically diagnosed cases of mental retardation are removed, two of the four regression coefficients differ significantly from zero; these are associated with the 8-15 and the 16-25 week age groups. The four coefficients continue to be significantly heterogeneous. The loss in IQ appears substantial -- 7 to 10 points for the 8-15 week group and 13 to 21 for the 16-25 week group per Gray of absorbed energy.

Table 6 gives the results of fitting a linear-quadratic model to these data. One or both regression coefficients are significantly different from zero only for the age group 8-15; this holds true whether the mentally retarded are or are not included. Moreover, within the four groups, it is only the age group 8-15 where the quadratic term is significantly different from zero. Both the linear and the quadratic terms are statistically heterogeneous but the quadratic terms are the more so. As we have seen, evidence of a radiation-related effect on mental retardation is confined to two age groups, 8-15 and 16-25 weeks; in this instance, the effect appears to be linear within the ages 8-15 and non-linear in the weeks 16-25 (Otake and Schull, 1984).

Table 5. The regression coefficients obtained when a linear model of test score on individual tissue absorbed dose is fitted to the data available on individuals within the clinical, the Revised PE-86 sample. The coefficients are expressed as change in IQ points per cGy of exposure.

Age Group (weeks)	Regression coefficient	Error of the coefficient	Significance	
a. All cases included:				
0-7	-0.0645	0.0598	1.16	n.s.
8-15	-0.0952	0.0259	13.51	.001
16-25	-0.2123	0.0437	23.60	.001
26+	-0.0373	0.0599	0.39	n.s.
All	-0.1114	0.0198	31.65	.001

Heterogeneity Chi Square = 46.25   df = 3   P < 0.001

b. After exclusion of clinically diagnosed cases of retardation				
0-7	-0.0645	0.0598	1.16	n.s.
8-15	-0.0692	0.0252	7.54	.01
16-25	-0.1387	0.0546	6.45	.01
26+	-0.0408	0.0590	0.48	n.s.
All	-0.0762	0.0206	13.68	.001

Heterogeneity Chi Square = 12.60   df = 3   P < 0.001

DISCUSSION

At least four sources of extraneous variation, possibly confounded here, could impinge on the findings we have described. These include (a) genetic variation, (b) nutrition, (c) bacterial and viral infections in the course of pregnancy, and lastly, since there is substantial evidence to suggest that the cerebrum and its adnexa are especially sensitive to oxygen deprivation, (d) an hypoxemia secondary to radiation damage to the haematopoietic systems of the mother and (or) her developing child. Assessment of the contribution each of these potential confounders made is formidable, for there is little direct evidence pertinent to any of these possibilities.

Table 6. The regression coefficients obtained when a linear-quadratic model of test score on individual tissue absorbed dose is fitted to the data available on the clinical, the Revised PE-86 sample. The coefficients are expressed as change in IQ points per cGy of exposure.

Age group (weeks)	Regression estimates					
	Linear coefficient	Standard error	P	Quadratic coefficient	Standard error	P

a. All cases included:

0-7	-0.1169	0.1636	n.s.	0.00045	0.00131	n.s.
8-15	-0.3407	0.0575	.001	0.00079	0.00017	.001
16-25	-0.1460	0.0903	n.s.	-0.00057	0.00068	n.s.
26+	-0.1262	0.1389	n.s.	0.00097	0.00137	n.s.
All	-0.2158	0.0349	.001	0.00046	0.00013	.001

Heterogeneity chi squares:

$31.43 \quad df = 3 \quad P < 0.001 \qquad 88.08 \quad df = 3 \quad P < 0.001$

b. After exclusion of clinically diagnosed cases of retardation

0-7	-0.1169	0.1636	n.s.	0.00045	0.00131	n.s.
8-15	-0.2676	0.0610	.001	0.00061	0.00017	.001
16-25	-0.0731	0.1292	n.s.	-0.00083	0.00148	n.s.
26+	-0.1363	0.1370	n.s.	0.00110	0.00140	n.s.
All	-0.1538	0.0364	.001	0.00033	0.00013	.01

Heterogeneity chi squares:

$15.95 \quad df = 3 \quad P < 0.001 \qquad 124.76 \quad df = 3 \quad P < 0.001$

Numerous genetic forms of mental retardation are known (McKusick, 1983). Most are recessively inherited and infrequent but collectively they have a significant impact on the frequency of this disorder. Rare, recessively inherited disorders are functionally related to the frequency of consanguineous marriages and at the time these survivors were conceived, such marriages were common in Hiroshima and Nagasaki, but especially so in the latter (Schull and Neel, 1965). This could explain the observed difference in the 'control' frequency of mental retardation in the two cities. Can genetic variation account for the apparent decline in intelligence test score with exposure? This depends upon a number of circumstances. Are the individuals heterozygous for the genes in question more vulnerable to environmental insults including ionizing radiation? Are such individuals non-randomly distributed with regard to distance from the hypocenter? The latter is possible in Nagasaki where the frequency of consanguineous marriages is inversely related to distance from the hypocenter within those distances where exposures of 10 cGy or more occurred (Schull, 1958). Here the frequency of heterozygotes could be roughly proportional to distance and dose could confound genetic variation. What form this might take is debatable. To recapitulate, genetic differences could account for some, possibly much of the intercity difference in the frequency of mental retardation but whether they contribute importantly to the shape of the dose-response curve in either city or in the various age groups is debatable.

The role of maternal malnutrition on the subsequent mental performance of the fetus is controversial, and evidence of the possible interaction of such malnutrition with radiation damage virtually non-existent. Some data show that maternal malnutrition may affect mental growth by decreasing DNA content or cell number (Winick, 1976, 1979; see also Rozovski and Winick, 1979). Marasmic infants of normal birthweight tend not to show these effects. The Dutch famine study (Stein et al., 1974), too, failed, in a previously well-nourished population, to show an effect of famine on mental retardation although social class distinctions were still clearly visible.

If the mental impairment stems largely from effects on neuronal number or migration, it seems unlikely that maternal malnutrition would restrict fetal growth as markedly in the second trimester as in the later, less protected, stages of gestation. Moreover, if, as Dobbing and Sands (1973; Dobbing, 1974) observe, malnutrition mostly interferes with the growth and establishment of neuronal connectivity, the effects of malnutrition will be largely postnatal since this phase of brain growth is predominantly postnatal. Special ration provisions were made in Japan in the war and in the postwar years for pregnant and recently parturient women. The fact of pregnancy could be registered at or subsequent to the 20th week of gestation and upon registration supplementary rations were made available. Every pregnant woman may not have availed herself of this opportunity, but evidence based upon the registration of pregnancies in these cities in the years 1948-1954 suggests that almost all did (Neel and Schull, 1956). Whether these supplementary rations were adequate to forestall fetal damage is unclear, for supplementation was based upon prevailing concepts of health needs and Japan's economic condition. There is, however, no report of underweight, marasmic infants (Committee, 1981). These were exceptional times and exceptional circumstances but whether a nutritional dependence, if indeed one existed, affected the dose-response other than additively is moot.

As earlier noted, there are other possible confounders including bacterial and viral infections, and an hypoxemia secondary to radiation damage to the haematopoietic systems of the mother and (or) her developing child. Mothers whose embryos or fetuses received absorbed doses of 0.5 Gray or more must have received 1 Gray or more themselves and experienced some degree of acute radiation illness. One possible consequence of the latter is an haematopoietic depression that sets in six weeks or so after exposure and persists for some time before a recovery occurs, if, of, course, the individual survives. Red blood cell counts fall to fifty or sixty percent of the normal value and haemoglobin values to 6-8 grams (see Committee, 1981, Figure 8.12). Whether this would give rise to a fetal hypoxemia is uncertain. Since the fall in red cells and haemoglobin is a gradual one, some form of cardiac or ventilatory compensation could occur. Moreover, women with sickle cell anemia who commonly have haemoglobin values in the range described above do not have an increased frequency of mentally retarded children. It can be argued too that even if an hypoxemia occurred it would have been only at higher maternal exposures, and should, therefore, contribute to a non-linear dose-response relationship. Studies of primates exposed in utero reveal that the Macaca mulatta fetus undergoes a haematopoietic depression at an exposure of 2 Gray or so (Ozzello and Rugh, 1965; Rugh et al., 1966). It seems probable, therefore, that among the in utero exposed in Hiroshima and Nagasaki who received 0.5 Gray or more some experienced a haematopoietic depression because of damage to their own bone marrow. Any hypoxemia that might result from direct damage to the fetus would appear inextricably confounded with a possible maternal effect. However, this again should enhance the likelihood of a non-linear effect.

Finally, there are the issues of sample bias and fortuity. Insofar as the former is concerned, it is reasonable to assume that those children who were not seen in the clinical facilities were, on average, more retarded than those who were; however, the decision to enroll a child involves sociologic judgments too and the fear of stigmatization may impinge on the enrollment of a child who might be able to perform, albeit at a subnormal level. This suggests that social values could prompt an underestimation of the biologic effects. Fortuity is another matter. Conventional statistical inference specifies the frequency of the so-called type I error -- the erroneous rejection of the hypothesis of no effect when, in fact, no effect occurred. This inferential basis fails, however, to incorporate prior knowledge, often unquantifiable but none the less real, that may suggest an effect. Only further evidence will resolve this issue.

Are the results biologically reasonable?

An answer to this question hinges ultimately upon an understanding of the molecular and cellular events that give rise to impaired intellectual performance and the identification of causes other than exposure to ionizing radiation that could be inadvertently confounded. Presently, too little is known to provide a compelling molecular and cellular model for radiation-related damage to the central nervous system. Individual conviction turns, then, on the ability to rule out other possible causal mechanisms. As we have attempted to indicate in the preceding paragraphs, this is difficultu to do. However, the correspondence in the findings for mental retardation and intellection generally strengthens the belief that the results are real, and not ascribable to fortuity, but this correspondence does not remove doubt as to the causal mechanism. Proof, if attainable, must come either from research on non-human primates, or through the accumulation of further evidence on sensitive periods and their relationship to exposure to ionizing radiation within this subset of survivors.

SUMMARY

Analysis of the occurrence of mental retardation and (or) intelligence test scores on individuals exposed in utero to the atomic bombings of Hiroshima and Nagasaki revealed the following: First, neither tests of skew nor graphical representation of the data suggest a commingling of distributions such as might arise through the inadvertent inclusion of a qualitatively different group of individuals, that is unrecognized cases of mental retardation. Indeed, the cumulative distribution suggests a general phenomenon, a shift in the distribution of scores with exposure. Second, there is no evidence of a radiation-related effect on mental retardation or intellection generally for those individuals exposed in the first eight weeks of life. Third, the mean test scores but not the variances are consistently significantly heterogeneous among exposure categories for those individuals exposed at 8-15 weeks after conception, and less heterogeneous for those groups exposed at 16-25, or 26 or more weeks of age. Fourth, regression analyses indicate that among those in utero individuals exposed either at 8-15 or 16-25 weeks of gestational age a significant decrease in intelligence test score occurs with increasing exposure. This obtains whether the eight clinically diagnosed cases of mental retardation to which allusion has been made are or are not included. However, the shape of the dose-response curves appears different; it is linear-

531

quadratic for the 8-15 week group and linear for the 16-25 week group. This is the opposite of the findings with respect to clinically diagnosed mental retardation in the Revised PE-86 sample. Finally, <u>fifth</u>, within the most sensitive group, that is, individuals exposed 8 to 15 weeks after conception, and with the better fitting model, the linear-quadratic, the diminution in intelligence score is 21-26 points per Gray of exposure, or about 0.2 points per cGy.

ACKNOWLEDGMENTS

This is one of a series of reports of a study conducted originally by the Atomic Bomb Casualty Commission (ABCC) in cooperation with the Japanese National Institute of Health of the Ministry of Health and Welfare (JNIH), and presently pursued by the successor to ABCC, the Radiation Effects Research Foundation (RERF). The ABCC was a research agency of the U.S. National Academy of Sciences-National Research Council and was supported by Contract AT-49-1-GEN-72 of the U.S. Atomic Energy Commission. The study is presently funded by the Japanese Ministry of Health and Welfare and by the National Academy of Sciences-National Research Council with support from Contract Ex-76-C-28-3161 from the Department of Energy.

REFERENCES

Anderson, A. M., 1982, The great Japanese IQ increase, <u>Nature</u>, 297:180.

Beebe, G. W. and Usagawa, M., 1968, The Major ABCC Samples, <u>Atomic Bomb Casualty Commission Technical Report</u>, 12-68.

Blot, W. J., 1975, Review of thirty years study of Hiroshima and Nagasaki atomic bomb survivors. II. Biological effects. C. Growth and development following prenatal and childhood exposure to atomic radiation, <u>J Radiat Res</u>, 16(Suppl):82.

Blot, W. J. and Miller, R. W., 1973, Mental retardation following in utero exposure to the atomic bombs of Hiroshima and Nagasaki, <u>Radiology</u>, 106:617.

Burrow, G. N., Hrubec, Z., and Finch, S. C., 1961, Background and status of clinical study to determine effects of in utero exposure, Hiroshima and Nagasaki, <u>Atomic Bomb Casualty Commission Technical Report</u>, 17-61.

Burrow, G. N., Hrubec, Z. and Hamilton, H. B., 1960,   Study of adolescents exposed in utero: Research plan, Atomic Bomb Casualty Commission Technical Report, 16-60.

Committee for the Compilation of Materials on Damage Caused by the Atomic Bombs in Hiroshima and Nagasaki, 1981, "Hiroshima and Nagasaki.   The Physical, Medical and Social Effects of the Atomic Bombings," Iwanami Shoten Publishers, Tokyo.

Dobbing, J., 1974,   The later development of the brain and its vulnerability, in, "Scientific Foundations of Pediatrics," J. A. Davis and J. Dobbing, ed, William Heinemann Medical Books, London.

Dobbing, J. and Sands, J., 1973,   Quantitative growth and development of human brain, Arch Dis Child, 48:757.

Fisher, R. A., 1950,   "Statistical Methods for Research Workers," 11th Edition, Oliver and Boyd, Edinburgh.

Hochberg, F. H. and Slotnick, B., 1980,   Neuropsychologic impairment in astrocytoma survivors, Neurology, 30:172.

Kerr, G. D., 1979,   Organ dose estimates for the Japanese atomic bomb survivors, Health Physics, 37:487.

Kerr, G. D., 1981,   Review of the dosimetry for the atomic bomb survivors, in, "Proceedings of the Fourth Symposium on Neutron Dosimetry, Gesellschaft fur Strahlen-und Umweltforschung, Munich-Neuherberg, June 1-5, 1981," Vol. 1, Office for Official Publications of the European Communities, Luxemburg.

Kerr, G. D. and Salomon, D. K., 1976,   The epicenter of Nagasaki weapon: A reanalysis of available data with recommended values, Oak Ridge National Laboratories,   ORNL-TM-5139.

Koga, Y., 1937,   Two intelligence test methods viewed in relation to evaluated intelligence. Collection of Reports in Commemoration of Dr. Matsumoto, Studies in Psychology and Arts, pp. 923-988. (In Japanese)

Koga, Y., 1956,   Some considerations of intelligence quotients, J Kurume Med Assoc, 19(1):117.

Loewe, W. E. and Mendelsohn, E., 1981,   Neutron and gamma doses at Hiroshima and Nagasaki, Lawrence Livermore Laboratory Publ, UCRL-86595.

Lynn, R., 1982, IQ in Japan and the United States shows a growing disparity, Nature, 297:222.

Martinez Martinez, P. F. A., 1982, "Neuroanatomy: Development and Structure of the Central Nervous System," W. B. Saunders, Philadelphia.

McKusick, V. A., 1983, "Mendelian Inheritance in Man: Catalogs of Autosomal Recessive, Autosomal Dominant and X-linked Phenotypes," The Johns Hopkins University Press, Baltimore.

Meadows, A. T., Gordon, J., Massari, D. J., Littman, P., Fergusson, J., and Moss, K., 1981, Declines in IQ scores and cognitive dysfunctions in children with acute lymphocytic leukaemia treated with cranial irradiation, Lancet, ii:1015.

Miller, R. W., 1956, Delayed effects occurring within the first decade after exposure of young individuals to the Hiroshima atomic bomb, Pediatrics, 18:1.

Miller, R. W. and Blot, W. J., 1972, Small head size after in utero exposure to atomic radiation, Lancet, ii:784.

Miller, R. W., and Mulvihill, J. J., 1976, Small head size after atomic irradiation, Teratology, 14:355.

Milton, R. C., and Shohoji, T., 1968, Tentative 1965 radiation dose estimation for atomic bomb survivors, Hiroshima and Nagasaki, Atomic Bomb Casualty Commission Technical Report, 1-68.

Neel, J. V. and Schull, W. J., 1956, "The Effect of Exposure to the Atomic Bombs on Pregnancy Termination in Hiroshima and Nagasaki," National Academy of Sciences Publ. No. 461, Washington, D. C.

Otake, M. and Schull, W. J., 1983, Mental retardation in children exposed in utero to the atomic bombs: A reassessment, Radiation Effects Research Foundation Technical Report, 1-83.

Otake, M. and Schull, W. J., 1984, "In utero exposure to A-bomb radiation and mental retardation: a reassessment, Brit J Rad, 57:409.

Ozzello, L. and Rugh, R., 1965, Acute pathological alterations in x-irradiated primate fetuses, Am J Roent Rad Ther Nucl Med, 93:209.

534

Plummer, G., 1952, Anomalies occurring in children exposed in utero to the atomic bomb in Hiroshima, Pediatrics, 10:687.

Raimondi, A. J. and Tomita, T., 1979, The advantages of total resection of medulloblastoma and disadvantages of full head post-operative radiation therapy, Childs Brain, 5:550.

Rakic, P., 1978, Neuronal migration and contact guidance in the primate telencephalon, Postgrad Med J, 54 (Suppl) 1:25.

Ron, E., Modan, B., Floro, S., Harkedar, I., and Gurewitz, R., 1982, Mental function following scalp irradiation during childhood, Am J Epidemiol, 116:149.

Rozovski, S. J., and Winick, M., 1979, Nutrition and cellular growth, in, "Nutrition: Pre and Postnatal Development," Plenum Press, New York.

Rugh, R., Duhamel, L., Skaredoff, L., and Somogyi, C., 1966, Gross sequellae of fetal x-irradiation of the monkey (Macaca mulatta). Effect on body and organ weights at 23 months, Atompraxix, 9:468.

Schull, W. J., 1958, A note on consanguineous marriages in the cities of Hiroshima and Nagasaki, Jap J Hum Genet, 3:33.

Schull, W. J. and Neel, J. V., 1965, "The effect of inbreeding on Japanese children," Harper and Row, New York.

Schull, W. J. and Otake, M., 1984, Intellection and in utero exposure to ionizing radiation, (Manuscript).

Sidman, R. L., and Rakic, P., 1982, Development of the human central nervous system, in, "Histology and Histopathology of the Nervous System," W. Haymaker and R. D. Adams, eds, C. C. Thomas, Springfield, Ill.

Stein, Z., Susser, M., Saenger, G., Marolla, F., 1974, "Famine and Human Development: The Dutch Hunger Winter 1944-1945," Oxford University Press, Oxford, England.

Tanaka, K., 1947, "Intelligence examination method of the Tanaka B test," Sekaisha, Tokyo. (In Japanese)

Tanaka, K., 1975, "Tanaka-Binet Intelligence Test," 29th Edition, Bunka Kagaku-sha, Tokyo. (In Japanese)

Tanebashi, M., 1972, Intelligence and Intelligence Tests, in, "Outline of Educational Psychology," 20th Edition, Tokyo.

Winick, M., 1976, "Malnutrition and Brain Development," Oxford University Press, New York.

Winick, M., 1979, Malnutrition and mental development, in, "Nutrition: Pre and Postnatal Development," Plenum Press, New York.

Wood, J. W., Johnson, K. G., Omori, Y., 1967, In utero exposure to the Hiroshima atomic bomb: Follow-up at 20 years, Pediatrics 39:385.

Wood, J. W., Johnson, K. G., Omori, Y., Kawamoto, S., and Keehn, R. J., 1967, Mental retardation in children exposed in utero to the atomic bomb in Hiroshima and Nagasaki, Amer J Public Health, 57:1381.

Yamazaki, J. N., Wright, S. W., Wright, P. M., 1954, Outcome of pregnancy in women exposed to the atomic bomb in Nagasaki, Am J Dis Child, 87:448.

UNANSWERED ISSUES IN LOW-LEVEL CHEMICAL POLLUTION: THE CASE OF DI-
OXINS AND RELATED COMPOUNDS

Paolo Bruzzi*, Paola Strigini*
Roberto Raschetti** and Luigi Bisanti**
*Department of Epidmiology, Instituto Nazionale per la
Ricera sul Cancro
Genova, Italy
**Department of Epidemiology, Instituto Superiore di Sanita,
Roma, Italy

INTRODUCTION

Over the last few decades, there has been increasing awareness
of the potential dangers associated with the introduction in the environment of new chemical substances, whose effects on man were poorly known. While chemical hazards for man are generally recognized
through animal experimentation, extrapolation from the latter is
often debatable and does not provide estimates of the actual risk
posed by chemicals to human populations. Furthermore, results from
animal experimentation may be missing, questionable or misleading:
the Thalidomide story[1] is considered an example of the limitations inherent in non-human testing systems for predicting adverse
health effects in man. As a consequence, epidemiological studies
have been regarded as the most reliable way of monitoring the effects
of environmental agents in order to detect and ban hazardous substances.

Their role, however, has been largely overstated: various kinds
of drawbacks, which are related to their observational nature, severely affect their ability to investigate the association between
environmental agents and diseases. Furthermore, massive chemical exposure in man is often linked to accidents, whose circumstances affect both the feasibility of epidemiologic studies and the behavioral biases to be taken into account.

Dioxins provide a good example of the limitations of the traditional epidemiological approach when applied to the study of the health effects of low-level environmental pollutants, particularly when these effects are neither acute nor specific. The objective of this discussion is to review the methodology of the studies of adverse pregnancy outcomes in the TCDD-polluted area of Seveso, Italy, in order to illustrate some of these limitations.

DIOXINS

Dioxins are extremely toxic substances at very low doses, and major concern was raised among the scientists and the public by the demonstration of their ability to cause cancer and congenital malformations in laboratory animals. (For extensive reviews see[2,3,4]). During the last decade, improvements in measurement techniques have made it possible to detect their presence in various occupational and environmental settings, usually as a consequence of industrial accidents or careless disposal of industrial wastes. Publication of many such reports and also of experimental TCDD studies has been fostered by the wide publicity given to the Seveso accident[5]. Yet, despite the number of instances in which human exposure to measurable amounts of these substances has taken place, and the efforts devoted to the study of the effects of such exposures, it has not been possible to clearly establish whether and under which exposure conditions, dioxins can cause cancer and/or congenital anomalies in man. As far as TCDD teratogenicity is concerned, the evidence from animal studies is solid. The defects which are found following administration during pregnancy vary depending on the species, and include cleft palate, renal and skeletal anomalies; embryolethality and growth retardation are also frequently observed. All these effects are seen at very low doses[6]. The evidence concerning human exposure is scanty, and based on studies which suffer from serious methodological flaws, which undermine the significance of their results. Among these are the studies of adverse pregnancy outcomes after the Seveso accident, which is one of the few instances in which exposure to TCDD of women in fertile age has taken place and has been extensively studied.

THE SEVESO ACCIDENT

The accident which took place in Seveso more than 8 years ago, has become one of the most cited examples of the dangers of industrialization and chemical pollution. Unfortunately, it became also an epidemiological nightmare, both for those who were directly involved in the subsequent studies, including the authors of the present review, and for those who try to draw some indication from the large amount of information accumulated in those studies, which, for various reasons, is still largely unpublished.

The accident occurred on July 10, 1976, in a chemical plant near Seveso, 15 miles from Milan, Italy, and has been already thoroughly described and discussed[7,8,9]. As a consequence of the accident, a toxic cloud containing several chemicals including 2,3,7,8,tetrachloro-di benzo-p-dioxin, and its isomers, spread over a wide, densely populated area: both the amount of TCDD which was produced in the accident and the quantity released through the safety valve into the atmosphere have been the subject of endless and unsettled arguments, projections ranging from few grams to several kilograms. The amount released in the environment has been estimated from 100 to 300 grams[10]. The patterns and the amount of pollution were assessed during the following weeks and months through systematic sampling and analysis of the soil, starting from the plant and proceeding in every direction as long as measurable amounts of TCDD were found. Three areas at decreasing level of pollution, referred to as A, B and R zones, were defined on the basis of this survey. Note that sampling density, hence reliability of the averages, decreases from zone A to zone R. The analytical results that contributed to the definition of the polluted zones are shown in table 1. The same table presents the size and the population of each zone. Most of the epidemiological studies encompassed a much larger reference area (S zone in tab.1), including 11 towns (3 Health Districts).

Table 1. Official Contamination Zones[11]

Zone	Population	Area (HA)	TCDD (mcg/m^3)			
			Mean	Max. Value	per cent neg. values	N° samples
Zone A	670	80	192.2	5.444	3.9	306
Zone B	4.855	269	3.0	43.8	24.5	106
Zone R	32.481	1.430	0.9	9.7	68.6	449
S	183.995	7.474	—	—	—	—
Total	222.001	9.381				

Within few days of the accident, vegetation, birds, courtyard animals had been seriously affected, and burn-like lesions had appeared on the exposed parts of the skin among inhabitants of the area. A chronic skin affection resembling juvenile acne which is quite specifically associated with exposure to halogenated compounds and therefore referred to as chloracne, was diagnosed mostly during the following year in several hundred individuals, partly because of spontaneous referral, partly through school screenings. A diagnosis of chloracne attributable to the accident was finally confirmed in 193 cases, mainly children.

While the heavily polluted A zone was evacuated and fenced off within 15-20 days of the accident, populations living in B and R zones were put under hygienic restrictions, such as that of avoiding locally grown vegetables, while all animals which were bred in the polluted area were sacrificed.

TCDD teratogenicity in laboratory animals was already known at that time, and the fear that pregnant women in the area could deliver defective children was widespread. In fact several pregnant women sought abortion (which was illegal at that time), and presumably many others avoided pregnancy. Several of these have been reported as spontaneous abortions.

In the aftermath of the accident, the local health services were overwhelmed by people seeking medical care or reassurance, and it took more than a year before any systematic research effort became possible.

SEVESO BIRTH DEFECTS REGISTRY (SBDR)

Birth defects reporting, in Italy and elsewhere, has always been quite erratic and unreliable. Birth defects are known to occur in 2-3% of all births, but in the area of Seveso, up to 1976, the number of congenital anomalies reported to the Health Authorities was 20 to 50 times below these figures (tab. 2). Thus, failure to detect an increase in the number of malformation reported in 1976 as compared to previous years[12] is meaningless. Equally meaningless is[5] the sharp increase observed in the years following 1976, which is likely to reflect the sharpened attention to birth defects on the part of the physicians and public health officers, due to the accident and to the operation of the Seveso Birth Defects Registry (SBDR)

SBDR was set up in 1978 to cover the whole population (220.000) of the 11 towns served by the 3 health districts involved with TCDD contamination. Population coverage became satisfactory during its second year of operation. Data concerning births of 1977 and 1978, however, were collected retrospectively through available medical records and subsequent ascertainments, thus proving less complete, especially for minor and mild defects. The task of SBDR, according to the emergency law enacted in 1977, was the collection of a complete and reliable record of the birth defects occurring in the monitored population for a number of years following the accident. Such a record was expected to make possible a subsequent analysis of the potential associations between TCDD exposure and specific BDs in the monitored population.

In short, SBDR operation can be summarized as follows: lists of newborns provided by each town were matched with clinical forms provided by local health services, which were alerted to cooperate in detecting BDs. Each newborn for whom the presence of some congenital anomaly - irrespective of an actual diagnosis - was not ruled out was subjected to further ascertainments by pediatricians of the SBDR team; in this case the available medical records were reviewed and new records established through new examinations, in order to establish a diagnosis. Such diagnoses were periodically further reviewed by a pediatrician and a medical epidemiologist of SBDR, with the referral, when needed, of a teratology consultant. Birth defects were recorded according to ICD 9; in addition, special codes were added to include hemangiomas in the survey. As a result of the above procedures, reasonably accurate and consistent diagnostic criteria were implemented, concerning the various BD types. Rates of birth defects in the monitored population in the 5 year period following 1976 fell within the ranges observed in national and international registries.

Table 2. Malformed Children reported to the local Health Authority in the Seveso area between 1973 and 1978

Year	Live births	Malformed children reported	SBDR*
1973	3783	2	—
1974	3656	5	—
1975	3516	3	
1976	3210	4	—
1977	2756	37	67
1978	2747	53	98

*Hemangiomas and other minor skin defects excluded.

EXPOSURE DEFINITION

The most important limitation of Seveso studies stems from the lack of reliable criteria for classifying pregnancies on the basis of TCDD exposure.

The population monitored by SBDR included newborns presumably exposed as well as unexposed to TCDD in utero. Using the date of last menstrual period (LMP) provided by the Seveso Pregnancy Registry, SBDR records were reorganized subsequently on the basis of LMP and the mother's residence at such date. Mother residence at delivery was also recorded and towns' population registries provided records for all persons' residence at the date of the accident.

The exposure which determines the TCDD risk for unfavourable pregnancy outcomes depends on the fate of the toxic taken in by the mother (or possibly by the father) and on the biological mechanisms of TCDD teratogenesis. Both are practically unknown in humans. Either only maternal exposure in (early) pregnancy is relevant (as implied in most experimental studies), or cumulative parental exposure up to (early) pregnancy is to be considered - because of TCDD persistence in the body or germinal cells damage. Only data relative to the former hypothesis are presented here, considering two extreme alternatives: 1) that the bulk of exposure took place shortly after the accident; 2) that exposure decreased slowly and gradually overtime.

The first alternative appears more plausible, as the probability for TCDD intake to occur was presumably highest for a short period after the accident and in its vicinity. Beyond such general statements, only an accurate and comprehensive exposure assessment is useful to better define the population at risk.

Exposure Assessment

The implementation of reliable devices for individual exposure assessment at Seveso would have probably entailed an intense effort of study design and planning soon after the accident, which was hardly feasible considering the size of and the turn-over in the epidemiologic team.

Direct measurements of dioxin intake and/or body burden had not been attempted by the time SBDR was established, two years after the accident. Attempts to indirect estimation of individual exposure had been done, before SBDR was established, by collecting various questionnaires, largely in zone A and B. Not only was the population cover covered outside zone B limited, but it was selected in part on a voluntary (non-randomized) basis; nor was it clear how to compare informations on potential exposure sources collected through different questionnaires. On the other hand, reclamation work in 1978 was well under way and considerable effort had been devoted to collect and assay TCDD soil samples in an area of about 15 square km.

Information thus available concerning environmental distribution of TCDD was considered sufficient to assess the probability of exposure at different levels for residents of the corresponding zones. Little refinement in the exposure assessment was expected from collecting, at high costs, further information on individual exposure circumstances, such as high risk (including consumption of locally grown food) or risk avoiding practices (including staying away from home) adopted by families.

In retrospect, such an argument appears to be based on the belief that substantial TCDD intake had occurred in the population living in the polluted area, which was shared by a number of epidemiologists for some time after the accident.

In any case, a cohort study design based on comparisons among zones was the easiest option open to the epidemiologic team that gathered at SBDR. Adoption of such a design involved not only relying on mothers' residence at some relevant period as the only exposure index, but also accepting the official pollution zones as the territorial basis to define average potential exposure in the corresponding cohorts of pregnancies. Zone average TCDD levels, which had been established on the basis of a preliminary analysis and incomplete evidence in a situation of emergency, did not prove consistent with the zone-specific chloracne rates. Not surprisingly, the inconsistency was apparent between the less polluted zone B and R, the latter showing a higher rate of chloracne. Unfortunately this inconsistency stirred an unnecessary, long and bitter controversy. Although alternative territorial assessments of potential exposure had been worked out by 1981, not until 1983 was SBDR allowed to redefine exposure according to the new evidence.

DIOXINS AND BIRTH DEFECTS AT SEVESO

Pregnancies started from April 1st, 1976 to December 31st, 1980 among women resident in the monitored area were included in a descriptive study, which SBDR reported to the local and national health authorities in 1983[13]. Pregnancy outcomes were analyzed according to the time and place of residence of the mother at LMP. According to alternative hypotheses concerning TCDD exposure (see above), the definition of the population at risk was either restricted to pregnancies started among potentially exposed women in the 2nd and 3rd trimesters of 1976, or in the whole period.

Some data concerning the former pregnancies are shown in table 3. Among the 431 pregnancies 1976-80 in zones A and B, only 22 (of which 3 terminated by spontaneous abortion) were initiated within the 2nd trimester of 1976, 9 (no abortion) within the 3rd trimester and 26 (5 abortions) in the 4th. No pregnancy resulted in still-birth or birth defect.

Among the 124 pregnancies started in zone R during the 2nd trimester of 1976, 16 spontaneous abortions and 5 cases of congenital anomalies occurred. 18 abortions, 1 still-birth and 4 malformations resulted from 96 pregnancies initiated in this zone in the 3rd trimester of 1976. The rate of congenital anomalies observed in zone S is lower than in zone R among II/76 pregnancies, but numbers are very small. Furthermore, birth defects rate among pregnancies initiated in 1976 observed at SBDR are much lower than in the following years, presumably due to low sensitivity of the register in its initial (retrospective) operation. No recurrence of specific birth defects, nor any obvious similarity, was noted among the outcomes of the pregnancies started in 1976 in the most polluted areas.

Statistical comparison between rates of birth defects occurring in "exposed" and "unexposed" pregnancies for various groups of congenital anomalies is only possible for the whole period. Relevant data are summarized in table 4. Clustering of specific defects or groups thereof in the most polluted areas was not detected, with the possible exception of hemangiomas.

As already mentioned, a different definition of the population at risk results from alternative territorial exposure assessment (based, for example, on chloracne distribution). In this case the ex-

Table 3. Abortions and Congenital Anomalies by Date and Zone at LMP in Seveso.

LMP	DATE ZONE	II/76	III/76	WHOLE PERIOD (II 76-IV 80)
SPONTANEOUS ABORTIONS	A + B	3	O	61
	R	16	18	265
	S	76	83	1.350
TOTAL* MALFORMA-TIONS	A + B	O	O	23
	R	5	4	90
	S	8	22	474
HEMANGIO-MAS	A + B	O	O	10
	R	2	1	37
	S	3	3	171
BIRTHS	A + B	19	9	370
	R	108	78	1.813
	S	546	486	9.178

*HEMANGIOMAS INCLUDED.

Table 4. Number of Cases Found and Expected by Malformation Type in Zone A+B+R.

GROUPS*	TOTAL NUMBER OF CASES MAPPED	NUMBER OF CASES IN AREA EXPECTED	FOUND
CNS	27	5.19	6
CNS + EYE	39	7.49	8
EAR/FACE/NECK	27	5.19	4
HEART	44	8.45	6
HEART/CIRCUL.	53	10.18	8
DIGESTIVE	14	2.69	3
HYPOSPADIAS	39	7.49	8
DISLOC./HIP	38	7.30	8
TALIPES	27	5.19	4
POLY/SYNDAC	16	3.07	3
OTHER MUS/SK	19	3.65	3
SKIN	30	5.76	6
ANGIOMAS/TUM	228	43.81	50
CHROMOSOMAL	27	5.19	4
OTHER	30	5.76	4
TOTAL	587		

*GROUPS ADAPTED FROM ICD 9.

cess of hemangiomas detected in "exposed" pregnancies is statistically significant[13] . Such excess is currently under study in order to ascertain a possible bias related to exposure, as more attention may have been paid to minor and mild defects in newborns from the most polluted areas.

An analogous significant excess of spontaneous abortions has been reported for "exposed" pregnancies following the accident[14] . In this case, bias may arise from selective reporting of voluntary abortions as "spontaneous." Occurance of such a bias is still under study, and has not yet been detected. Indeed, the true number of voluntary abortions is obviously relevant also to define fertility changes related to the accident. A time-adjusted analysis has been performed for abortion rates and is underway for hemangiomas. An integrated analysis of unfavourable pregnancy outcomes requires overcoming theoretical and practical difficulties.

METHODOLOGICAL CONSIDERATIONS

The generally negative results of Seveso BD studies could be expected if their statistical power were analyzed. Relevant to statistical power are both uncertainties in exposure definition and relatively small size of the exposed population as compared to the rarity and multiplicity of the outcomes to be considered. As previously outlined, the level of TCDD exposure during a critical period of pregnancy is not adequately described by the time and place of residence at LMP, not to mention the presumable inadequacy of zoning for epidemiological purposes.

Difficulties arising from the probabilistic nature and inaccuracy of the exposure assessment are compounded in the definition of the exposed groups. Had been the exposed groups restricted, for example, to pregnancies started in A zone during the 3 months preceeding the accident, only a handful of pregnancies with high probability of exposure would have to be considered at risk. Conversely loose criteria, such as those adopted in table 3 and 4, lead to include a large proportion of pregnancies with presumably little or no exposure, in the group at risk.

Rarity and multiplicity of birth defects in a limited population raise further difficulties affecting statistical power.

Most known teratogens have been shown to cause only a limited

number of anomalies[1], which represent a small fraction of the overall
birth defect rate. Consequently comparison of overall rates can obscure differences limited to few anomalies. On the other hand, single
defects have extremely low prevalences at birth, ranging from 1% downward. In order to avoid the statistical problems of multiple comparisons of rare events in a sample of limited size (insufficient power
and risk of falsely positive results due to chance), anomalies have
to be lumped together in groups, according to some meaningful criteria.
Since no information of the possible defects caused by TCDD in humans
was available, in SBDR anomalies were grouped by organ or apparatus,
which, in the light of the present general embriological knowledge, is
little better than random grouping.

Thus, those carried out in SBDR are little more than ecological
comparisons, since the various cohorts are only on the average at different levels of exposure. The choice of this study design, which has
little sensitivity unless the effects of exposure are very strong or
specific, reflects the expectation, common in the early years after
the accident, that major increases in birth defect rates were occurring in the polluted areas.

As a matter of fact, sensible analyses were possible only for
those pregnancy outcomes: abortions and hemangiomas, with frequencies
greater than 1%. On the other hand, such outcomes - as already mentioned - are most easily affected by potential biases. If the latter
can be ruled out, the Seveso studies would provide evidence for some
reproductive effects of TCDD in humans.

CONCLUSIONS

The results of Seveso birth defect studies clearly indicate that
the Seveso accident did not cause any major change in the pattern or
in the frequency of congenital anomilies among newborns in the polluted areas. They do not provide evidence in favour of, or against TCDD
teratogenicity, nor do they permit to rule out that TCDD pollution has
caused, under specific exposure circumstances, congenital anomalies
in a limited number of children.

Indeed, the Seveso epidemiologic study is paradigmatic, in the
sense that TCDD pollution sprang from a single source in space and
time, related acute effects were observed in humans and animals and
health monitoring of a large population was relatively timely and accurate. In spite of these circumstances, the study design was flawed

548

by uncertainties in the exposure assessment which resulted in an inaccurate probabilistic definition of the population at risk.

Similar weaknesses are apparent in other studies investigating TCDD related risk in pregnant women[6]. In such studies pollution was due to agricultural or military spraying with herbicides of wide areas, and the attempts to correlate the spatial and temporal distribution of toxics with birth defect rates were based on environmental monitoring and/or territorial assessment of potential exposure. On the other hand, studies of occupational or military groups refer mainly to males and their negative results could be due to a weak mutagenic or cytogenetic effect of these substances or to undetected reduction of fertility besides exposure uncertainty.

Thus, epidemiologic studies concerning TCDD reproductive effects should be based on an exposure assessment as direct and accurate as possible. Since this is hardly feasible in large cohorts, a case/control design should be given priority, including carefully designed and detailed questionnaires , as well as objective exposure indicators, such as direct measurements of body burden or biological tests. Otherwise epidemiological studies are likely to provide negative results, unless TCDD exposure is massive, or the relative risk for specific birth defects is very high, or the excess risk for some adverse pregnancy outcome is large.

Environmental monitoring for early detection and removal of hazardous substances by means of epidemiologic studies cannot be regarded as an acceptable strategy. Use of negative results from epidemiologic studies as an argument against TCDD reproductive risk is unwarranted or even dangerous, in light of their limitations. Epidemiologic studies should not be used as an alibi for failure to adopt reasonable preventive measures in environmental health.

REFERENCES
1. R. B. Kurzel, C. L. Ctrulo, The effect of environmental pollutants on human reproduction, including birth defects. Env. Sc. Tech., 15/6/:626 (1981).

2. R. J. Kociba, and B. A. Schwetz, Toxicity of 2,3,7,8,tetrachloro-dibenzo-p-dioxin (TCDD), Drug.Metab.Rev.,13/3:387, (1974).

3. M. P. Esposito, T. O. Tiernan, and F. E. Dryden,"Dioxins", Industrial Environmental Research Laboratory, EPA 600/2-80-197, (1980).

4. Veterans Administration,"Review of the literature on herbicides, Including phenoxy Herbicides and associated dioxins", Veterans Administration, Washington, D.C. (1981).

5. G. Tognoni, and A. Bonaccorsi, Epidemiological Problems with TCDD (a critical view), Drug Metab. Rev., 13/3:447, (1982).

6. J. M. Friedman, Does Agent Orange cause Birth Defects? Teratology, 29:193, (1984);

7. A. Hay, "The chemical scythe-lessons of 2,4,5,T and dioxins" Plenum Press, New York, (1982).

8. F. Pocchiari et al., Environmental impact of accidental release of TCDD at Seveso, Italy, in "Accidental exposure to dioxins" F. Coulston and F. Pocchiari eds., Academic Press, New York (1983)

9. P. Strigini, The industrial chemical industry and the case of Seveso, UNEP Industry and Environment, 6/4:16, (1983).

10. F. Pocchiari, Discussion in "Accidental exposure to dioxins", F. Coulston and F. Pocchiari eds., Academic Press, New York (1983).

11. L. Bisanti, et al., Experiences from the accident of Seveso, Acta Morphol. Acad. Sci. Hung., 28:139, (1980).

12. G. Reggiani, Acute human exposure to TCDD in Seveso, Italy,Toxicol Environ. Health, 6:27, (1980).

13. Registro delle Malformazioni dell'Ufficio Speciale di Seveso, "Rapporto conclusivo sui difetti congeniti ed altri esiti sfavo-revoli di gravidanza rilevati nella popolazione dell'area di Seveso interessata all'inquinamento da TCDD il 10.7.1976" Seveso, (1983).

14. G. Remotti, W. Bianco and L. Meazza, Spontaneous abortion studies, paper presented at the Scientific Congress "5 years of epidemio-logic studies in Seveso area", Milano, Italy, 1981

RADIATION EXPOSURE AND LEVELS OF OCCUPATIONAL SAFETY

Edward E. Pochin

National Radiological Protection Board
Chilton, Didcot
Oxfordshire OX11 ORQ. England

ABSTRACT

In any review of the safety or risk of occupational exposures
to radiation, it is important to compare the risk involved with
those resulting from other hazards in existing industries. A
simple but obviously incomplete comparison can be based on the
death rate by injury or disease attributable to occupational causes,
per worker-year at risk, provided that account is taken of the
nature of death and the ages at which such deaths would occur.
The comparison should, however, be more broadly based, so as to
recognise the differing severity of detriment from different forms
of injury and disease. Such comparisons could be related
quantitatively to the total periods of time lost, either from
normal health and activity during temporary or permanent incapacity,
or by loss of life expectancy from fatal injury or disease.

INTRODUCTION

Occupational exposure to radiation was clearly recognised as
causing tissue damage and an increased cancer mortality in early
radiologists[1]; and the increased frequency of bone sarcoma in dial
painters was related to the radiation delivered by ingested radium
in 1931[2]. Much earlier - indeed 400 years earlier - pitchblende
miners were reported to suffer from a greatly increased frequency
of fatal lung disease[3], now understandable as due to lung cancer
resulting from high radon concentrations in the mines. In general,
however, the occupational risks of radiation exposure are not
regularly identified in annual industrial records, in the way that
accidental risks and those from a few other occupational diseases
are recorded. This is inevitable, particularly at the low dose

currently received in most occupations, since cancers induced by
radiation are indistinguishable clinically and microscopically from
the cancers of the same types which occur naturally, and the
detection of any excess depends upon detailed statistical comparisons with cancer rates in comparison populations.

This difficulty, which is common to various other kinds of
occupational disease, contrasts with the ease with which industrial
accident rates for most forms of industry can be examined and
compared, from records extending over many years in many countries.
In most cases, estimates of the number of workers at risk in each
industrial group are, or can be made, available. In consequence
the risks of accidental deaths at work per worker-year can be
compared in various ways: for example between industries in one
country, between years in one industry, or between countries in
comparable industries. Such comparisons depend upon the criteria
used in attributing deaths to occupational causes being similar in
different industries, years or countries; and upon uniform
standards being adopted for inclusion of injuries in the total of
accidents - for example by including all injuries involving more
than 3 days off work.

It is not difficult, however, to derive quantitative estimates
of the risks of a large number of industries from recorded accident
rates; just as it is possible to make quantitative estimates of the
risks of occupational exposure to radiation - from epidemiological
evidence in a few occupations, or predictively in others by knowledge of the types and levels of exposure and of the risks to be
expected from such exposures.

In comparing the risk from such radiation exposures with
other occupational risks, both these types of quantitative assessment are obviously necessary. It is necessary also, however, to
develop some way of comparing the different kinds of risks which
may occur in different industries, and of aggregating the contributions of such different kinds of risk when they occur in the same
industry. This is the more difficult because the comparison of
risks should not depend only on the magnitude of the risks, but
also on the relative weight that people attach to different kinds
of risk. Any suggested ways of comparing the total harm of
different industries will inevitably be tentative and somewhat
arbitrary in nature, although of potential value in seeking to
develop valid quantitative criteria of industrial safety.

COMPARISON OF MORTALITY RATES

A simple, although manifestly incomplete, criterion of
occupational risk can be obtained by expressing the total number of
deaths attributable to each year of work as a fatality rate, for
example per 100,000 workers at risk. If this is done, the rates of

deaths from occupational injuries are found to vary very widely in different industries, from less than one, to more than 200 such deaths per year per 100,000 workers (Tables 1 and 2). In most industries deaths from injuries greatly outnumber deaths from recorded industrial diseases.

Table 1

Fatal accident rates (annual deaths at work per 100,000 employed) in industries in the UK (average rates for years 1974-1978 except as stated)

Manufacture of clothing and footwear	0.5
Manufacture of vehicles	1.5
Manufacture of timber, furniture, etc.	4.0
Manufacture of bricks, pottery, etc.	6.5
Chemical and allied industries	8.5
Shipbuilding and marine engineering	10.5
Agriculture (employees)	11
Construction industries	15
Railway staff	18
Coal miners	21
Quarries	29
Non-coal miners	75
Offshore oil and gas (1967-76)	165
Deep sea fishing (accidents at sea only, 1959-68)	280

Reproduced, with permission, from "Risk Assessment: A study group report", Royal Society, London[4]

In occupations involving radiation exposure, the frequency with which fatal cancers might be induced by the radiation doses received annually could similarly be expressed as a mortality attributable to each year's exposure.

Deaths due to radiation exposure at work cannot however be regarded as equivalent to deaths resulting from industrial injuries. On the one hand, a death from an induced cancer, which may be preceded by a prolonged period of suffering and distress, clearly may involve greater detriment to the victim and to his family than an immediate or early death following severe injury. On the other hand, the long average latent interval between a radiation exposure and the development of a cancer resulting from it, implies that such deaths are likely to occur at an average age 20 or more years older than that at which accidental deaths from injuries occur. And it is not self-evident which should, or would,

Table 2
Fatal accident rates (annual deaths at work per 100,000
employed) in industry groups in the USA

	1955	1961	1968	1974	1980
Trade	12	9	7	6	6
Manufacturing	12	11	9	8	8
Service and	15	(13	12	10	7
Government		(13	13	13	11
Transport and					
public utilities	34	43	38	34	28
Agriculture	55	60	65	54	61
Construction	75	74	74	63	45
Mining and					
quarrying	104	108	117	71	50

Based on review of data derived from Accident Facts[5]

be regarded as involving the greater detriment – deaths from disease
at an average age of 60, or deaths from injury at an average age of
40. The weighting that would be given to two alternative forms of
risk would necessarily influence the comparison between the fatality
rates from occupational injuries and from occupational radiation
exposure.

Table 3 summarises the dose rates recorded for a large number
of occupations in the most recent report in 1982, of the United
Nations Scientific Committee on the Effects of Atomic Radiation
(UNSCEAR), in most cases giving rates recorded to 1978[6].

The mean rates quoted, although not based on comprehensive or
properly weighted sampling, show rates for most occupational groups
as lying between 1 and 2 mSv per year, with a minority extending up
to about 10 mSv per year, as of 1980. The mean of all occupational
exposure rates in the UK in 1984 is estimated to be 1.5 mSv per
year[7] (effective dose equivalent).

The rate at which fatal cancers are believed to be induced
differs according to whether it is postulated that cancers may occur
– after a period of 5 or 10 years – at a constant rate during the
remaining lifetime, or at a rate proportional to the rate at which
cancers normally develop at increasing ages. On the former, the
"absolute risk predictive hypothesis", a mean induction rate of
$1.25 \ 10^{-5} \ mSv^{-1}$ has been estimated[8]. On the latter, the "relative
risk predictive hypothesis", a 1.7 times greater rate has been

Table 3

Mean rates of occupational exposure

Annual dose equivalents for different categories of workers

Occupational group	Data from:- No. of countries	No. of sub-groups	Table(s) ref.*	Mean dose rate $(mSv.y^{-1})$
Nuclear power production				
Uranium mining	3	3	(2)	9.3
Fuel processing	3	5	(3-5)	1.0
Reactor operation	4	20	(6,7,10, 12,13, 15,16)	4.3
Fuel reprocessing	4	4	(22,24, 27,28)	6.8
Nuclear research	8	9	(29-32)	2.2
Medical				
Diagnostic radiol.	6	16	(41)	0.7
Nuclear medicine	3	7	(36,44)	1.6
Radiotherapy	3	7	(45)	1.5
Dental	5	5	(43)	0.2
General	9	21	(37-40,46)	1.1
Other				
Industrial radiog.	5	7	(47)	1.6
Luminisers	4	5	(48)	8.0
Other industrial	4	11	(49)	1.1
Research activities	9	21	(50-52)	1.6

*Data as given in Annex H of UNSCEAR 1982[6]; the values used are those for the latest year quoted, usually 1978.

estimated for exposures received during the period of a working lifetime[9].

The annual number of deaths attributable to a dose rate of 1.5 mSv per year would thus be about 2 per 10^5 at risk on the former hypothesis, and 4 per 10^5 on the latter. For a dose rate of 10 mSv per year the estimates would be of 12 and 20 such deaths per 10^5 at risk.

On this important but insufficient basis, therefore, of comparing numbers of deaths attributable to occupational causes, the radiation exposures involved in the majority of occupations may be responsible for a fatality rate which is numerically equal to that in the safer manufacturing processes noted in Table 1. (Or, otherwise expressed, such exposures, if continued for a 50 year working lifetime, would raise a normal risk of dying from cancer from 20% to between 20.1 and 20.2%.) In a few occupations such as uranium mining, a higher radiation dose rate of 10 mSv per year (corresponding to current average exposures of 1 WLM per year) would entail a radiation risk numerically equal to that from accidental injuries currently recorded in construction work or in coal mining in the UK.

COMPARISON OF PERIODS OF TIME LOSS

Comparison of the risks of different industries, including those involving radiation exposure, ought however to be made on a wider basis than on the annual risk of death alone; non-fatal accidents or diseases and other factors contribute to the total risk of harm. Nor can deaths from accidents be simply equated to deaths from disease, or deaths at different ages be regarded as equal in detriment to the worker or to his family.

One potentially helpful step in assessing and aggregating the detriment resulting from different fatal and non-fatal effects of occupational injuries and diseases, occurring at different ages and involving different periods of disability, may be to take account of time lost: of the total duration of health and activity impaired by non-fatal conditions, and the length of normal life expectancy lost as a result of fatal ones[10]. Again, different weight should clearly be attached to equal periods of time lost through repeated minor injuries, serious diseases, permanent disabilities, or death. The weighting factors that people would consider applicable to time and health lost i1 such different ways would properly be based on opinion about the different forms or severities of harm, rather than on any simple objective criterion. But then, the need to compare the safety of different industries must in any case include considerations of perceived, as well as objective, risk. Any review of safety and risk should surely avoid an assessment based only on numerical levels of different risks regardless of the kinds of risk involved, just as it should avoid judgements based only on the types of risk, regardless of whether these risks were large or small.

The following sections therefore review, first, such estimates as can be made of the time losses, from health or life, that result from industrial injuries. An attempt is then made to make a similar estimate of the time losses that would result from carcinogenic, genetic and developmental effects of occupational

556

exposure to radiation, at a typical dose rate (of 1.5 mSv per year),
using current estimates of the frequency with which such effects
are caused at low dose rates. The intention here can only be to
present a simple numerical intercomparison between the frequency of
different effects and the time losses that they involve, so that
the equivalence between a given dose rate and the accident rate in
different industries can be considered. No claim can be made to
precision in such estimates, and they are given in detail in later
Tables (Tables 4 and 6) only to suggest the likely relative magni-
tudes of the various types of detriment as assessed by time loss.
The severity of different types of detriment cannot, in any case,
be compared only on a numerical basis, although this basis should
enter into the comparison. So, how do current risks of occupational
injury compare with those of radiation exposure?

TIME LOSS IN CONVENTIONAL INDUSTRIES

In attempting to base some kind of index of total harm in
different industries on the lengths of time lost in various ways,
valid information on the effect of injuries is ordinarily more
accessible than that on most occupational diseases. This is in
part because of uncertainty as to what diseases are occupational
in origin, or are admitted to be so and included in records; and
the recognition of particular diseases as occupational in origin
may vary at different times and in different countries, and
occasionally as new carcinogenic or other effects of industrial
exposure are identified.

In terms of time lost, however, the contribution to detriment
from recognised occupational disease is, in most industries, small
compared to that from injuries[10].

Occupational injuries

The average lengths of time lost owing to industrial
injuries can be assessed as the total of components from three
sources.

(a) non-fatal injuries which do not cause permanent
     disability. Records are commonly available of
     the annual frequency of these injuries, eg. per
     thousand workers at risk, and of the average
     numbers of days off work that such temporary
     disabilities involve[11]. An estimate of the
     (calendar) years of disability per thousand
     worker-years can therefore be derived (Table
     4).

Table 4

Time loss estimate (years per 1000 worker-years)
for an industry with annual fatal accident rate of 10
per 100,000 at risk; rounded values based on 4 national surveys

Accidents causing:	No. per 1000 worker yrs.	years per accident	weighting per year lost	Product (years)
death	0.1	30	1	3
permanent disability	0.07	30	say 0.75	1.6
temporary disability	40	0.05	say 0.2	0.4

(b) injuries causing a greater or less degree of permanent
disability. Data are often recorded on the number of
new injuries occurring annually which are judged to
cause permanent disability, or inability to work in
the industry. The degree of disability will vary,
however, from slight limitation in performing some
types of work, to a complete incapacity to continue
work at all. The degree of disability is sometimes
recorded in individual cases as a fraction of a
complete disability or as a percentage of the pension
that would be awarded in a case of complete disability;
and in some countries (eg. in the Federal Republic of
Germany) uniform criteria apply in all industries to
the fraction of complete disability that is attributed
to particular types of injury. When this is done, the
frequency of permanent disabilities may then be
expressed as the equivalent number of cases of complete
disability occurring per year. If this frequency is
combined with the mean expectation of life at the mean
age (and sex) at which such injuries occur, an
approximate figure can again be obtained of the years
of normal activity lost annually per thousand workers
at risk, the degree of disability being equivalent to
that of complete loss of working capacity in the
industry concerned (Table 4).

The estimate of this component of industrial harm is
sensitive to the procedures adopted in different
countries and industries for compensation and

therefore for the weighting for different degrees
of injury. It at least allows a rough assessment,
however, of the time losses from permanent
disabilities to be compared with those from purely
temporary ones and from fatal accidents.

(c)   fatal accident rates are regularly recorded in
most industries, and the mean age at which they
occur differs little from the mean age of the
working population at risk, although commonly
exceeding it by a year or two owing to a somewhat
lower risk in younger than in older workers. If
the ages at which accidental deaths occur are
related to the expectation of life at these ages,
fatal industrial accidents usually involve an
average loss of about 30 years of life expectancy[10],
although this figure may be increased in countries
and industries in which the work of older members
of the industry differs substantially from that of
younger workers.

In records of industries in a number of countries, the total
time loss due to injuries causing temporary incapacity has been
somewhat less than (ie. about 0.6 times) that from fatal injuries.
That due to permanent incapacities has been much more variable,
but again rather less than from fatal injuries (on average about
0.7 times). If it were considered that life with an injury
equivalent to permanent incapacity to work had a detriment approaching that of loss of life over the same period of time, but that an
equal total period of temporary disabilities (typically averaging
about 20 days off work) caused a substantially lower detriment, it
would suggest that fatal injuries were on average the greatest
contributor to harm, and that the other two categories together
contributed an equal or rather smaller total detriment (eg. as in
Table 4). If so, it would not seem useful or necessary to seek
any closer definition of the size of weighting factor for equal
periods of time loss from the three categories of accidental
injury.

These data correspond to findings in the aggregate of all
national industries in various economically developed countries
from which relevant records were available. The results are known
to vary, however, in different individual industries within these
countries, and may differ in other and developing countries.

In this discussion, injuries during travel to and from work
have been omitted. These vary with country and industry, but in
some cases make a contribution to harm approaching that sustained
while at work. (In 5 countries for which comprehensive records
are available, fatal accidents at work cause an average of 14

deaths annually per 100,000 workers, with a further 6 deaths annually per 100,000 in travel to and from work.)

In terms of time loss, the risks of industrial injuries can therefore be provisionally summarised as follows:-

1. A fatal accident involves an average loss of life expectancy of about 30 years. In an industry with a fatal accident rate of 10 per 100,000 worker-years, therefore, the time-loss from this cause would amount to 3 years per thousand worker-years.

2. Accidents causing temporary disability occur with several hundred to a thousand times the frequency of fatal accidents, and involve an average of a few weeks of disability each. Relative to the 3 years absolute loss of life from fatal accidents referred to in the previous paragraph, the workers in industry would sustain a roughly comparable number of years of moderate disability per thousand worker years although a substantially lower weighting would probably be thought to apply to each such year.

3. Accidents causing some degree of permanent disability are more difficult to summarise, owing to the very varying degrees of disability involved, the dependence of records upon individual assessment and weighting of these degrees of severity, and probably also considerable differences in weight attaching to such disabilities in different industries and countries. As stated above, however, the average total of time loss in industries for which an assessment has been possible is rather lower than that from fatal accidents, and similar to the total from accidents causing temporary disability only.

These figures are obviously very tentative and in fact the ratios of the contributions to time loss from accidents causing fatal, permanent and temporary effects are found to vary with the general level of hazard in the industry concerned - temporary disabilities contributing a smaller proportion of the total in industries in which the accidental death rate is high. However, they indicate a possibility of making a rough aggregation of consequences of industrial injuries in terms of the weight that would probably be attached to different categories of life or health lost. Thus, if for example the weight attached to each year of permanent disability was judged to be rather less than that of a year of absolute loss of life, and if the weight given to each year of temporary disability was substantially less than that of a year of being dead, and industry with an annual fatality rate of

10 per 100,000 workers at risk, could be regarded as having an
annual detriment from occupational injuries equivalent to about
5 years' loss of life expectancy per thousand worker-years (Table 4).

Occupational diseases

Before considering the way in which the available estimates
of radiation risk may be interpreted in terms of time loss, it
should be noted that occupational diseases - apart from any that
may be caused by radiation - ordinarily appear to increase the
total time loss due to injuries by only a few per cent[10]. In
certain industries, such as coal mining and probably also in some
chemical industries, the contribution from disease to time loss is
substantially higher. Also in some sections of industries in the
past, high rates of fatal cancer induction, ordinarily from
exposure to chemicals, have been identified (Table 5); and the

Table 5

Cancer mortalities attributed to occupational exposures
to chemical agents

Industry, or sections of industry	Year reported	Types of cancer	Fatal cancers (per 100,000 per yr.)
Shoe making (press and finishing rooms)	1970	nasal	13
Printing trade	1972	lung and bronchus	20
Work with cutting oils (Arve District)	1971	scrotal	40
Asbestos workers (males, smokers)	1972	lung	75
Rubber mill workers	1965	bladder	340
Mustard gas manufacture (Japan, 1929-45)	1968	bronchus	1040
Nickel workers (pre-1925)	1970	lung and nasal	2200
Beta naphthylamine manufacture	1954	bladder	2400

Based, with permission, on data reviewed in Community
Health[12]

corresponding mean losses of life expectancy will have been considerable. Epidemiological surveys continue to detect significantly raised mortalities from particular types of cancer in certain industries; and even a raised annual cancer rate detectable at only 10 per 100,000 workers at risk, causing death at a mean age of 55, would involve a total annual life loss of about 2 years per 1000 worker-years.

While, therefore, the average time loss due to recognised occupational diseases across all industries is unlikely to add significantly to the estimates of life loss from all industrial injuries, in a few industries the totals from induced disease and from injury may be similar; and, in the past, the former will occasionally have greatly exceeded the latter.

TIME LOSS FROM RADIATION EXPOSURE

In attempting a similar analysis and aggregation of time loss from all effects of occupational exposure to radiation, it is necessary to take account of the rate with which fatal and non-fatal cancers may be induced by the annual doses received, and the corresponding lengths of life lost, and of illness prior to cure or during cure. As regards inherited, or "genetic", disease induced by these exposures, it is necessary to estimate the frequency with which different forms of such diseases are induced; and, as far as possible, the average durations of both disability and loss of life expectancy that are caused by these types of disease. In addition, when women are liable to be occupationally exposed to radiation during pregnancy, estimates should be included to cover the period of disability and loss of life expectancy of children born with disease or defects attributable to any exposure that they received in utero.

It is unlikely, however, that any significant component of time loss will result from any so-called non-stochastic effects of normal occupational exposure. Except for accidents at work causing high doses to the body or to particular organs or parts of the body, the amounts of tissue damage from annual exposures are most unlikely to cause thresholds for impairment of organ functions to be exceeded, even after prolonged exposure received continuously at the dose limit. The threshold dose levels for causing damage to skin, the lens of the eye, or to body organs, could be exceeded occasionally in relatively severe accidents which caused obvious disability to the individual exposed, but which were too infrequent to affect significantly the mean risk of detriment as averaged through the occupation as a whole.

Fatal cancer induction

The average loss of life expectancy due to the induction of

562

cancers which prove fatal depends upon four ascertainable figures.

(a) the mean dose rate (Table 3). The occupational
     exposure of the body to external radiation is
     regularly monitored in exposed individuals.
     Internal exposure of different organs by
     radionuclides taken into the body can usually
     be assessed, although more approximately, in
     working conditions in which such intake may
     occur.

(b) the frequency with which cancers may be
     induced by these doses, and the probability
     that the types of cancer induced may prove
     fatal. The epidemiological data described
     in earlier papers given in this meeting give
     a basis for estimating these risks approxi-
     mately, at least for the organs in which
     the majority of induced fatal cancers occur.

(c) the average interval between the radiation
     exposure of an organ, and the time at which
     a cancer attributable to that exposure
     develops and becomes detectable. For two
     types of malignancy - leukaemia and sarcoma
     of bone - which probably form about 20% of
     all malignancies induced by whole body
     irradiation, this average "latency" is of
     about 13 years. For other malignancies, the
     mean interval is likely to be about twice
     this, or perhaps more.

(d) the mean age at which radiation exposure
     occurs, which appears usually to be at or
     about the mean age of the workforce, or a
     few years later[10].

Given an average age at exposure of about 40 years, therefore,
and the development of induced cancers at an average of 25 years
after exposure, the mean loss of life expectancy and of illness
preceding death for an induced cancer which proves to be fatal
would be between 10 and 13 years.

For an industrial group having a dose rate of 1.5 mSv per
year of whole body exposure (the current average rate of all
groups occupationally exposed in the UK[7]), and assuming an
induction rate for all fatal cancers of 2×10^{-5} per mSv, the
annual time loss by death, and by a period of illness preceding
death, would then amount to about 0.35 years per 1000 exposed
worker-years.

The main uncertainties involved in this estimate depend upon the mean age at development of induced cancers, and the risk of fatal cancers per millisievert; the mean age at receipt of doses is unlikely to be in error by more than a few years. If however the induction rate of cancers were greater at young occupational ages than in old (and the reverse is more likely to be true), the mean age at development of cancer would be younger and the average loss of life expectancy greater. The same would hold if latencies were shorter in the young than in the old.

Similarly the induction rate per millisievert differs according to the two hypotheses referred to above.

(a) on the so-called absolute risk predictive hypothesis, the risks of fatal cancer per 100,000 exposed are taken to be of 1 per mSv in males and 1.5 in females[8]. The relative risk hypothesis, however, postulates that induced cancers will appear at all ages after exposure in numbers proportional to the numbers of "naturally occurring" cancers which develop at these ages. This hypothesis predicts that, following exposures received at the ages of a normal working lifetime, the number of cancers will be about 1.7 times the numbers indicated by the absolute risk hypothesis[9]. This would imply annual numbers of fatal cancers induced, per 100,000 exposed at 1 mSv per year, of 1.7 in males and 2.6 in females.

Table 6

Time loss estimates (years per 1000 worker-years)
from occupational exposure at 1.5 mSv per year)

Cancer Induction	Men		Women	
	on predictive risk hypothesis:-			
	Absolute, or relative		Absolute, or relative	
Fatal cancer	0.2	0.35	0.3	0.5
Curable cancer	0.05	0.1	0.07	0.12
Genetic effects	0.2		0.15	
Effects on a fetus				
Preimplantation			0.08	
Developmental			0.24	
Cancer induction			0.08	
	0.45 to 0.65		0.9 to 1.15	

On these bases, the time loss of 0.35 years per
1000 worker years derived from a risk of 2 per
100,000 per mSv, might lie between 0.2 and 0.5
years, according to the sex distribution of the
working population and the risk predictive
hypothesis adopted (Table 6). The age
distribution of the population would be unlikely
to affect this range considerably unless
consisting of predominantly old or young members.

(b) On both hypotheses, the risk rates quoted depend
on the assumption of the same risk per unit dose
at low dose as is observed epidemiologically at
higher dose. For the radiations of low "linear
energy transfer" (LET) which predominate in most
forms of occupational exposure, this derivation
is more likely to overestimate the risk at low
dose, although perhaps only by a factor of 2 or
3, than to underestimate it. For any component
of high LET radiation (from neutrons or alpha
particles), the linear derivation of risk at low
dose is more likely to be correct, or possibly
to under-estimate the true risk by a factor of
2 or 3.

Induction of curable cancers

The frequency with which cancers are induced, which are
curable by operation or other treatment, is less commonly estimated
in epidemiological surveys than the frequency of fatal cancers,
since it is often more reliable to obtain comprehensive records of
causes of death than of causes of illness or reasons for operations.
The frequency can, however, be inferred from that of fatal cancers,
since it can probably be assumed that induced cancers, of a given
organ and microscopic type, and developing in a given age group and
sex, have the same likelihood of successful cure as naturally
occurring cancers of the same type. On this basis, and from
statistics of the long term (eg. 15 years) symptom-free survival of
different types of cancer after treatment, it is probable that
about twice as many cancers are induced which can be cured, as the
numbers which will prove fatal (Table 7).

This figure includes cancers of the skin of the types
induced by radiation (ie. of the basal and the squamous cell
types). These are so readily and regularly removed by simple
operation that few reliable records exist of the overall cure rate.
This cure rate is probably about 98 or 99% with adequate medical
treatment.

Table 7

Estimated number of cancers induced (per 100
persons exposed to 1 Sv, whole body radiation)

Organ	No. of fatal cancers		No. of curable cancers		weighting for curable cancers	Curable cancers as equivalent no. of fatal cancers	
	M	F	M	F		M	F
Breast	0.0	0.5	0.0	0.3	0.6	0.0	0.18
Bone marrow	0.2		0.01		0.95	0.01	
Lungs	0.2		0.01		0.95	0.01	
Thyroid	0.05		1.0		0.05	0.05	
Bone	0.05		0.01		0.75	0.01	
Skin	0.01		1.0		0.01	0.01	
Remainder	0.5		0.15		0.75	0.11	
	1.0	1.5	2.2	2.5		0.2	0.4

Weighting for severity of curable cancers is set equal
to mortality of each cancer type despite treatment.
On this basis, mean severity of a cured cancer (of
0.3/2.35) appears as one eighth that of a fatal cancer.

The time loss and the amount of detriment due to all curable
cancers depends not only on the frequency of their induction but
also on the period of illness or amount of suffering, hardship,
and anxiety involved in their cure, and any detriment or anxiety
continuing after their cure. Here there is an obvious gradation
between the ease with which the skin cancers can usually be cured,
with limited surgery or subsequent surveillance and probably
limited anxiety, and the substantial periods of illness, suffering,
treatment and subsequent follow-up and inevitable anxiety in the
case of many cancers, and disabilities following extensive surgery
in some.

Within this range, the types of thyroid cancer that are
induced by radiation have an intermediate position, with a
considerable majority being removable by relatively simple initial
surgery, and many of the remainder being effectively treated by
means of radioactive iodine even though already disseminated
through the body.

Pending the collection of comprehensive data on the lengths of time, and assessment of the amounts of hardship, involved in the successful treatment of different proportions of the cancers of different types, some approximate estimate can be made of the total detriment resulting from the induction of cancers which can be cured. The lengths of time that are typically required in the treatment and close surveillance of most of the skin cancers is of a few days or weeks, with few or no symptoms from the cancer before its treatment. For the thyroid cancers, the corresponding period is of weeks or a few months - again usually with little or no discomfort or disability before treatment. For many other cancers, suffering and disability precede and accompany the process of cure to a variable extent; and the period of such disability, cure, and close subsequent surveillance is commonly of a few years rather than of months. In this sense, the ease of cure corresponds roughly with the probability of cure being effective. If this very approximate criterion were adopted for the types of curable cancer that are induced, it would suggest that the average detriment from a fatal cancer, of the types and numbers likely to be induced by radiation, would be about 8 times that of one that could be cured; and that the total detriment from all curable induced cancers was about one quarter of that from the fatal ones (Table 7).

The quantitative bases for these figures are clearly extremely tenuous. In terms of perceived risk, however - which is ultimately the criterion required - it is obvious that cure of an existing cancer is greatly preferable to failure of cure - whether the "preference" was judged to correspond to a factor of 8 or not. If so, and with the frequency of curable cancers likely to be less than 3 times that of fatal ones, it seems improbable that a time loss estimate of the annual detriment from all cancer induction would be raised by more than about one quarter (as in Table 6) by inclusion of the detriment due to curable cancers.

Genetic effects

The attempt at estimating the time loss detriment of radiation induced inheritable disease has been greatly helped by the work of geneticist members of UNSCEAR, following a question put to the late Professor Cedric Carter, an experienced human geneticist working on that Committee. Estimates had been published in earlier UNSCEAR reports on the numbers of genetic diseases of various types that were likely to be induced, and expressed in later generations, by radiation exposure of parents. In the Committee's 1982 report[6], however, further data were included on the main abnormalities contributing to the genetic effects of radiation exposure. For each such type of abnormality, records were sought showing the average age at which symptoms of the abnormality started to appear, and the average age at death of sufferers from the abnormality. Given the frequency with which

567

each abnormality was induced per unit exposure prior to conception of the child, an approximate figure could thus be derived of the resulting years of impaired, and of lost, life per million children.

In a population of working ages exposed to 1.5 mSv per year of whole body radiation, including the germinal tissues at this dose rate, some estimate can therefore be given of the years of impaired or lost life that will be expressed in subsequent generations, as a result of each year's exposure of the working population. The result can be stated in the same way as for cancer induction: namely as years of life lost or impaired as a result of the annual exposure of 1000 members of the total work-force to one millisievert. The figures differ slightly for women and for men, since it is only the radiation received prior to conception of children which can have genetic effects in the children, and the mean age at conception of children is rather lower in females (about 26 years) than in males (29 years, on UK data for 1977[13]). For women, the total of years of life impaired plus years of life lost would be estimated at 0.15 years per 1000 female worker-years, about 0.03 years being expressed in the first two generations. For men, the corresponding figures would be 0.2 years, with 0.04 years in the first two generations. (Data are emerging[6] that genetic defects are less frequently induced per unit dose by irradiation of females than of males, so this disparity may in fact be greater.)

On this criterion, however, and giving equal weight to years of lost life in the offspring as to years of the impairment of their health, which is commonly severe in these inherited conditions, the average genetic detriment of between 0.15 and 0.2 years in all posterity is rather less than the corresponding estimate of between 0.25 and 0.5 years detriment resulting annually (Table 6) from fatal cancer induction in 1000 workers exposed at 1.5 mSv per year.

Effects of exposure during pregnancies

It is finally necessary to assess the possible detriment due to exposure of the developing child during work involving radiation exposures during pregnancies. The following estimates are made with the maximising but simplifying assumptions that all women continue at work during the whole of all pregnancies, that pregnancies occur in the workforce at the same rate as in the population as a whole, and that the dose to the fetus is the same as that recorded for the mother, although in general it will be somewhat less for most qualities of radiation. To derive average values of risk, as previously, it is further assumed that the dose rate of 1.5 mSv per year is received at a uniform rate during pregnancy.

Three kinds of effect need to be reviewed.

(a)   death of the fertilized ovum or conceptus,
        prior to its implantation in the uterine wall

(b)   developmental abnormalities caused by exposure
        of the embryo at certain stages of its growth

(c)   induction of cancers, which subsequently
        develop during the first ten years of life.

In estimating, as previously, the detriment due to each year's exposure of 1000 (female) workers, the frequency of pregnancies is based on the assumption that each woman will have an average of 2 pregnancies during a working life of from age 18 to 65; therefore with 42.5 pregnancies occurring in every 1000 female worker-years.

The conceptus is vulnerable to the cell killing effects of radiation, probably without a significant threshold dose below which damage does not occur, during the short period - of about 8 days after conception - before it becomes implanted into the uterine wall. The detriment of any such cell death is not expressed in harm to a liveborn child, and is recognisable to the mother only as the missing of a menstrual period. If, however, the event is treated as the loss of 70 years of life expectancy, and has a risk of occurrence of 8×10^{-4} per mSv (a risk based on animal data, in the absence of adequate quantitative information in man), then the contribution to time loss would be estimated at about 0.08 years (combining 8 days of exposure at 1.5 mSv per year, 42.5 pregnancies per 1000 worker years, 70 years life loss and the stated risk per mSv).

The major identified developmental abnormality in man is that of mental retardation induced in children in Hiroshima and Nagasaki exposed to radiation from atomic bombs during a 7 week period in pregnancy when the cortex of the brain was developing[14]. The data give no evidence of a threshold, but do not exclude the existence of a threshold of up to a few tens of millisieverts. If however, no threshold is assumed, a time loss detriment of 0.24 years could be estimated from this cause, assuming the detriment to last during 70 years of life, to be induced with a rate of about 4×10^{-4} per mSv, and with the same frequency of pregnancies and constancy of dose rate during the 7 week period as assumed above.

A number of other types of developmental anomalies occur spontaneously in man, but no evidence has been obtained of their induction by radiation at low dose or of what their rate of induction might be at such doses.

Most developmental defects, however, are likely to be due to the killing of a number of cells, and therefore to result from radiation exposure only if a threshold dose is exceeded. This is in contrast to genetic effects depending on the survival of a single damaged germ cell, for which no threshold can be expected. At the very low doses delivered during the relevant brief periods of development, usually of a few days only which are critical for each anomaly, it must be uncertain whether any developmental anomalies which depend upon multiple cell killing might be induced when the average dose rate is only 1.5 mSv per year.

The third type of detriment which may be induced during pregnancy is the induction of cancer in the developing fetus. Here there is some evidence suggesting that the induction rate, per unit dose, may be somewhat greater than, and perhaps twice, that in the adult. The risk is uncertain: firstly because the doses delivered to the fetus (by x rays of the mother's pelvis during pregnancy) could only be assessed retrospectively from knowledge of radiological practises at the relevant time; and secondly, because a more extensive survey showed only about half the relative risk of cancer after exposure of the fetus. The estimated time loss detriment from this effect is small, with a value of 0.08 years per 1000 female worker-years, even if the higher induction rate is assumed (of 2.3×10^{-5} per mSv[15]) with a 70 year loss of life expectancy per cancer and 40 weeks exposure at the rate of 1.5 mSv per year.

Combining the time loss detriments estimated for the forms of harm identified above as inducable in the developing child exposed during pregnancy, a total is reached of about 0.4 years from the annual exposure of a female workforce of 1000.

TIME LOSS DETRIMENTS FROM OCCUPATIONAL INJURIES OR RADIATION EXPOSURE

The estimates of time loss detriment that have been made in this paper may be more useful in suggesting the possibility of developing comparisons between different types and levels of occupational risk, than in providing any definitive quantitative grading of the risk or safety of different occupations.

The need, in any case, is to present for review a clear estimate of the occupational risks of radiation and of other industrial hazards. The present discussion of the differences in weight that might be placed on periods of life lost or impaired may clarify the suitability of accepting or modifying these weighting factors.

In fact it emerges from the estimates of the risks of different kinds, that there is little need for developing precise numerical weighting factors, if it is assumed that about equal weight should be given to periods of life lost, or of active disease or permanent substantial disability, in exposed individuals or in their descendants; and that substantially lower weighting should be given to equal periods of temporary disability of a few weeks duration from accidental injuries.

It seems useful, however, to consider the numerical values derived above, to review the comparisons to which they lead, and to form a basis for improving the weaker estimates and assumptions in the light of closer study.

Industrial injuries were estimated to involve a time loss detriment of about 5 years annually per 1000 workers, in an industry with an accidental mortality rate of 10 per 100,000 worker years.

Radiation exposure at a rate of 1.5 mSv per year is estimated to involve a total time loss detriment of about 0.5 years annually per 1000 male workers, and about 1 year in a female workforce working throughout all pregnancies (Table 6).

If it is assumed, as has been done above, that the time loss detriment from occupational injuries is proportional to the fatal accident rate in the industry, the detriment attributable to radiation exposure at a rate of 1.5 mSv per year would correspond to that from injuries in an industry with an annual fatality rate of between 1 and 2 per 100,000 workers at risk: rates recorded in the safer manufacturing processes (Table 1). At the highest rates of radiation exposure noted in Table 3 of about 10 mSv per year in uranium miners, the detriment in males would be comparable to that from injuries in the manufacture of bricks and pottery in the UK, and in trade, manufacture, service and government in the United States.

It is obvious from the inadequacies of the present analysis that this subject of aggregation and comparison of occupational risks needs further study and development. It is also obvious that similar methods could be applicable to public exposures to radiation, and to occupational exposures to other potentially harmful agents.

It is equally important, however, that an informed and responsible societal perspective on environmental risks in general is necessary but cannot reasonably be expected unless the sources and types of detriment can be summarised, and suitable methods developed for their quantitative intercomparison.

REFERENCES

1. L.I. Dublin and M. Spiegelmann. Mortality of medical
    specialists 1938-1942. J. Amer. med. Assoc., 137:1519
    (1948).
2. H.S. Martland. The occurrence of malignancy in radioactive
    persons. Amer. J. Cancer 15:2435 (1931).
3. Agricola (Georg Bauer) "De re metallica", Froben, Basle, (1556).
4. "Risk assessment: a study group report", Royal Society,
    London (1983).
5. "Accident Facts", U.S. National Safety Council, Chicago
    (1956-1981).
6. United Nations Scientific Committee on the Effects of Atomic
    Radiation "Ionizing Radiation: sources and biological
    effects". 1982 report to the General Assembly, United
    Nations, New York (1982).
7. J.S. Hughes and G.C. Roberts. The radiation exposure of the
    UK population - a further review. (UK) National
    Radiological Protection Board report. In course of
    publication. NRPB, Chilton, Oxfordshire (1984).
8. "Recommendations of the International Commission on
    Radiological Protection", ICRP Publication 26. Annals
    of the ICRP 1 (3):1 (1977).
9. Committee on the Biological Effects of Ionizing Radiation.
    "The effects on populations of exposure to low levels
    of ionizing radiation". National Academy Press,
    Washington D.C. (1980).
10. "Problems involved in developing an index of harm", ICRP
    Publication 27. Annals of the ICRP 1 (4):1 (1977).
11. "Work Injury and Illness Rates", (US) National Safety
    Council, annual publications, Chicago.
12. E.E. Pochin. "Occupational and other fatality rates".
    Community Health 6:2 (1974).
13. Office of Population Censuses and Surveys, "Birth Statistics"
    Series FM 4, HMSO, London (1979).
14. M. Otake and W.J. Schull. In utero exposure to A-bomb
    radiation and mental retardation: a reassessment.
    Brit. J. Radiology 57:509 (1984).
15. United Nations Scientific Committee on the Effects of Atomic
    Radiation, "Ionizing Radiation: levels and effects"
    Vol. II: Effects, Annex H. 1972 Report to the General
    Assembly. United Nations, New York (1972).

INDEX

mutation induction, 188
myc oncogene, 169, 467
myelodisplastic syndromes, 501

N-acetoxy-2-acetylaminofluorene, 239
nasal cancer, 313, 322
natural radiation, 10, 339, 363, 368
neoplastic transformation, 163
nervous system microwave effects, 445
Nevada test, 419
Nevi natural history, 216
nevoid basal cell carcinoma syndrome, 215
neurastenic syndrome, 444
neurablastoma, 230
neurofibromatosis, 390
neuronal migration, 529
neutron
    exposure, 385
    kerma, 422
    RBE, 167
    residual radiation, 413
NIH/3T3 cells, 460
nickel, 18, 302
nickel refinery workers, 180
nine parameters formula, 424
nigrogen mustard, 503
4-Nitroquinolin d-oxide, 221, 239, 246, 260
N-methyl-N1-nitro-N-nitrosoguani-dine, 246
N-methyl-N-nitrosourea, 247
  age increasing toxicity, 251
non-stocastic processes, 206
N-ras oncogene, 226
nuclear reactors releases, 370

Occupational
  injuries, 552
  surveillance, 334
  toxicity, 310
ocular effects of microwave, 447
odds ratio, 39
oncogenes, 168
onc-proteins, 462

optimization of dose, 347
organ dose, 53, 58, 127, 136, 344, 350, 366, 374, 420
organochlorine contaminants, 302
ORNL studies, 97
osteosarcoma, 273, 280
over-exposed workers management, 354
ovarian cancer, 506
ovaries x-irradiated, 70

Pace-Marcum dosymetry, 425
particulate-x-emitters, 128
p21 coding sequences, 228
personal dosimetry, 47
phosphoglucomutase, 393
photoreactivation, 206, 241
Pierce model, 111
pneumoconiosis, 307
point mutation, 229
polycythemia vera, 511
polyoma virus, 159, 169
    middle T gene, 169
    large T gene, 169
power density of microwave, 434
pregnancy
    loss, 20
    outward rate, 387
premature death, 384
probability of causation
    tables, 49
    cancers, 59
procarbazine, 503
prompt radiation, 421
protein kinase, 462
protein molecules abnormaities, 392
prato oncogenes, 225, 459
p 28 sis processing, 463
pyrimidine dimers, 190, 206, 237, 376

radiation
    DNA synthesis depression, 258
    hormones synergism, 282
    induced menopause, 70
    interactions, 82

580

radiation (continued)
  occupational exposure, 339
  smoking interaction, 57
  total population exposure, 64
radiation carcinogenesis
  animal studies, 94
  epidemiological studies, 3
  tissue factors, 136
Radiation Effects Research
    Foundation, 383, 414, 516
radiactive nuclides repositories,
    364
radiologists, 68, 145
radionuclides, 4
radiofrequency bands, 435
radioresistance increased in
    cancer prone families, 257
radiotherapy
  ankilosing spondylitis, 71
  cervix cancer, 71
  non- malignant diseases, 6
radiowave sickness, 444
radium, 224, 128, 273
radium dial painters, 9
radon, 8, 551
  daughter products, 9, 128, 400
  indoor exposure, 41, 368, 370,
    402
  miners' exposure, 41
  quantitative risk, 406
ras oncogene, 169, 225, 472
  in human cells/tumors, 131,
    230
rat brain tumor, 157
rat mammary tumor, 157
Rous sarcoma virus, 167, 459
RBE, 342, 419
reference levels, 350
refractory anemia, 501
repair (DNA-repair)
  aberrant, 242
  alkyl repair in smokers, 211
  alkyl transfer, 206
  and cancer susceptibility, 207
  bulky lesion-repair complex,
    244
  cell cycle dependence, 197
  daughter strand, 237

repair (continued)
  deficiency and breast cancer,
    485
  deficient cells, 187
  in AT cells, 246
  incision step, 239
  in microbial systems, 240
  in XP cells, 242
  levels in tissues, 378
  mechanisms, 98, 206
  O^6-methylguanine, 198, 247,
    375
  4 NQO lesions, 246
  nucleotide excision, 206, 239,
    245
  rate in human cells, 380
  time available, 195
  transformation, 187
  variation, 207
respiratory volume, 25
retinol binding protein, 20
retinablastoma, 215, 389
retroviruses, 225
Rh locus, 219
risk
  absolute, 53
  acceptance/acceptability, 182,
    367
  by age, 427
  bone marrow irradiation, 7
  coefficients, 53
  comparison, 352, 551
  evaluation and duration, 73
  estimation, 393
  extropolation, 428
  genetic, 383
  linear quadratic, 52
  liver irradiation, 7
  of CMM, 218
  of death in sport, 308
  perception, 182
  quantification, 4, 218
  relative risk model, 55
RNA tumor viruses, 162
Rossi-counters, 130
Rothmund Thomson syndrome, 253

safety levels, 2
safety of chemicals, 311
sampling, 151, 298
sensitivity individual organ, 4
sentinel phenotypes, 384, 390
sequencial cloning assay, 163
Seveso accident, 538
Seveso birth defect registry, 540
sex dependent differences in kinetics, 294
sickle cell anemia, 530
Simian sarcoma virus, 459
single gene disorders, 213
sis oncogene, 459
sister chromatid exchange, 391
skeletal dose, 275
skin cancer, 12, 569
SK-H-SH cells, 230
smoking
  alkyl acceptor levels, 211
  and arsenic trioxide, 320
  and radon, 403
  as behavioural factor, 33
  by miners, 8, 87
  influence on lung cancer, 400
  in probability of causation, 57
  insulation workers, 177
  mesothelioma, 177
  mucous stimulation, 409
  radiation interaction, 57
smoke detectors, 371, 373
soft x-rays, 356
solid tumors following chemotherapy, 510
somatic cell mutation, 160
specific absorbtion rate, 435
src oncogene, 167
(non) stochastic effects, 341, 366
stomach cancer, 9, 59, 322
streptomyces griseus, 241
streptozotocin, 508
study/ies
  base, 34
  case-control, 142, 500
  cause direct, 22, 296
  cohort, 142, 499
  design choice, 144

study/ies (continued)
  disease oriented, 143
  exposure oriented, 142
  individual direct, 22
  observational, 142
  situation direct, 22, 296
susceptibility (see cancer susceptibility)
SW 1271 cells, 230
SW 480 cells, 230

T4 bacteriophage, 239
T24 bladder carcinoma cells, 226, 241
T24/EJ bladder tumor oncogene, 228
TCDD, 26
TCDD teratogenicity, 538
T65 (Oak Ridge) dosimetry, 138, 385, 414, 424, 517
testicular cancer, 323, 509
thalidomide, 532
6-thioguamine, 188
thorium, 7
thorotrast, 7,
Three Mile Island, 47
threshold dose, 3, 130, 181
thyroid cancer, 4, 12, 51, 416, 566
thyroid gland, 47
time loss industrial injuries, 556
timepiece luminous, 372
tinea capitis, 515
tissue dose, 343, 523
toluene, 26
Tort law, 45
toxic effects recognizing, 310
toxicokinetics, 293
trace metals, 40
training, 353
transformation (in vitro)
  anchorage independence, 157, 165, 185
  assay, 159, 162
  DNA repair, 187
  efficiency, 460
  frequency, 160
  morphological, 161
  partial, 168
  proteins, 459